IMPORTANT:

HERE IS YOUR REGISTRATION CODE TO ACCESS
YOUR PREMIUM McGRAW-HILL ONLINE RESOURCES.

For key premium online resources you need THIS CODE to gain access. Once the code is entered, you will be able to use the Web resources for the length of your course.

If your course is using **WebCT** or **Blackboard**, you'll be able to use this code to access the McGraw-Hill content within your instructor's online course.

Access is provided if you have purchased a new book. If the registration code is missing from this book, the registration screen on our Website, and within your WebCT or Blackboard course, will tell you how to obtain your new code.

Registering for McGraw-Hill Online Resources

TO gain access to your McGraw-Hill web resources simply follow the steps below:

1. USE YOUR WEB BROWSER TO GO TO: **http://www.mhhe.com/thompson15e**
2. CLICK ON **FIRST TIME USER**.
3. ENTER THE REGISTRATION CODE* PRINTED ON THE TEAR-OFF BOOKMARK ON THE RIGHT.
4. AFTER YOU HAVE ENTERED YOUR REGISTRATION CODE, CLICK **REGISTER**.
5. FOLLOW THE INSTRUCTIONS TO SET-UP YOUR PERSONAL UserID AND PASSWORD.
6. WRITE YOUR UserID AND PASSWORD DOWN FOR FUTURE REFERENCE.
   KEEP IT IN A SAFE PLACE.

TO GAIN ACCESS to the McGraw-Hill content in your instructor's **WebCT** or **Blackboard** course simply log in to the course with the UserID and Password provided by your instructor. Enter the registration code exactly as it appears in the box to the right when prompted by the system. You will only need to use the code the first time you click on McGraw-Hill content.

Thank you, and welcome to your McGraw-Hill online Resources!

* YOUR REGISTRATION CODE CAN BE USED ONLY ONCE TO ESTABLISH ACCESS. IT IS NOT TRANSFERABLE.
0-07-292178-1 T/A THOMPSON: MANUAL OF STRUCTURAL KINESILOGY, 5/E

ONLINE RESOURCES

SO-ASN-662

REGISTRATION CODE

rigorously-74791870

Higher Education

Manual of Structural Kinesiology

Clem W. Thompson, Ph.D., F.A.C.S.M., who died in 1990, helped shape the field of physical education for his students and colleagues alike. Dr. Thompson wrote the fourth through the eleventh editions of *Manual of Structural Kinesiology*. He published many research papers, articles, and presentations, but he considered this book to be his most important professional accomplishment.

Dr. Thompson was a professor emeritus of physical education at Mankato State University in Mankato, Minnesota, where he served on the faculty for 25 years. He had taught at the University of Arkansas and Boston University before coming to MSU and retired from teaching in 1984. Dr. Thompson was a member of The American Alliance for Health, Physical Education, Recreation and Dance and served on various governing boards of the American Heart Association.

Dr. Thompson received his undergraduate degree from Knox College in Galesburg, Illinois, in 1938, his master's degree from the University of Illinois in 1941, and his doctorate from the University of Iowa in 1950.

Dr. Thompson was a pioneer in the campaign against smoking when it was more popular to smoke than to denounce it. He was a leader in the efforts to awaken Americans to the need to be healthy. His own outstanding personal example of physical fitness touched the lives of thousands of students and hundreds of his colleagues. His legacy of a commitment to a fit and healthy life will be perpetuated in the professional careers of them all.

Manual of Structural Kinesiology

R. T. Floyd EdD, ATC, CSCS
Director of Athletic Training and Sports Medicine
Professor of Physical Education and Athletic Training
Chair, Department of Physical Education and
    Athletic Training
The University of West Alabama
    (formerly Livingston University)
Livingston, Alabama

Clem W. Thompson Ph.D., F.A.C.S.M.
(deceased)
Professor Physical Education, Emeritus
Mankato State University
Mankato, Minnesota

FIFTEENTH EDITION

with 249 illustrations

Boston   Burr Ridge, IL   Dubuque, IA   Madison, WI   New York   San Francisco   St. Louis
Bangkok   Bogotá   Caracas   Kuala Lumpur   Lisbon   London   Madrid   Mexico City
Milan   Montreal   New Delhi   Santiago   Seoul   Singapore   Sydney   Taipei   Toronto

Higher Education

MANUAL OF STRUCTURAL KINESIOLOGY, FIFTEENTH EDITION

Published by McGraw-Hill, a business unit of The McGraw-Hill Companies, Inc., 1221 Avenue of the Americas, New York, NY 10020. Copyright © 2004, 2001, 1998, 1994, 1989, 1985, 1981, 1977, 1973, 1969, 1965, 1961, 1956, 1951, 1948 by The McGraw-Hill Companies, Inc.

Some ancillaries, including electronic and print components, may not be available to customers outside the United States.

This book is printed on acid-free paper.

1 2 3 4 5 6 7 8 9 0 QPD/QPD 0 9 8 7 6 5 4 3

ISBN   0-07-255891-1

Vice president and editor-in-chief: *Thalia Dorwick*
Publisher: *Jane E. Karpacz*
Executive editor: *Vicki Malinee*
Developmental editor: *Lynda Huenefeld*
Senior marketing manager: *Pamela S. Cooper*
Project manager: *Richard H. Hecker*
Production supervisor: *Enboge Chong*
Media technology producer: *Lance Gerhart*
Designer: *George Kokkonas*
Art editor: *Emma Ghiselli*
Senior supplement producer: *David A. Welsh*
Compositor: *Interactive Composition Corporation*
Typeface: *10.5/12.5 Garamond*
Printer: *Quebecor World Dubuque, IA*

The credits section for this book begins on page 346 and is considered an extension of the copyright page.

Library of Congress Cataloging-in-Publication Data

Floyd, R. T.
      Manual of structural kinesiology / R. T. Floyd, Clem W. Thompson.-- 15th ed.
        p. cm.
      Includes index.
      ISBN 0-07-255891-1 (alk. paper)
      1. Kinesiology. 2. Human locomotion. 3. Muscles. I. Thompson, Clem W. II. Title.

QP303.T58 2004
612.7'6--dc21

                                                                2003045231

This text was based on the most up-to-date research and suggestions made by individuals knowledgeable in the field of athletic training. The authors and publisher disclaim any responsibility for any adverse effects or consequences from the misapplication or injudicious use of information contained within this text. It is also accepted as judicious that the coach and/or athletic trainer performing his or her duties is, at all times, working under the guidance of a licensed physician.

To

my family,
Lisa, Robert Thomas, Jeanna, Rebecca, and Kate
who understand, support, and allow me to
pursue my profession

and to my parents,
Ruby and George Franklin,
who taught me the importance of a strong work ethic
with quality results

R.T.F.

Contents

Preface

In revising this edition I have attempted to further refine the chapters for consistency and to improve the overall completeness and accuracy of the text. As with previous revisions, I have attempted to maintain the successful presentation approach the late Dr. Clem Thompson established from 1961 through 1989. I first used this book as an undergraduate and later in my teaching over the years. Having developed great respect for this text and Dr. Thompson's style, it is my intention to continue to preserve the effectiveness of this time-honored text, while adding material pertinent to the professions working with today's ever-growing physically active population. Hopefully, I have maintained a clear, concise, and simple presentation method supplemented with applicable information gained through my career experiences.

This text, now in its 57th year, has undergone many revisions over the years. My goal continues to be to make the material as applicable as possible to everyday physical activity and to make it more understandable and easier to use for the student. With this in mind, numerous tables and illustrations have been added to this edition. I challenge kinesiology students and professionals to immediately apply the content of this text to physical activities with which they are individually familiar. I hope that the student will simultaneously palpate his or her own moving joints and contracting muscles to gain application. Concurrently, I encourage students to palpate the joints and muscles of fellow students to gain a better appreciation of the wide range of normal anatomy and, when possible, appreciate the variation from normal found in injured and pathological musculoskeletal anatomy.

Audience

This text is designed for students in an undergraduate structural kinesiology course after completing courses in human anatomy and physiology. While primarily utilized in physical education, exercise science, athletic training, physical therapy, and massage therapy curriculums, it is often used as a continuing reference by other clinicians and educators in addressing musculoskeletal concerns of the physically active. Applied kinesiologists, athletic trainers, athletic coaches, physical educators, physical therapists, health club instructors, strength and conditioning specialists, personal trainers, massage therapists, physicians, and others who are responsible for improving and maintaining the muscular strength, endurance, flexibility, and overall health of individuals will benefit from this text.

With the tremendous growth in the number of participants in an ever-increasing spectrum of physical activity, it is imperative that medical, health, and education professionals involved in providing instruction and information to the physically active be correct in and accountable for the teachings that they provide. The variety of exercise machines, techniques, strengthening and flexibility programs, and training programs is continuously expanding and changing, but the musculoskeletal system is constant in its design and architecture. Regardless of the goals sought or the approaches used in exercise activity, the human body is the basic ingredient and must be thoroughly understood and considered to maximize performance capabilities and minimize undesirable results. Most advances in exercise science continue to result from a better understanding of the body and how it functions. I believe that an individual in this field can never learn enough about the structure and function of the human body.

Those who are charged with the responsibility of providing instruction to the physically active will find this text a helpful and valuable resource in what I hope is their never-ending quest for knowledge and understanding of human movement.

New to this edition

Major changes to this edition include the replacement of several illustrations and the addition of others, as well as numerous tables added in each chapter. Content relative to understanding the structure and function of bones, joints, muscles, and nerves and their individual and combined contribution to human movement has been expanded.

Chapter 1, "Foundations of Structural Kinesiology," has been divided into two chapters. Chapter 1 retains the foundations related to bones and joints, with additions regarding bony features, bone growth, bone markings, bone properties, and joint movements, including discussion related to physiological movements and accessory motions. The new Chapter 2, "Neuromuscular Fundamentals," contains the previous edition's information on neuromuscular function, with substantial additions regarding muscle nomenclature, muscle shape and fiber arrangement, muscle tissue properties, determination of muscle action, lines of pull, neural control of voluntary movement, proprioception and kinesthesis, muscle length–tension and muscle force–velocity relationships, and angle of pull. Chapter 12 from the previous edition, "Basic Biomechanical Factors and Concepts," has been moved to Chapter 3 to allow coverage of these important concepts prior to addressing the muscles of each joint in the subsequent chapters. Some concepts has been expanded, including types of machines found in the body, friction, and mechanical loading basics. In the eight chapters that address specific body parts, tables have been added to clearly detail the origin, insertion, action, plane of motion, palpation, and innervation for each muscle. All palpations have been carefully reviewed and revised, with an emphasis placed on combining movement with palpation in many cases. Illustrations detailing the ranges of motion have been added, as well as a section on the nerves involved, with related illustrations. Chapter 5, "The Shoulder Joint," and Chapter 9, "The Hip and Pelvic Girdle," now have illustrations to depict the ligaments of the glenohumeral and acetabularfemoral joints, respectively. The movement analysis examples in Chapters 8 and 13 have been reworked, with the analyses broken down by phases and placed in tables for clearer understanding.

The Glossary has been essentially doubled in volume and contains well over 100 terms new to this edition. The definitions of several other terms have been revised. Finally, the listings of web sites included at the end of each chapter have been updated. A third appendix has been added to include a listing of the more commonly used exercises for strengthening selected muscles.

Ancillaries

Image Presentation CD-ROM
ISBN 0-07-284288-1

The Image Presentation CD-ROM is an electronic library of visual resources. The CD-ROM comprises images from the text displayed in Power-Point, which allows the user to view, sort, search, use, and print catalog images. It also includes a complete, ready-to-use PowerPoint presentation, which allows users to play chapter-specific slide shows.

Online Learning Center
www.mhhe.com/floyd15e

The Online Learning Center to accompany this text offers a number of additional resources for both students and instructors. Visit this website to find useful materials such as these:

For the instructor:
- Downloadable PowerPoint presentations
- Interactive web activities
- Chapter-specific interactive animations
- Links to professional resources
- PowerWeb access

For the student:
- Self-scoring chapter quizzes
- Anatomy flashcards and crossword puzzles for learning key terms and their definitions
- Chapter-specific interactive animations
- Learning objectives
- Interactive labeling activities
- PowerWeb access

PowerWeb

PowerWeb is a reservoir of course-specific articles and current events. Students can access PowerWeb articles to take a self-scoring quiz, complete an interactive exercise, click through an interactive glossary, or check the daily news. An expert in each discipline analyzes the day's news to show students how it relates to their field of study. PowerWeb articles are available on the Online Learning Center that accompanies this text.

Acknowledgments

I am very appreciative of the excellent comments, ideas, and suggestions provided by the ten reviewers. These reviews have been an extremely helpful guide in this revision. These reviewers are

Rebekah Bower
Wright State University

Salome Brooks
Sacred Heart University

Laura Clark
Western Illinois University

Mike Daniel
Texas A&M University, Kingsville

Erika Goodwin
Wilmington College

J. Ty Hopkins
Illinois State University

Dean Jacks
Winston-Salem State University

Mike Lester
Idaho State University

Kenneth Sarubbi
DePaul University

Vassilios Vardaxis
Indiana University

I would also like to thank Brad Montgomery, MAT, ATC; Karen Straub, MS, ATC; and the kinesiology/athletic training students of The University of West Alabama for their advice and input throughout this revision. Their assistance and suggestions have been most helpful. I also acknowledge Mr. John Hood and Mrs. Lisa Floyd of Birmingham and Livingston, Alabama, respectively, for the fine photographs. Special thanks to Mrs. Linda Kimbrough of Birmingham, Alabama, for her superb illustrations and insight. I appreciate the models for the photographs: Mr. David Whitaker, Miss Kala Peak, Mr. Marcus Shapiro, Mrs. Zina Pruitt, and Mr. Darrell Locket. My thanks also go to Lynda Huenefeld, Carlotta Seely, Vicki Malinee, and Rick Hecker of the McGraw-Hill staff, who have been most helpful in their assistance and suggestions in preparing the manuscript for publication.

R.T. Floyd

Chapter 1

Foundations of Structural Kinesiology

Objectives

- To review the anatomy of the skeletal system

- To review and understand the terminology used to describe body part locations, reference positions, and anatomical directions

- To review the planes of motion and their respective axes of rotation in relation to human movement

- To describe and understand the various types of bones and joints in the human body and their characteristics

- To describe and demonstrate the joint movements

Online Learning Center Resources

Visit *Manual of Structural Kinesiology's* **Online Learning Center** at **www.mhhe.com/floyd15e** for additional information and study material for this chapter, including:

- *Self-grading quizzes*
- *Anatomy flashcards*
- *Animations*

Structural kinesiology is the study of muscles as they are involved in the science of movement. Both skeletal and muscular structures are involved. Bones are different sizes and shapes—particularly at the joints, which allow or limit movement. Muscles vary greatly in size, shape, and structure from one part of the body to another.

More than 600 muscles are found in the human body. In this book, an emphasis is placed on the larger muscles that are primarily involved in movement of the joints. Details related to many of the small muscles located in the hands, feet, and spinal column are provided to a lesser degree.

However, anatomists, coaches, strength and conditioning specialists, personal trainers, nurses, physical educators, physical therapists, physicians, athletic trainers, massage therapists, and others in health-related fields should have an adequate knowledge and understanding of all the large muscle groups, so they can teach others how to strengthen, improve, and maintain these parts of the human body. This knowledge forms the basis of the exercise programs that should be followed to strengthen and maintain all of the muscles. In most cases, exercises that involve the larger primary movers also involve the smaller muscles.

Fewer than 100 of the largest and most important muscles, primary movers, are considered in this text. Some small muscles in the human body, such as the multifidus, plantaris, scalenus, and serratus posterior, are omitted, since they are exercised with other, larger primary movers. In addition, most small muscles of the hands and feet are not given the full attention provided to the larger muscles. Many small muscles of the spinal column are not considered in full detail.

Kinesiology students frequently become so engrossed in learning individual muscles that they lose sight of the total muscular system. They miss the "big picture"—that muscle groups move joints in given movements necessary for bodily movement and skilled performance. Although it is vital to learn the small details of muscle attachments, it is even more critical to be able to apply the information to real-life situations. Once the information can be applied in a useful manner, the specific details are usually much easier to understand and appreciate.

Skeletal systems

Fig. 1.1 shows anterior and posterior views of the skeletal system. Two hundred six bones make up the skeletal system, which provides support and protection for other systems of the body and provides for attachments of the muscles to the bones by which movement is produced. Additional skeletal functions are mineral storage and hemopoiesis, which involves blood cell formation in the red bone marrow. The skeleton may be divided into the appendicular and the axial skeleton. The

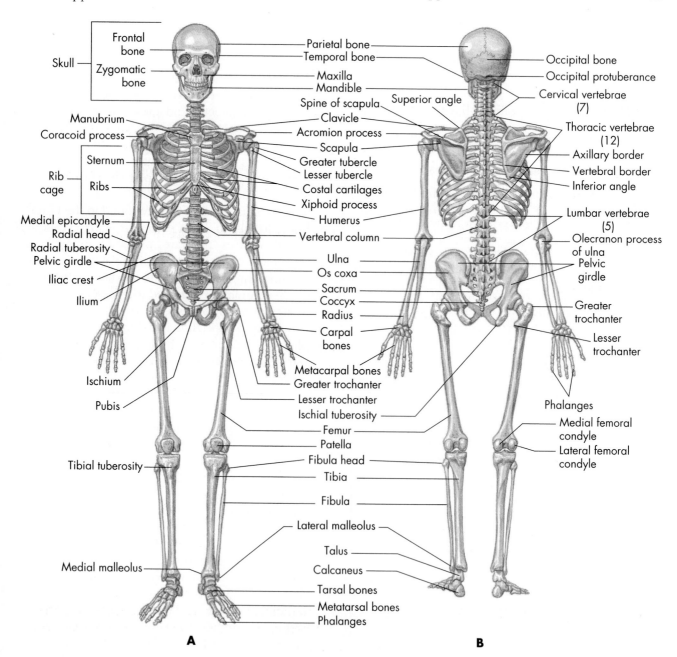

A, Anterior view; **B**, posterior view.

FIG. 1.1 ● Skeleton. **A,** Anterior view; **B,** posterior view.

Modified from Van De Graaff KM: *Human anatomy,* ed 5, New York, 2000, McGraw-Hill.

appendicular skeleton is composed of the appendages, or the upper and lower extremities, and the shoulder and pelvic girdles, while the axial skeleton consists of the skull, vertebral column, ribs, and sternum. Most students who take this course will have had a course in human anatomy, but a brief review is desirable before beginning the study of kinesiology. Other chapters provide additional information and more detailed illustrations of specific bones.

Reference positions

It is crucial for kinesiology students to begin with a reference point in order to better understand the musculoskeletal system, its planes of motion, joint classification, and joint movement terminology. Two reference positions may be used as a basis from which to describe joint movements. The *anatomical position* is the most widely used and accurate for all aspects of the body. Fig. 1.2 demonstrates this reference position, with the subject standing in an upright posture, facing straight ahead, feet parallel and close, and palms facing forward. The *fundamental position* is essentially the same as the anatomical position, except that the arms are at the sides and facing the body.

Anatomical directional terminology FIG. 1.2

Anterior
In front or in the front part

Anteroinferior
In front and below

Anterolateral
In front and to the outside

Anteromedial
In front and toward the inner side or midline

Anteroposterior
Relating to both front and rear

Anterosuperior
In front and above

Caudal
Below in relation to another structure; inferior

Cephalic
Above in relation to another structure; higher, superior

Contralateral
Pertaining or relating to the opposite side

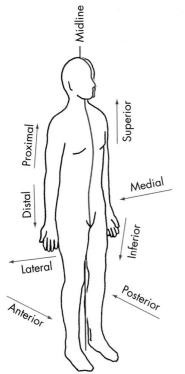

FIG. 1.2 ● Anatomical position and Anatomical directions. Anatomical directions refer to the position of one body part in relation to another.

From Prentice WE: *Arnheim's principles of athletic training,* ed 11, New York, 2003, McGraw-Hill.

Deep

Beneath or below the surface; used to describe relative depth or location of muscles or tissue

Distal

Situated away from the center or midline of the body, or away from the point of origin

Dorsal

Relating to the back; posterior

Inferior

(infra) Below in relation to another structure; caudal

Inferolateral

Below and to the outside

Inferomedial

Below and toward the midline or inside

Ipsilateral

On the same side

Lateral

On or to the side; outside, farther from the median or midsagittal plane

Medial

Relating to the middle or center; nearer to the medial or midsagittal plane

Palmar

Relating to the palm or volar aspect of the hand

Posterior

Behind, in back, or in the rear

Posteroinferior

Behind and below; in back and below

Posterolateral

Behind and to one side, specifically to the outside

Posteromedial

Behind and to the inner side

Posterosuperior

Behind and at the upper part

Prone

Face downward position of the body; stomach lying

Proximal

Nearest the trunk or the point of origin

Superficial

Near the surface; used to describe relative depth or location of muscles or tissue

Superior

(supra) Above in relation to another structure; higher, cephalic

Superolateral

Above and to the outside

Superomedial

Above and toward the midline or inside

Supine

Lying on the back; face upward position of the body

Ventral

Relating to the belly or abdomen

Volar

Relating to palm of the hand or sole of the foot

Planes of motion

When studying the various joints of the body and analyzing their movements, it is helpful to characterize them according to specific planes of motion (Fig. 1.3). A plane of motion may be defined as an imaginary two-dimensional surface through which a limb or body segment is moved.

There are three specific, or *cardinal,* planes of motion in which the various joint movements can be classified. The specific planes that divide the body exactly into two halves are often referred to as cardinal planes. There are an infinite number of planes within each half that are parallel to the cardinal planes. This is best understood in the following examples of movements in the sagittal plane. Sit-ups involve the spine, and as a result, are performed in the cardinal sagittal plane, which is also known as the *midsagittal* plane. Biceps curls and knee extensions are performed in

parasagittal planes, which are parallel to the midsagittal plane. Even though these examples are not in the cardinal plane, they are thought of as movements in the sagittal plane.

Although each specific joint movement can be classified as being in one of the three planes of motion, our movements are usually not totally in one specific plane, but occur as a combination of motions from more than one plane. These movements from the combined planes may be described as occurring in diagonal, or oblique, planes of motion.

Sagittal, anteroposterior, or AP plane

The sagittal, anteroposterior, or AP plane bisects the body from front to back, dividing it into right and left symmetrical halves. Generally, flexion and extension movements such as biceps curls, knee extensions, and sit-ups occur in this plane.

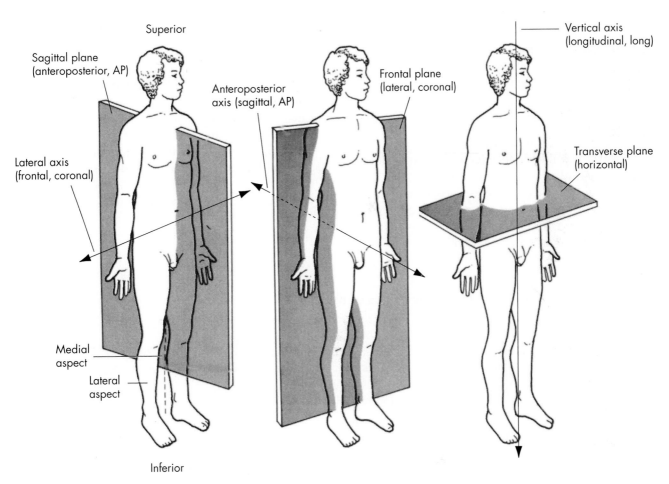

FIG. 1.3 ● Planes of motion and axes of rotation.

Modified from Booher JM, Thibodeau GA: *Athletic injury assessment,* ed 4, New York, 2000, McGraw-Hill.

Frontal, lateral, or coronal plane

The frontal plane, also known as the lateral or coronal plane, bisects the body laterally from side to side, dividing it into front and back halves. Abduction and adduction movements such as jumping jacks and spinal lateral flexion occur in this plane.

Transverse or horizontal plane

The transverse plane divides the body horizontally into superior and inferior halves. Generally, rotational movements such as pronation, supination, and spinal rotation occur in this plane.

Diagonal or oblique plane

The diagonal or oblique plane is a combination of more than one plane. In reality, most of our movements in sporting activities fall somewhere less than parallel or perpendicular to the previously described planes and occur in a diagonal plane.

Axes of rotation

As movement occurs in a given plane, the joint moves or turns about an axis that has a 90-degree relationship to that plane. The axes are named in relation to their orientation (Fig. 1.3). Table 1.1 lists the planes of motion with their axes of rotation.

Frontal, lateral, or coronal axis

If the sagittal plane runs from anterior to posterior, then its axis must run from side to side. Since this axis has the same directional orientation as the frontal plane of motion, it is named similarly. As the elbow flexes and extends in the sagittal plane when performing a biceps curl, the forearm is actually rotating about a frontal axis that runs laterally through the elbow joint.

Sagittal or anteroposterior axis

Movement occurring in the frontal plane rotates about a sagittal axis. This sagittal axis has the same directional orientation as the sagittal plane of motion and runs from front to back at a right angle to the frontal plane of motion. As the hip abducts and adducts during jumping jacks, the femur rotates about an axis that runs front to back through the hip joint.

Vertical or longitudinal axis

The vertical axis, also known as the longitudinal or long axis, runs straight down through the top of the head and is at a right angle to the transverse plane of motion. As the head rotates or turns from left to right when indicating disapproval, the skull and cervical vertebrae are rotating around an axis that runs down through the spinal column.

Osteology

The adult skeleton, consisting of approximately 206 bones, may be divided into the axial skeleton and the appendicular skeleton. The axial skeleton contains 80 bones, which include the skull, spinal column, sternum, and ribs. The appendicular skeleton contains 126 bones, which include all of the bones of the upper and lower extremities. The pelvis is sometimes classified as being part of the axial skeleton due to its importance in linking the axial skeleton with the lower extremities of the appendicular skeleton. The exact number of bones as well as their specific features occasionally vary from person to person.

TABLE 1.1 • Planes of motion and their axes of rotation

Plane	Description of plane	Axis of rotation	Description of axis	Common movements
Sagittal (anteroposterior or AP)	Divides the body into right and left halves	Frontal (lateral or coronal) (medial-lateral)	Runs medial/lateral	Flexion, extension
Frontal (lateral or coronal)	Divides the body into anterior and posterior halves	Sagittal (anteroposterior or AP)	Runs anterior/posterior	Abduction, adduction
Transverse (horizontal)	Divides the body into superior and inferior halves	Vertical (longitudinal or long)	Runs superior/inferior	Internal rotation, external rotation

Skeletal functions

The skeleton has five major functions:

1. protection of vital soft tissues such as the heart, lungs, and brain
2. support to maintain posture
3. movement by serving as points of attachment for muscles and acting as levers
4. storage for minerals such as calcium and phosphorus
5. hemopoiesis, which is the process of blood formation that occurs in the red bone marrow located in the vertebral bodies, femur, humerus, ribs, and sternum.

Types of bones

Bones vary greatly in shape and size, but can be categorized in five major categories (Fig. 1.4).

Long bones

Composed of a long cylindrical shaft with relatively wide, protruding ends; serve as levers. The shaft contains the medullary canal. Examples include phalanges, metatarsals, metacarpals, tibia, fibula, femur, radius, ulna, and humerus.

Short bones

Small, cube-shaped, solid bones that usually have a proportionally large articular surface in order to articulate with more than one bone. Short bones provide some shock absorption and include the carpals and tarsals.

Flat bones

Usually having a curved surface and varying from thick (where tendons attach) to very thin. Flat bones generally provide protection and include the ilium, ribs, sternum, clavicle, and scapula.

Irregular bones

Irregular shaped bones serving a variety of purposes and including the bones throughout the entire spine and the ischium, pubis, and maxilla.

Sesamoid bones

Small bones embedded within the tendon of a musculotendinous unit that provide protection as well as improve the mechanical advantage of musculotendinous units. In addition to the patella, there are small sesamoid bones within the flexor tendons of the great toe and the thumb.

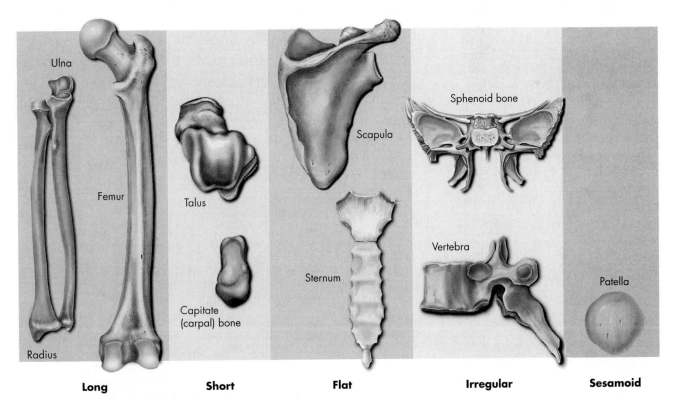

Long   **Short**   **Flat**   **Irregular**   **Sesamoid**

FIG. 1.4 ● Classification of bones by shape.

Modified from Booher JM, Thibodeau GA: *Athletic injury assessment*, ed 4, New York, 2000, McGraw-Hill and Shier D, Blutler J, Lewis R: *Hole's Human anatomy & physiology*, ed 9, New York, 2002, McGraw-Hill.

Typical bony features

Long bones possess features that are typical of bones in general as illustrated in Fig. 1.5. Long bones have a shaft or *diaphysis,* which is the long cylindrical portion of the bone. The diaphysis wall, formed from hard, dense compact bone, is the *cortex*. The outer surface of the diaphysis is covered by a dense, fibrous membrane known as the *periosteum*. A similar fibrous membrane known as the *endosteum* covers the inside of the cortex. Between the walls of the diaphysis lies the *medullary* or marrow cavity, which contains yellow or fatty marrow. At each end of a long bone is the *epiphysis,* which is usually enlarged and specifically shaped to join with the epiphysis of an adjacent bone at a joint. The epiphysis is formed from spongy or *cancellous* or *trabecular*

bone. During bony growth the diaphysis and the epiphysis are separated by a thin plate of cartilage known as the *epiphyseal plate,* commonly referred to as a growth plate. As skeletal maturity is reached, on a timetable that varies from bone to bone as detailed in Table 1.2, the plates are replaced by bone and are closed. To facilitate smooth, easy movement at joints, the epiphysis is covered by articular or *hyaline* cartilage, which provides a cushioning effect and reduces friction.

Bone growth

Bones continue to grow longitudinally as long as the epiphyseal plates are open. These plates begin closing around adolescence and disappear. Most close by age 18, but some may be present until 25. Growth in diameter continues throughout life. This is done by an internal layer of periosteum building new concentric layers on old layers. Simultaneously, bone around the sides of the medullary cavity is resorbed so that the diameter is continually increased. New bone is formed by specialized cells known as *osteoblasts,* whereas the cells that resorb new bone are *osteoclasts.*

FIG. 1.5 ● Major parts of a long bone.

From Shier D, Butler J, Lewis R: *Hole's human anatomy & physiology,* ed 9, New York, 2002, McGraw-Hill.

TABLE 1.2 • **Epiphyseal closure timetables**

Approximate age	Bones
7–8	Inferior rami of pubis and ischium (almost complete)
15–17	Scapula, lateral epicondyle of humerus, olecranon process of ulna
18–19	Medial epicondyle of humerus, head and shaft of radius
About 20	Humeral head, distal ends of radius and ulna, distal ends of femur and fibula, proximal end tibia
20–25	Acetabulum in pelvis
25	Vertebrae and sacrum, clavicle, proximal end of fibula, sternum and ribs

Adapted from Goss CM: *Gray's anatomy of the human body,* ed 29, Philadelphia, 1973, Lea & Febiger.

Bone properties

Calcium carbonate, calcium phosphate, collagen, and water are the basis of bone composition. About 60% to 70% of bone weight is made up of calcium carbonate and calcium phosphate, with water making up approximately 25% to 30% of bone weight. Collagen provides some flexibility and strength in resisting tension. Aging causes progressive loss of collagen and increases bone brittleness, resulting in increased likelihood of fractures.

Most outer bone is cortical; cancellous is underneath. Cortical bone is harder and more compact, with only about 5% to 30% of its volume being porous, with nonmineralized tissue. In contrast, cancellous bone is spongy, with around 30% to 90% of its volume being porous. Cortical bone is stiffer; it can withstand greater stress, but less strain, than cancellous bone. Due to its sponginess, cancellous bone can undergo greater strain before fracturing.

Bone size and shape are influenced by the direction and magnitude of forces that are habitually applied to them. Bones reshape themselves based upon the stresses placed upon them and their mass increases over time with increased stress.

Bone markings

Bones have specific markings that exist to enhance their functional relationship with joints, muscles, tendons, nerves and blood vessels. Many of these markings serve as important bony landmarks in determining muscle location and attachments and joint function. Essentially, all bone markings may be divided into

1. processes (including elevations & projections), which either form joints or serve as a point of attachment for muscles, tendons or ligaments; and

2. cavities (depressions), which include openings and grooves that contain tendons, vessels, nerves, and spaces for other structures. Detailed descriptions and examples of many bony markings are provided in Table 1.3.

Types of joints

The articulation of two or more bones allows various types of movement. The extent and type of movement determine the name applied to the joint. Bone structure limits the kind and amount of movement in each joint. Some joints have no movement, others are only very slightly moveable, and others are freely moveable with a variety of movement ranges. The type and range of movements are similar in all humans; but the freedom, range, and vigor of movements are limited by ligaments and muscles.

Articulations may be grouped according to the structure or function. Classification by structure places joints into one of three categories: fibrous, cartilaginous, or synovial. Functional classification also results in three categories: synarthrodial, amphiarthrodial, and diarthrodial. In both cases, there are subcategories in each classification. Due to the strong relationship between structure and function, there is significant overlap between the classification systems. That is, there is more similarity than difference between the two members in each of the following pairs: fibrous and synarthrodial joints, cartilaginous and amphiarthrodial joints, and synovial and diarthrodial joints. However, not all joints fit neatly into both systems. Since this text is concerned primarily with movement, the more functional system (synarthrodial, amphiarthrodial, and diarthrodial joints) will be used throughout, following a brief explanation of structural classification.

Fibrous joints are joined together by connective tissue fibers and are generally immovable. Subcategories are sutures and gomphosis, which are immovable, and syndesmosis, which allow a slight amount of movement. Cartilaginous joints are joined together by hyaline cartilage or fibrocartilage, which allows very slight movement. Subcategories include synchondrosis and symphysis. Synovial joints are freely movable and generally are diarthrodial. Their structure and subcategories are discussed in detail under diarthrodial joints.

The articulations are grouped into three classes based primarily on the amount of movement possible, with consideration given to their structure.

TABLE 1.3 • **Bone markings**

	Marking	Description	Examples
Processes that form joints	Condyle	Large, rounded projection that usually articulates with another bone	Medial or lateral condyle of femur
	Facet	Small, flat or nearly flat surface	Articular facet of vertebra
	Head	Prominent, rounded projection of the proximal end of a bone, usually articulating	Head of femur Head of humerus
Processes to which muscles, tendon, or ligaments attach	Crest	Prominent, narrow, ridgelike projection	Iliac crest of pelvis
	Epicondyle	Projection located above a condyle	Medial or lateral epicondyle of humerus
	Line	Ridge of bone less prominent than a crest	Linea aspera of femur
	Process	Any prominent projection	Acromion process of scapula, Olecranon process of humerus
	Spine (spinous process)	Sharp, slender projection	Spinous process of vertebra, Spine of scapula
	Suture	Line of union between bones	Sagittal suture between parietal bones of skull
	Trochanter	Very large projection	Greater or lesser trochanter of femur
	Tubercle	Small rounded projection	Greater and lesser tubercles of humerus
	Tuberosity	Large rounded or roughened projection	Radial tuberosity, tibial tuberosity
Cavities (depressions)	Facet	Flatted or shallow articulating surface	Intervertebral facets in cervical, thoracic, anf lumbar spine
	Foramen	Rounded hole or opening in bone	Foramen magnum in base of skull
	Fossa	Hollow, depression, or flattened surface	Supraspinatus fossa, iliac fossa
	Fovea	Very small pit or depression	Fovea capitis of femur
	Meatus	Tubelike passage within a bone	External auditory meatus of temporal bone
	Sinus	Cavity or hollow space within a bone	Frontal sinus
	Sulcus (groove)	Furrow or groovelike depression on a bone	Intertubercular (bicipital) groove of humerus

Synarthrodial (immovable) joints   FIG. 1.6

Found in the sutures of the cranial bones and sockets of the teeth. The sutures of the skull are truly immovable beyond infancy. The socket of a tooth is often referred to as a gomphosis (type of joint in which a conical peg fits into a socket). Normally, there should be an absolutely minimal amount of movement of the teeth in the mandible or maxilla.

Amphiarthrodial (slightly movable) joints   FIG. 1.7

Structurally, these articulations are divided into three types:

Syndesmosis

Type of joint held together by strong ligamentous structures that allow minimal movement between the bones. Examples are the coracoclavicular joint and the inferior tibiofibular joint.

Symphysis

Type of joint separated by a fibrocartilage pad that allows very slight movement between the bones. Examples are the symphysis pubis and the intervertebral discs.

Synchondrosis

Type of joint separated by hyaline cartilage that allows very slight movement between the bones. Examples are the costochondral joints of the ribs with the sternum.

FIG. 1.6 ● Synarthrodial joints.

Modified from Booher JM, Thibodeau GA: *Athletic injury assessment,* ed 4, New York, 2000, McGraw-Hill.

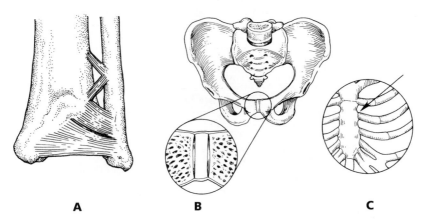

A   **B**   **C**

FIG. 1.7 ● Amphiarthrodial joints. **A,** Syndesmosis joint; **B,** symphysis joint; **C,** synchondrosis joint.

Modified from Booher JM, Thibodeau GA: *Athletic injury assessment,* ed 4, New York, 2000, McGraw-Hill.

Diarthrodial (freely movable) joints   FIG. 1.8

Diarthrodial joints, also known as synovial joints, are freely movable. A sleevelike covering of ligamentous tissue known as the *joint capsule* surrounds the bony ends forming the joints. This ligamentous capsule is lined with a thin vascular synovial capsule that secretes synovial fluid to lubricate the area inside the joint capsule, known as the *joint cavity*. In certain areas the capsule is thickened to form tough, nonelastic ligaments that provide additional support against abnormal movement or joint opening. These ligaments vary in location, size, and strength depending upon the particular joint.

In many cases, additional ligaments, not continuous with the joint capsule, provide further support. The articular surfaces on the ends of the bones inside the joint cavity are covered with layers of articular or *hyaline cartilage*. This resilient cartilage absorbs shock to protect the bone it covers. When the joint surfaces are unloaded or distracted, this articular cartilage slowly absorbs a slight amount of the joint synovial fluid, only to slowly secrete it during subsequent weight bearing and compression. Additionally, some diarthrodial joints have a fibrocartilage disk between their articular surfaces. Structurally, this type of articulation can be divided into six groups, as shown in Fig. 1.9.

Diarthrodial joints have motion possible in one or more planes. Those joints having motion possible in one plane are said to have one degree of freedom of motion, whereas joints having motion in two or three planes of motion are described as having two and three degrees of freedom of motion, respectively. Refer to Table 1.4 for a comparison of diarthrodial joint features by subcategory.

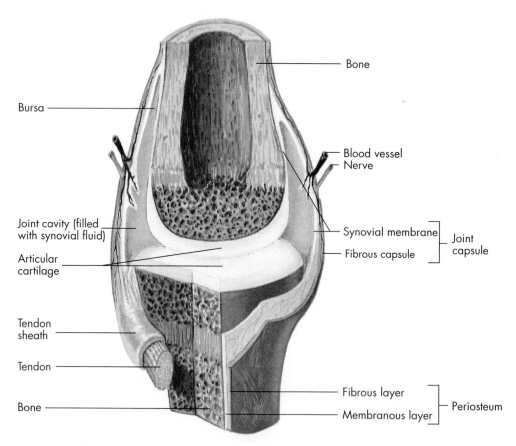

FIG. 1.8 ● Structure of a diarthrodial synovial joint.

From Seeley RR, Stephens TD, Tate P: *Anatomy & physiology,* ed 6, New York, 2000, McGraw-Hill.

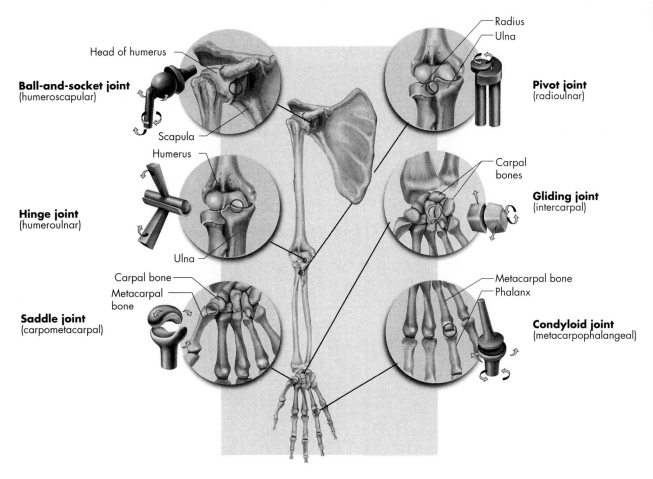

FIG. 1.9 ● Types of diarthrotic or synovial joints.

From Booher JM, Thibodeau GA: *Athletic injury assessment,* ed 4, New York, 2000, McGraw-Hill.

Arthrodial (gliding, plane) joint

This joint type is characterized by two flat, or plane, bony surfaces that butt against each other. This type of joint permits limited gliding movement. Examples are the carpal bones of the wrist and the tarsometatarsal joints of the foot.

Condyloidal (ellipsoid, ovoid, biaxial ball and socket) joint

This is a type of joint in which the bones permit movement in two planes without rotation. Examples are the wrist between the radius and the proximal row of the carpal bones or the second, third, fourth, and fifth metacarpophalangeal joints.

Enarthrodial (spheroidal, multiaxial ball-and-socket) joint

This is a type of joint that permits movement in all planes. Examples are the shoulder (glenohumeral) and hip joints.

Ginglymus (hinge) joint

This is a type of joint that permits a wide range of movement in only one plane. Examples are the elbow, ankle, and knee joints.

Sellar (saddle) joint

This type of reciprocal reception is found only in the thumb at the carpometacarpal joint and permits ball-and-socket movement, with the exception of rotation.

Trochoidal (pivot, screw) joint

This is a type of joint with a rotational movement around a long axis. An example is the rotation of the radius at the radioulnar joint.

TABLE 1.4 • Diarthrodial joint classification

Classification name	Number of axes	Degrees of freedom	Typical movements	Joint examples	Plane for examples	Axis for examples
Ginglymus (hinge)	Uniaxial	One	Flexion, extension	Elbow joint (humeroulnar)	Sagittal	Frontal
Trochoid (pivot, screw)			Internal rotation, external rotation	Proximal and distal radioulnar joint	Transverse	Vertical
Condyloid (ellipsoid, ball-and-socket, ovoid)	Biaxial	Two	Flexion, extension, Abduction, adduction	2nd–5th metacarpophalangeal joints	Sagittal / Frontal	Frontal / Sagittal
Arthrodial (gliding, plane)	Multiaxial	Three	Flexion, extension, Abduction, adduction, Internal rotation, external rotation	Transverse tarsal joint	Variable Frontal	Variable Sagittal
Enarthrodial (ball-and-socket, spheroidal)				Glenohumeral joint	Sagittal Frontal Transverse	Frontal Sagittal Vertical
Sellar (saddle)				1st carpometacarpal joint	Sagittal Frontal Transverse	Frontal Sagittal Vertical

Movements in joints

In many joints, several different movements are possible. Some joints permit only flexion and extension; others permit a wide range of movements, depending largely on the joint structure. The specific amount of movement possible in a joint may be measured by using an instrument known as a *goniometer* to compare the change in joint angles. The goniometer axis, or hinge point, is placed even with the axis of rotation at the joint line. As the joint is moved, both arms of the goniometer are held in place either along or parallel to the long axis of the bones on either side of the joint. The joint angle can then be read from the goniometer, as shown in Fig. 1.10. As an example, we could measure the angle between the femur and tibia in full knee extension (which would usually be zero) and then ask the person to flex the knee as far as possible. If we measured the angle again upon reaching full knee flexion, we would find a goniometer reading of around 140 degrees.

FIG. 1.10 • Goniometric measurement of hip joint flexion.

From Prentice WE: *Arnheim's principles of athletic training,* ed 11, New York, 2003, McGraw-Hill.

14   www.mhhe.com/floyd15e

Please note that the normal range of motion for a particular joint varies to some degree from person to person. Appendixes 1 and 2 provide the average normal ranges of motion for all joints.

When using movement terminology it is important to understand that the terms are used to describe the actual change in position of the bones relative to each other. That is, the angles between the bones change, whereas the movement occurs between the articular surfaces of the joint. We may say, in describing knee movement, "flex the knee"; this movement results in the leg moving closer to the thigh. Some describe this as leg flexion occurring at the knee joint and may say "flex the leg," meaning flex the knee. Additionally, movement terms are utilized to describe movement occurring throughout the full range of motion or through a very small range. Using the knee flexion example again, we may flex the knee through the full range by beginning in full knee extension (zero degrees of knee flexion) and flexing it fully, so that the heel comes in contact with the buttocks; this would be approximately 140 degrees of flexion.

We may also begin with the knee in 90 degrees of flexion and then flex it 30 degrees more; this movement results in a knee flexion angle of 120 degrees, even though the knee only flexed 30 degrees. In both examples, the knee is in different degrees of flexion. We may also begin with the knee in 90 degrees of flexion and extend it 40 degrees, which would result in a flexion angle of 50 degrees. Even though we extended the knee, it is still flexed, only less so than before.

Some movement terms may be used to describe motion at several joints throughout the body, whereas other terms are relatively specific to a joint or group of joints (Fig. 1.11). Rather than list the terms alphabetically, we have chosen to group them according to the body area and pair them with opposite terms where applicable. Additionally, prefixes such as *hyper-* or *hypo-* may be combined with these terms to emphasize excessive or reduced motion, respectively. Of these combined terms, *hyperextension* is the most commonly used.

A

B

C

FIG. 1.11 ● Joint movements. **A,** illustrates examples of sagittal plane movements; **extension** of left toes, ankle (plantar flexion), knee, hip, shoulder, elbow, wrist, fingers, and cervical spine; **flexion** of right toes, ankle (dorsiflexion), knee, hip, shoulder, elbow, wrist, and fingers. **B,** illustrates examples of lateral plane movements; **abduction** of left transverse tarsal/subtalar joints (eversion), shoulder, wrist, fingers, and shoulder girdle upward rotation, cervical spine (lateral flexion to left), and right hip; **adduction** of right transverse tarsal/subtarsal joints (inversion), shoulder, wrist, fingers, and shoulder girdle downward rotation. **C,** illustrates examples of transverse plane movements; **internal rotation** of right hip, left shoulder, radioulnar joints (pronation); **external rotation** of left knee, hip, right shoulder, radioulnar joints (supination), and cervical spine (right rotation).

Terms describing general movements

Abduction

Lateral movement away from the midline of the trunk in the frontal plane. An example is raising the arms or legs to the side horizontally.

Adduction

Movement medially toward the midline of the trunk in the frontal plane. An example is lowering the arm to the side or the thigh back to the anatomical position.

Flexion

Bending movement that results in a decrease of the angle in a joint by bringing bones together, usually in the sagittal plane. An example is the elbow joint when the hand is drawn to the shoulder.

Extension

Straightening movement that results in an increase of the angle in a joint by moving bones apart, usually in the sagittal plane. Using the elbow, an example is when the hand moves away from the shoulder.

Circumduction

Circular movement of a limb that delineates an arc or describes a cone. It is a combination of flexion, extension, abduction, and adduction. Sometimes referred to as circumflexion. An example occurs when the shoulder joint and the hip joint move in a circular fashion around a fixed point.

Diagonal abduction

Movement by a limb through a diagonal plane away from the midline of the body.

Diagonal adduction

Movement by a limb through a diagonal plane toward and across the midline of the body.

External rotation

Rotary movement around the longitudinal axis of a bone away from the midline of the body. Occurs in the transverse plane and is also known as rotation laterally, outward rotation, and lateral rotation.

Internal rotation

Rotary movement around the longitudinal axis of a bone toward the midline of the body. Occurs in the transverse plane and is also known as rotation medially, inward rotation, and medial rotation.

Terms describing ankle and foot movements

Eversion

Turning the sole of the foot outward or laterally in the frontal plane; abduction. An example is standing with the weight on the inner edge of the foot.

Inversion

Turning the sole of the foot inward or medially in the frontal plane; adduction. An example is standing with the weight on the outer edge of the foot.

Dorsal flexion (dorsiflexion)

Flexion movement of the ankle that results in the top of the foot moving toward the anterior tibia bone in the sagittal plane.

Plantar flexion

Extension movement of the ankle that results in the foot and/or toes moving away from the body in the sagittal plane.

Terms describing radioulnar joint movements

Pronation

Internally rotating the radius in the transverse plane so that it lies diagonally across the ulna, resulting in the palm-down position of the forearm.

Supination

Externally rotating the radius in the transverse plane so that it lies parallel to the ulna, resulting in the palm-up position of the forearm.

Terms describing shoulder girdle and shoulder joint movements

Depression

Inferior movement of the shoulder girdle in the frontal plane. An example is returning to the normal position from a shoulder shrug.

Elevation

Superior movement of the shoulder girdle in the frontal plane. An example is shrugging the shoulders.

Horizontal abduction

Movement of the humerus in the horizontal plane away from the midline of the body. Also known as horizontal extension or transverse abduction.

Horizontal adduction

Movement of the humerus in the horizontal plane toward the midline of the body. Also known as horizontal flexion or transverse adduction.

Protraction (abduction)

Forward movement of the shoulder girdle in the horizontal plane away from the spine. Abduction of the scapula.

Retraction (adduction)

Backward movement of the shoulder girdle in the horizontal plane toward the spine. Adduction of the scapula.

Rotation downward

Rotary movement of the scapula in the frontal plane with the inferior angle of the scapula moving medially and downward. Occurs primarily in the return from upward rotation. The inferior angle may actually move upward slightly as the scapula continues in extreme downward rotation.

Rotation upward

Rotary movement of the scapula in the frontal plane with the inferior angle of the scapula moving laterally and upward.

Terms describing spine movements

Lateral flexion (side bending)

Movement of the head and/or trunk in the frontal plane laterally away from the midline. Abduction of the spine.

Reduction

Return of the spinal column in the frontal plane to the anatomic position from lateral flexion. Adduction of the spine.

Terms describing wrist and hand movements

Dorsal flexion (dorsiflexion)

Extension movement of the wrist in the sagittal plane with the dorsal or posterior side of the hand moving toward the posterior side of the forearm.

Palmar flexion

Flexion movement of the wrist in the sagittal plane with the volar or anterior side of the hand moving toward the anterior side of the forearm.

Radial flexion (radial deviation)

Abduction movement at the wrist in the frontal plane of the thumb side of the hand toward the forearm.

Ulnar flexion (ulnar deviation)

Adduction movement at the wrist in the frontal plane of the little finger side of the hand toward the forearm.

Opposition of the thumb

Diagonal movement of the thumb across the palmar surface of the hand to make contact with the fingers.

Reposition of the thumb

Diagonal movement of the thumb as it returns to the anatomical position from opposition with the hand and/or fingers.

These movements are considered in detail in the chapters that follow as they apply to the individual joints.

Combinations of movements can occur. Flexion or extension can occur with abduction, adduction, or rotation.

Physiological movements versus accessory motions

Movements such as flexion, extension, abduction, adduction, and rotation occur by the bones moving through planes of motion about an axis of rotation at the joint. These movements may be referred to as physiological movements. The motion of the bones relative to the three cardinal planes resulting from these physiological movements is referred to *osteokinematic* motion. In order for these osteokinematic motions to occur, there must be movement between the actual articular surfaces of the joint. This motion between the articular surfaces is known as *arthrokinematics,* and includes three specific types of *accessory motion.* These accessory motions, named specifically to describe the actual change in relationship between the articular surface of one bone relative to another, are *roll, spin,* and *glide* (Fig. 1.12).

Roll is sometimes referred to as rock or rocking, whereas glide is sometimes referred to as slide or translation. If accessory motion is prevented from occurring, then physiological motion cannot occur to any substantial degree other than by joint compression or distraction. Because most diarthrodial joints in the body are composed of a concave surface articulating with a convex surface, roll and glide must occur together to some degree. For example, as illustrated in Fig. 1.13, as a person stands from a squatting position, in order for the knee to extend, the femur must roll forward and simultaneously slide backward on the tibia. If not for the slide, the femur would roll off the front of the tibia, and if not for the roll, the femur would slide off the back of the tibia.

FIG. 1.12 ● Joint arthrokinematics. **A,** Spin; **B,** Roll; **C,** Glide.

From Prentice WE: *Rehabilitation techniques in sports medicine,* ed 3, Dubuque, IA, 1999, WCB/McGraw-Hill.

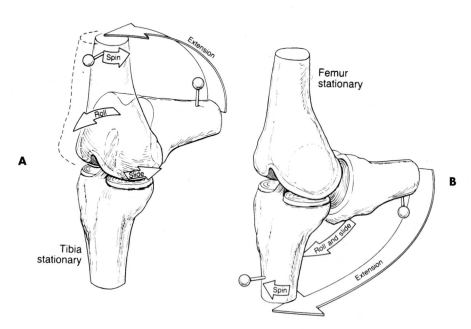

FIG. 1.13 ● Knee joint arthrokinematics. **A,** Standing from squatting; **B,** flexing from non-weightbearing position.

Modified from Prentice WE: *Rehabilitation techniques in sports medicine,* ed 3, Dubuque, IA, 1999, WCB/McGraw-Hill.

TABLE 1.5 • Accessory motion

Accessory motion	Anatomical joint example	Analogy	
Roll (rocking)	Knee extension occurring from femoral condyles rolling forward on tibia as a person stands from squatted position	Tire rolling across a road surface, as in normal driving with good traction	*Combination of roll & glide:* Tire spinning on slick ice (i.e., poor traction), but still resulting in movement across the road surface
Glide (slide or translation)	Knee extension occurring from femoral condyles sliding backward on tibia as a person stands from squatted position	Tire skidding across a slick surface with the brakes locked	
Spin	Radioulnar pronation/ supination occurring from spinning of radial head against humeral capitulum	Point of a toy top spinning around in one spot on the floor	

Spin may occur in isolation or in combination with roll and glide, depending upon the joint structure. To some degree, spin occurs at the knee as it flexes and extends. In the squatting to standing example, the femur spins medially or internally rotates as the knee reaches full extension. Table 1.5 provides examples of accessory motion.

Roll (rock)

A series of points on one articular surface contacts with a series of points on another articular surface.

Glide (slide, translation)

A specific point on one articulating surface comes in contact with a series of points on another surface.

Spin

A single point on one articular surface rotates about a single point on another articular surface. Motion occurs around some stationary longitudinal mechanical axis in either a clockwise or a counterclockwise direction.

Web site

Anatomy & Physiology Tutorials:

www.gwc.maricopa.edu/class/bio201/index.htm

Worksheet exercises

As an aid to learning, for in-class or out-of-class assignments, or for testing, tear-out worksheets are found at the end of the text (see pp. 322 and 323).

Posterior skeletal worksheet (no. 1)

On the posterior skeletal worksheet, list the names of the bones and all of the prominent features of each bone.

Anterior skeletal worksheet (no. 2)

On the anterior skeletal worksheet, list the names of the bones and all of the prominent features of each bone.

Laboratory and review exercises

1. Locate the various types of joints on a human skeleton and palpate their movements on a living subject.
2. Individually practice the various joint movements, on yourself or with another subject.
3. The specific body area joint movement terms arise from the basic motions in the three specific planes: flexion/extension in the sagittal plane, abduction/adduction in the frontal plane, and rotation in the transverse plane. With this in mind, complete the joint movement terminology chart on p. 21.
4. Determine which joints have movements possible in each of the following planes:
   a. Sagittal
   b. Frontal
   c. Transverse
5. Determine the planes in which the following activities occur. Also, use a pencil to visualize the axis for each of the following activities.
   a. Walking up stairs
   b. Turning a knob to open a door
   c. Nodding the head to agree
   d. Shaking the head to disagree
   e. Shuffling the body from side to side
   f. Looking over your shoulder to see behind you
6. Choose several different locations at random on your body and specifically describe the locations, using the correct anatomical directional terminology.
7. Stand facing a closed door. Reach out and grasp the knob. Turn it and open the door widely toward you. Determine all of the joints involved in this activity and list the movements for each joint.
8. Utilize a goniometer to measure the joint ranges of motion for several students in your class for each of the following movements. Compare your results with the average ranges provided in Appendixes 1 and 2.
   a. External and internal rotation of the shoulder with the shoulder in 90 degrees of abduction while supine
   b. Elbow flexion in the supine position
   c. Wrist extension with the forearm in neutral and the elbow in 90 degrees of flexion
   d. Hip external and internal rotation in the sitting position with the hip and knee each in 90 degrees of flexion
   e. Knee flexion in the prone position
   f. Ankle dorsiflexion with the knee in 90 degrees of flexion versus knee in full extension

Joint type, movement, and plane with axes of motion chart

Joint	Type	Planes of motion		
		Sagittal	Frontal	Transverse
Scapulothoracic joint				
Glenohumeral joint				
Elbow				
Radioulnar joint				
Wrist				
Metacarpophalangeal and metatarsophalangeal joints				
Proximal interphalangeal joints				
Distal interphalangeal joints				
Cervical spine				
Lumbar spine				
Hip				
Knee				
Ankle				

Joint position chart

Multiple joint movement	Joints and respective position of each
Reach straight over the superior aspect of your head to touch the contralateral ear	
Place the toe of one foot against the posterior aspect of the contralateral calf	
Reach behind the back and use your thumb to touch a spinous process	
Pull the knee as far as possible to the ipsilateral shoulder	
Place the plantar aspect of both feet against each other	

9. Complete the joint type, movement, and plane of motion chart (p. 20) by
   a. Filling in the type of diarthrodial joint
   b. Listing the movements of the joint under the plane of motion in which they occur
10. Using proper terminology, complete the joint position chart above by listing the name of each joint involved and its position upon completion of the multiple joint movement.

Joint movement terminology chart

For each specific motion in the left column, provide the basic motion that it represents in the right column by using *flexion, extension, abduction, adduction,* or *rotation (external* or *internal).*

Specific motion	Basic motion
Eversion	
Inversion	
Dorsal flexion	
Plantar flexion	
Pronation	
Supination	
Lateral flexion	
Radial flexion	
Ulnar flexion	

References

Anthony C, Thibodeau G: *Textbook of anatomy and physiology,* ed 10, St. Louis, 1979, Mosby.

Booher JM, Thibodeau GA: *Athletic injury assessment,* ed 4, New York, 2000, McGraw-Hill.

Goss CM: *Gray's anatomy of the human body,* ed 29, Philadelphia, 1973, Lea & Febiger.

Hamilton N, Luttgens K: *Kinesiology: scientific basis of human motion,* ed 10, New York, 2002, McGraw-Hill.

Lindsay DT: *Functional human anatomy,* St. Louis, 1996, Mosby.

Logan GA, McKinney WC: *Anatomic kinesiology,* ed 3, Dubuque, IA, 1982, Wm. C. Brown.

National Strength and Conditioning Association; Baechle TR, Earle RW: *Essentials of strength training and conditioning,* ed 2, Champaign, IL, 2000, Human Kinetics.

Neumann, DA: *Kinesiology of the musculoskeletal system: foundations for physical rehabilitation,* St. Louis, 2002, Mosby.

Northrip JW, Logan GA, McKinney WC: *Analysis of sport motion: anatomic and biomechanic perspectives,* ed 3, Dubuque, IA, 1983, Brown.

Prentice WE: *Rehabilitation techniques in sports medicine,* ed 3, New York, 1999, McGraw-Hill.

Stedman TL: *Stedman's medical dictionary,* ed 23, Baltimore, 1976, Williams & Wilkins.

Steindler A: *Kinesiology of the human body,* Springfield, Ill, 1970, Charles C Thomas.

Van De Graaff KM: *Human anatomy,* ed 5, New York, 2000, McGraw-Hill.

Van De Graaff KM, Fox SI, LaFleur KM: *Synopsis of human anatomy & physiology,* Dubuque, IA, 1997, Wm. C. Brown.

Chapter 2

Neuromuscular Fundamentals

Objectives

- To review the basic anatomy and function of the muscular and nervous systems

- To review and understand the basic terminology used to describe muscular locations, arrangements, characteristics, and roles, as well as neuromuscular functions

- To learn and understand the different types of muscle contraction and the factors involved in each

- To learn and understand basic neuromuscular concepts in relation to how muscles function in joint movement and work together to achieve motion

- To develop a basic understanding of the neural control mechanisms for movement

---

Online Learning Center Resources

Visit *Manual of Structural Kinesiology's* Online Learning Center at **www.mhhe.com/floyd15e** for additional information and study material for this chapter, including:

- *Self-grading quizzes*
- *Anatomy flashcards*
- *Animations*

Skeletal muscles are responsible for movement of the body and all of its joints. Muscle contraction produces the force that causes joint movement in the human body. In addition to the function of movement, muscles also provide protection, contribute to posture and support, and produce a major portion of total body heat. There are over 600 skeletal muscles, which constitute approximately 40% to 50% of body weight. Of these, there are 215 pairs of skeletal muscles. These pairs of muscles usually work in cooperation with each other to perform opposite actions at the joints they cross. In most cases, muscles work in groups rather than independently to achieve a given joint motion. This is known as *aggregate muscle action*.

Muscle nomenclature

In attempting to learn the skeletal muscles, it is helpful to have an understanding of how they are named. Muscles are usually named because of one or more distinctive characteristics, such as their visual appearance, anatomical location, or function. Examples of skeletal muscle naming are as follows:

Shape—deltoid, rhomboid
Size—gluteus maximus, teres minor
Number of divisions—triceps brachii
Direction of its fibers—external oblique
Location—rectus femoris, palmaris longus
Points of attachment—coracobrachialis, extensor hallucis longus, flexor digitorum longus
Action—erector spinae, supinator, extensor digiti minimi
Action and shape—pronator quadratus
Action and size—adductor magnus
Shape and location—serratus anterior

Location and attachment—brachioradialis
Location and number of divisions—biceps femoris

In discussions regarding the muscles they are often grouped together for brevity of conversation and clearer understanding. The naming of muscle groups follows a similar pattern. Next are some muscle groups according to different naming rationales.

Shape—hamstrings
Number of divisions—quadriceps, triceps surae
Location—peroneals, abdominal, shoulder girdle
Action—hip flexors, rotator cuff

The total superficial muscular system is shown in Figs. 2.1 and 2.2. Any figure is limited, since many muscles are not surface muscles. Still, these

Frontalis
Orbicularis oculi
Masseter
Sternocleidomastoid
Sternothyroid
Deltoid (anterior)
Pectoralis major
Coracobrachialis
Latissimus dorsi
Serratus anterior
Brachioradialis
Rectus sheath
Extensor carpi radialis longus
Palmaris longus
Tensor fasciae latae
Sartorius

Quadriceps femoris {
Rectus femoris
Vastus lateralis
Vastus medialis
Vastus intermedius (not shown)
}

Tibialis anterior
Peroneus longus
Extensor digitorum longus
Peroneus brevis
Tendon extensor hallucis longus

Orbicularis oris
Sternohyoid
Trapezius
Triceps brachii
Biceps brachii
Brachialis
Pronator teres
External oblique
Rectus abdominis
Flexor carpi radialis
Iliopsoas
Pectineus
Adductor longus
Gracilis
Adductor magnus
Gastrocnemius
Soleus

FIG. 2.1 ● Superficial muscles of the human body, anterior view from anatomical position.

From Thibodeau GA: *Anatomy and physiology,* St. Louis, 1987, Mosby.

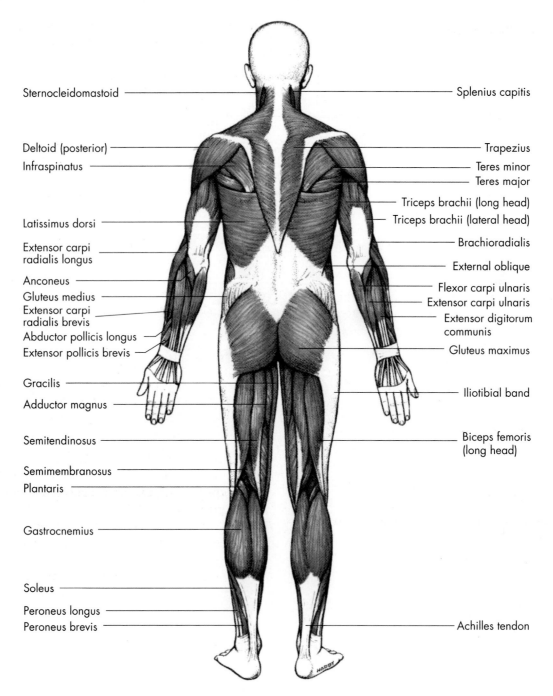

Sternocleidomastoid

Deltoid (posterior)

Infraspinatus

Latissimus dorsi

Extensor carpi radialis longus

Anconeus

Gluteus medius

Extensor carpi radialis brevis

Abductor pollicis longus

Extensor pollicis brevis

Gracilis

Adductor magnus

Semitendinosus

Semimembranosus

Plantaris

Gastrocnemius

Soleus

Peroneus longus

Peroneus brevis

Splenius capitis

Trapezius

Teres minor

Teres major

Triceps brachii (long head)

Triceps brachii (lateral head)

Brachioradialis

External oblique

Flexor carpi ulnaris

Extensor carpi ulnaris

Extensor digitorum communis

Gluteus maximus

Iliotibial band

Biceps femoris (long head)

Achilles tendon

FIG. 2.2 ● Superficial muscles of the human body, posterior view.

From Thibodeau GA: *Anatomy and physiology,* St. Louis, 1987, Mosby.

figures will help provide a better overview of the entire superficial muscular structure.

Muscles shown in these figures, and many other muscles, will be studied in more detail as

each joint of the body is considered in other chapters of this book.

Shape of muscles and fiber arrangement

Various muscles have different shapes, and their fibers may be arranged differently in relation to each other and to the tendons to which they join. The shape and fiber arrangement play a role in the muscle's ability to exert force and the range through which it can effectively exert force onto the bones to which it is attached. A factor in the ability of a muscle to exert force is its cross-section diameter. Keeping all other factors constant, a muscle with a greater cross-section diameter will be able to exert a greater force. A factor in the ability of a muscle to move a joint through a large range of motion is its ability to shorten. Generally, longer muscles can shorten through a greater range and therefore are more effective in moving joints through large ranges of motion.

Essentially, all skeletal muscles may be grouped into two major types of fiber arrangements: parallel and pennate. Each may be subdivided further according to shape.

Parallel muscles have their fibers arranged parallel to the length of the muscle. Generally, parallel muscles will produce a greater range of movement than similar-sized muscles with a pennate arrangement. Parallel muscles are categorized into the following shapes:

Flat muscles are usually thin and broad, originating from broad, fibrous, sheet-like aponeuroses that allow them to spread their forces over a broad area. Examples include the rectus abdominus and external oblique.

Fusiform muscles are spindle-shaped with a central belly that tapers to tendons on each end; this allows them to focus their power onto small, bony targets. Examples are the brachialis and the brachioradialis.

Strap muscles are more uniform in diameter with essentially all of their fibers arranged in a long parallel manner. This also enables a focusing of power onto small, bony targets. The sartorius is an example.

Radiate muscles are also described sometimes as being triangular, fan-shaped, or convergent. They have the combined arrangement of flat and fusiform muscles, in that they originate on broad aponeuroses and converge onto a tendon such as the pectoralis major or trapezius.

Sphincter or circular muscles are technically endless strap muscles which surround openings and function to close them upon contraction. An example is the orbicularis oris, surrounding the mouth.

Pennate muscles have shorter fibers that are arranged obliquely to their tendons in a structure similar to that of a feather. This arrangement increases the cross-sectional area of the muscle, thereby increasing the power. Pennate muscles are categorized based upon the exact arrangement between the fibers and the tendon.

Unipennate muscle fibers run obliquely from a tendon on one side only. Examples are seen in the biceps femoris, extensor digitorum longus, and tibialis posterior.

Bipennate muscle fibers run obliquely on both sides from a central tendon, as in the rectus femoris and flexor hallucis longus.

Multipennate muscles have several tendons with fibers running diagonally between them, as in the deltoid.

Type and Description	Appearance
Parallel—straplike; long excursion (contract over a great distance); good endurance; not especially strong; e.g., sartorius and rectus abdominis muscles	
Radiate—fan-shaped; force of contraction focused onto a single point of attachment; stronger than parallel type; e.g., deltoid and pectoralis major	
Sphincteral—fibers concentrically arranged around a body opening (orifice); act as a sphincter when contracted; e.g., orbicularis oculi and orbicularis oris	
Pennate—many fibers per unit area; strong muscles; short excursions; highly dexterous; tire quickly; three types: (a) unipennate, (b) bipennate, and (c) multipennate	A B C

FIG. 2.3 ● Muscle shapes and fiber arrangement.

Modified from Van de Graaff KM: *Human anatomy,* ed 6, Dubuque, IA, 2002, McGraw-Hill.

Bipennate and unipennate produce strongest contraction. Review Fig. 2.3 regarding muscle shapes and fiber arrangements.

Muscle tissue properties

Skeletal muscle tissue has four properties related to its ability to produce force and movement about joints. *Irritability* refers to the muscle property of being sensitive or responsive to chemical, electrical, or mechanical stimuli. *Contractility* refers to the ability of muscle to contract and develop tension or internal force against resistance when stimulated. *Extensibility* refers to the ability of muscle to be stretched back to its original length following contraction. *Elasticity* refers to

the ability of muscle to return to its original length following stretching.

Muscle terminology

Locating the muscles, their proximal and distal attachments, and their relationship to the joints they cross is critical to determining the effects that muscles have on the joints. It is also necessary to understand certain terms as body movement is considered.

Intrinsic

Pertaining usually to muscles within or belonging solely to the body part on which they act. The small intrinsic muscles found entirely within the hand are examples.

Extrinsic

Pertaining usually to muscles that arise or originate outside of (proximal to) the body part on which they act. The forearm muscles that attach proximally on the distal humerus and insert on the fingers are examples.

Action

The specific movement of the joint resulting from a concentric contraction of a muscle which crosses the joint. An example is the biceps brachii, which has the action of flexion at the elbow. In most cases a particular action is usually caused by a group of muscles working together. Any of the muscles in the group can be said to cause the action, even though it is usually an effort of the entire group. A particular muscle may cause more than one action either at the same joint or at a different joint, depending upon the characteristics of the joints crossed by the muscle and the exact location of the muscle and its attachments in relation to the joint(s).

Innervation

The segment of the nervous system defined as being responsible for providing a stimulus to muscle fibers within a specific muscle or portion of a muscle. A particular muscle may be innervated by more than one nerve, and a particular nerve may innervate more than one muscle or portion of a muscle.

Amplitude

Range of muscle fiber length between maximal and minimal lengthening.

Gaster (belly or body)

The central, fleshy portion of the muscle that generally increases in diameter as the muscle contracts. It is the contractile portion of the muscle.

When a particular muscle contracts, it tends to pull both ends toward the *gaster,* or middle, of the muscle. Consequently, if neither of the bones to which a muscle is attached were stabilized, then both bones would move toward each other upon contraction. The more common case, however, is that one bone is more stabilized by a variety of factors, and as a result, the less stabilized bone usually moves toward the more stabilized bone upon contraction.

Origin

Proximal attachment, generally considered the least movable part or the part that attaches closest to the midline or center of the body.

Insertion

Distal attachment, generally considered the most movable part or the part that attaches farthest from the midline or center of the body.

As an example, in the biceps curl exercise the biceps brachii muscle in the arm has its origin (least movable bone) on the scapula and its insertion (most movable bone) on the radius. In some movements this process can be reversed. An example of this reversal can be seen in the pull-up, where the radius is relatively stable and the scapula moves up. The biceps brachii would be an extrinsic muscle of the elbow, whereas the brachialis would be intrinsic to the elbow. For each muscle studied, the origin and insertion are indicated.

Types of muscle contraction

All muscle contractions can be classified as being either isometric or isotonic. An isometric contraction occurs when tension is developed within the muscle but the joint angles remain constant. Isometric contractions may be thought of as static contractions, because a significant amount of tension may be developed in the muscle to maintain the joint angle in a relatively static or stable position.

Isotonic contractions involve the muscle developing tension to either cause or control joint movement. They may be thought of as dynamic contractions, because the varying degrees of tension in the muscles are causing the joint angles to change. The isotonic type of muscle contraction is classified further as being either concentric or eccentric on the basis of whether shortening or lengthening occurs. In Fig. 2.4, *A* and *B* illustrate isotonic and *C* demonstrates isometric contractions.

It is also important to note that movement may occur at any given joint without any muscle contraction whatsoever. This movement is referred to as passive, and is solely due to external forces such as those applied by another person, object, or resistance, or the force of gravity in the presence of muscle relaxation.

Concentric contractions involve the muscle developing tension as it shortens, whereas eccentric contractions involve the muscle lengthening under tension. Actually, the term *contraction* is somewhat contradictory in regard to eccentric muscle activity, since the muscle is really lengthening while maintaining considerable tension. Eccentric muscle action is perhaps more correct.

Concentric contraction

Involves the muscle developing tension as it shortens, and occurs when the muscle develops enough force to overcome the applied resistance. Concentric contractions may be thought of as causing movement against gravity or resistance and are described as positive contractions. The force developed by the muscle is greater than that of the resistance. This results in the joint angle being changed in the direction of the applied muscular force and causes the body part to move against gravity or external forces.

Eccentric contraction (muscle action)

Involves the muscle lengthening under tension, and occurs when the muscle gradually lessens in tension to control the descent of the resistance. The weight or resistance may be thought of as overcoming the muscle contraction, but not to the point that the muscle cannot control the descending movement. Eccentric muscle actions control movement with gravity or resistance and are described as negative contractions. The force developed by the muscle is less than that of the resistance; this results in a change in the joint angle in the direction of the resistance or external force, and causes the body part to move with gravity or external forces (resistance). Some authorities refer to this as a muscle action instead of a contraction, since the muscle is lengthening as opposed to shortening.

Muscle contracts with force greater than resistance and shortens (concentric contraction)

Movement

Muscle contracts with force less than resistance and lengthens (eccentric contraction)

Movement

Muscle contracts but does not change length (isometric contraction)

No movement

A　　　　　　　　　**B**　　　　　　　　　**C**

FIG. 2.4 ● Isotonic and isometric contractions. **A,** concentric contraction; **B,** Eccentric contraction; **C,** Isometric contractions, occurring when a muscle contracts but does not shorten.

Modified from Shier David; Butler Jackie; Lewis Ricki: *Hole's human anatomy & physiology,* ed 9, Dubuque, IA, 2002, McGraw-Hill.

Table 2.1 explains the various types of contraction and resultant joint movements. The terminology utilized in defining and describing these actions is included.

Various exercises may use any one or all of these contraction types for muscle development.

Development of exercise machines has resulted in another type of muscle exercise known as *isokinetics*. Isokinetics is not another type of contraction, as some authorities have mistakenly described; rather, it is a specific technique that may

TABLE 2.1 • Muscle contraction and movement matrix

Definitive and descriptive factors	Types of contraction			Movement without contraction
	Isometric	Isotonic		
		Concentric	Eccentric	
Agonist muscle length	No appreciable change	Shortening →←	Lengthening ←→	Dictated solely by gravity and/or external forces
Antagonist muscle length	No appreciable change	Lengthening ←→	Shortening →←	Dictated solely by gravity and/or external forces
Joint angle changes	No appreciable change	In direction of force	In direction of external force (resistance)	Dictated solely by gravity and/or external forces
Direction of body part	Against immovable object or matched external force (resistance)	Against gravity and/or other external force (resistance)	With gravity and/or other external force (resistance)	Consistent with gravity and/or other external forces
Motion	Pressure (force) applied, but no resulting motion	Causes motion	Controls motion	Either no motion or passive motion occurs as a result of gravity and/or other external forces
Description	Static Fixating	Dynamic shortening Positive work	Dynamic lengthening Negative work	Passive Relaxation
Applied muscle force versus resistance	Force = resistance	Force > resistance	Force < resistance	No force, all resistance
Speed relative to gravity or applied resistance including inertial forces	Equal to speed of applied resistance	Faster than the inertia of the resistance	Slower than the speed of gravity or applied inertial forces	Consistent with inertia of applied external forces or the speed of gravity
Acceleration/deceleration	Zero acceleration	Acceleration ↗	Deceleration ↘	Either zero or acceleration consistent with applied external forces
Descriptive symbol	(=)	(+)	(−)	(0)

use any or all of the different types of contractions. Isokinetics is a type of dynamic exercise usually using concentric and/or eccentric muscle contractions in which the speed (or velocity) of movement is constant and muscular contraction (ideally, maximum contraction) occurs throughout the movement. Biodex, Cybex, Lido, and other new types of apparatuses are engineered to allow this type of exercise.

Students well educated in kinesiology should be qualified to prescribe exercises and activities for the development of large muscles and muscle groups in the human body. They should be able to read the description of an exercise or observe an exercise and immediately know the most important muscles being used. Descriptive terms of how muscles function in joint movements follow.

Role of muscles

Agonist FIG. 2.5

Generally described as muscles that, when contracting concentrically, cause joint motion through a specified plane of motion; known as primary or prime movers, or muscles most involved.

Antagonist FIG. 2.5

Muscles that are usually located on the opposite side of the joint from the agonist and have the opposite concentric action; known as contralateral muscles, they work in cooperation with agonist muscles by relaxing and allowing movement, but when contracting concentrically, they perform the opposite joint motion of the agonist.

FIG. 2.5 ● Agonist–antagonist relationship. **A,** Biceps is agonist in flexing the elbow while triceps is antagonist; **B,** Triceps is agonist in extending the elbow while biceps is antagonist.

Modified from Shier David; Butler Jackie; Lewis Ricki: *Hole's human anatomy & physiology,* ed 9, Dubuque, IA, 2002, McGraw-Hill.

Stabilizers

Muscles that surround the joint or body part and contract to fixate or stabilize the area to enable another limb or body segment to exert force and move; known as fixators, they are essential in establishing a relatively firm base for the more distal joints to work from when carrying out movements.

Synergist

Muscles that assist in the action of agonists but are not necessarily prime movers for the action; known as guiding muscles, they assist in refined movement and rule out undesired motions.

Neutralizers

Muscles that counteract or neutralize the action of other muscles to prevent undesirable movements such as inappropriate muscle substitutions; referred to as neutralizing, they contract to resist specific actions of other muscles.

Tying roles of muscles all together

When a muscle with multiple agonist actions contracts, it attempts to perform all of its actions. Muscles cannot determine which of their actions are appropriate for the task at hand. The resulting actions actually performed depend upon several factors, such as the motor units activated, joint position, muscle length, and the relative contraction or relaxation of other muscles acting on the joint. In certain instances, two muscles may work in synergy by counteracting their opposing actions to accomplish a common action.

As discussed, agonist muscles are primarily responsible for a given movement, such as that of hip flexion and knee extension during kicking a ball. In this example, the hamstrings are antagonistic and relax to allow the kick to occur. This does not mean all other muscles in the hip area are uninvolved. The preciseness of the kick depends upon the involvement of many other muscles. As the lower extremity swings forward, its route and subsequent angle at the point of contact depend upon a certain amount of relative contraction or relaxation in the hip abductors, adductors, internal rotators, and external rotators. These muscles act in a synergistic fashion to guide the lower extremity in a precise manner. That is, they are not primarily responsible for knee extension and hip flexion, but they do contribute to the accuracy of the total movement. These guiding muscles assist in refining the kick and preventing extraneous motions. Additionally,

the muscles in the contralateral hip and pelvic area must be under relative tension to help fixate or stabilize the pelvis on that side in order to provide a relatively stable pelvis for the hip flexors on the involved side to contract against. In kicking the ball, the pectineus and tensor fascia latae are adductors and abductors, respectively, in addition to flexors. The actions of abduction and adduction are neutralized by each other and the common action of the two muscles results in hip flexion.

From a practical point of view, it is not essential that individuals know the exact force exerted by each of the elbow flexors—biceps, brachialis, and brachioradialis—in chinning. It is important to understand that this muscle group is the agonist or primary mover responsible for elbow joint flexion. Similarly, it is important to understand that these muscles contract concentrically when the chin is pulled up to the bar and that they contract eccentrically when the body is lowered slowly. Antagonistic muscles produce actions opposite those of the agonist. For example, the muscles that produce extension of the elbow joint are antagonistic to the muscles that produce flexion of the elbow joint. It is important to understand that specific exercises need to be given for the development of each antagonistic muscle group. The return movement to the hanging position at the elbow joint after chinning is elbow joint extension, but the triceps and anconeus are not being strengthened. A concentric contraction of the elbow joint flexors occurs, followed by an eccentric contraction of the same muscles.

Reversal of muscle function

A muscle group that is described to perform a given function can contract to control the exact opposite motion. Fig. 2.5, *A* illustrates how the biceps is an agonist by contracting concentrically to flex the elbow. The triceps is an antagonist to elbow flexion, and the pronator teres is considered to be a synergist to the biceps in this example. If the biceps were to slowly lengthen and control elbow extension, it would still be the agonist, but it would be contracting eccentrically. Fig. 2.5, *B* illustrates how the triceps is an agonist by contracting concentrically to extend the elbow. The biceps is an antagonist to elbow extension in this example. If the triceps were to slowly lengthen and control elbow flexion, it would still be the agonist, but it would be eccentrically contracting. In both of these examples, the deltoid, trapezius, and various other shoulder muscles are serving as stabilizers of the shoulder area.

Determination of muscle action

The specific action of muscle may be determined through a variety of methods. These include reasoning in consideration of anatomical lines of pull, anatomical dissection, palpation, models, electromyography, and electrical stimulation.

With an understanding of a muscle's line of pull relative to a joint, one may determine the muscle's action at the joint. (See lines of pull later in this chapter.) Although not available to all students, cadaver dissection of muscles and joints is an excellent way to further understand muscle action.

For most of the skeletal muscles, *palpation* is a very useful way to determine muscle action. This is done through using the sense of touch to feel or examine a muscle as it is contracted. Palpation is limited to superficial muscles, but is also helpful in furthering one's understanding of joint mechanics. Models such as long rubber bands may be used to facilitate understanding of lines of pull and simulate muscle lengthening or shortening as joints move through various ranges of motion.

Electromyography (EMG) utilizes either surface electrodes that are placed over the muscle or fine wire/needle electrodes placed into the muscle. As the subject then moves the joint and contracts the muscles, the EMG unit detects the action potentials of muscles and provides an electronic readout of the contraction intensity and duration. EMG is the most accurate way of detecting the presence and extent of muscle activity.

Electrical muscle stimulation is somewhat a reverse approach of electromyography. Instead of electricity being to detect muscle action, it is used to cause muscle activity. Surface electrodes are placed over a muscle and then the stimulator causes the muscle to contract. The joint's actions may then be observed to see the effect of the muscle's contraction on it.

Lines of pull

Combining the knowledge of a particular joint's functional design and diarthrodial classification with an understanding of the specific location of a musculotendinous unit as it crosses a joint is extremely helpful in understanding its action on the joint. For example, knowing that the rectus femoris has its origin on the anterior inferior iliac spine and its insertion on the tibial tuberosity via the patella, you can then determine that the muscle must have an anterior relationship to the knee and hip. Combining this knowledge with knowing that both joints are capable of sagittal plane movements such as flexion/extension, then you can determine that when the rectus femoris contracts concentrically that it should cause the knee to extend and the hip to flex.

Furthermore, knowing that the semitendinosus, semimembranosus, and biceps femoris all originate on the ischial tuberosity and that the semitendinosus and semimembranosus cross the knee posteromedially before inserting on the tibia but that the biceps femoris crosses the knee posterolaterally before inserting on the fibula head, you may determine that all three muscles have posterior relationships to the hip and knee which would enable them to be hip extensors and knee flexors upon concentric contraction. The specific knowledge related to their distal attachments and the knee's capability to rotate when flexed would allow you to determine that the semitendinosus and semimembranosus would cause internal rotation, whereas the biceps femoris would cause external rotation. A knowledge of the knee's axes of rotation being only frontal and vertical, but not sagittal enables you to determine that even though the semitendinosus and semimembranosus have a posteromedial line of pull and the biceps femoris has a posterolateral line of pull, they are not capable of adduction and abduction, respectively.

You also apply this concept in reverse. For example, if the only action of a muscle such as the brachialis is known to be elbow flexion, then you should be able to determine that its line of pull must be anterior to the joint. Additionally, you would know that the origin of the brachialis must be located somewhere on the anterior humerus and the insertion must be somewhere on the anterior ulna.

Consider all of the following factors and their relationships as you study movements of the body to have a more thorough understanding.

1. Exact locations of bony landmarks to which muscles attach proximally and distally and their relationship to joints

2. The planes of motion through which a joint is capable of moving

3. The muscle's relationship or line of pull relative to the joint's axes of rotation

4. As a joint moves through a particular range of motion, the ability of the line of pull of a particular muscle to change and even result in the muscle having a different or opposite action than in the original position

5. The potential effect of other muscles' relative contraction or relaxation on a particular muscle's ability to cause motion

6. The effect of a muscle's relative length on its ability to generate force (See muscle length–tension relationship and active/passive insufficiency.)

7. The effect of the position of other joints on the ability of a biarticular or multiarticular muscle to generate force or allow lengthening (See biarticular/multiarticular muscles.)

Neural control of voluntary movement

When we discuss muscular activity we should really state it as neuromuscular activity, since muscle cannot be active without nervous innervation. All voluntary movement is a result of both the muscular and nervous systems working together. All muscle contraction occurs as a result of stimulation from the nervous system. Ultimately, every muscle fiber is innervated by a somatic motor neuron, which, when an appropriate stimulus is provided, results in a muscle contraction. Depending upon a variety of factors, this stimulus may be processed in varying degrees at different levels of the *central nervous system* (CNS), which, for the purposes of this discussion, may be divided into five levels of control. This listing, in order from the most general level of control and the most superiorly located to the most specific level of control and the most inferiorly located, includes the cerebral cortex, the basal ganglia, the cerebellum, the brain stem, and the spinal cord.

The *cerebral cortex* is the highest level of control. It provides for the creation of voluntary movement as aggregate muscle action, but not as specific muscle activity. Sensory stimuli from the body also are interpreted here to a degree for the determination of needed responses.

The *basal ganglia* is the next level. It controls the maintenance of postures and equilibrium and learned movements such as driving a car. Sensory integration for balance and rhythmic activities is controlled here.

Third, the *cerebellum* is a major integrator of sensory impulses and providing feedback relative to motion. It controls the timing and intensity of muscle activity to assist in the refinement of movements.

Next, the *brain stem* integrates all central nervous system activity through excitation and inhibition of desired neuromuscular actions and functions in arousal or maintaining a wakeful state.

The *spinal cord* is the common pathway between the CNS and the *peripheral nervous system* (PNS), which contains all the remaining nerves throughout the body. It has the most specific control and integrates various simple and complex spinal reflexes, as well as cortical and basal ganglia activity, with various classifications of spinal reflexes.

Functionally, the PNS can be divided into sensory and motor divisions. The sensory or *afferent* nerves bring impulses from receptors in the skin, joints, muscles, and other peripheral aspects of the body to the CNS, while the motor or *efferent* nerves carry impulses to the outlying regions of the body.

The spinal nerves, illustrated in Fig. 2.6, also provide both motor and sensory function for their respective portions of the body, and are named for the locations from which they exit the vertebral column. From each side of the spinal column, there are 8 cervical nerves, 12 thoracic nerves, 5 lumbar nerves, 5 sacral, and 1 coccygeal nerve. Cervical nerves 1 through 4 form the cervical plexus, which is generally responsible for sensation from the upper part of the shoulders to the back of the head and front of the neck. The cervical plexus supplies motor innervation to several muscles of the neck. Cervical nerves 5 through 8, along with thoracic nerve 1, form the brachial plexus, which supplies motor and sensory function to the upper extremity and most of the scapula. Thoracic nerves 2 through 12 run directly to specific anatomical locations in the thorax. All of the lumbar, sacral, and coccygeal nerves form the lumbosacral plexus, which supplies sensation and motor function to the lower trunk and the entire lower extremity and perineum.

One aspect of the sensory function of spinal nerves is to provide feedback to the CNS regarding

FIG. 2.6 ● Spinal nerve roots and plexuses.

Modified from Booher JM; Thibodeau GA: *Athletic injury assessment,* ed 4, Dubuque, IA, 2000, McGraw-Hill.

skin sensation. A defined area of skin supplied by a specific spinal nerve is known as a *dermatome*. Regarding motor function of spinal nerves, a *myotome* is defined as a muscle or group of muscles supplied by a specific spinal nerve. Certain spinal nerves are also responsible for reflexes. See Table 2.2 regarding the specific spinal nerve functions.

The basic functional units of the nervous system responsible for generating and transmitting impulses are nerve cells known as *neurons*. Neurons consist of a *neuron cell body,* one or more branching projections known as *dendrites* which transmit impulses to the neuron and cell body, and an *axon,* which is an elongated projection that transmits impulses away from neuron cell bodies. Neurons are classified into three types, according to the direction in which they transmit impulses. *Sensory neurons* transmit impulses to the spinal cord and brain from all parts of the body, whereas *motor neurons* transmit impulses away from the brain and spinal cord to muscle and glandular tissue. *Interneurons* are central or connecting neurons that conduct impulses from sensory neurons to motor neurons.

TABLE 2.2 • **Spinal nerve root dermatomes, myotomes, reflexes, and functional application**

	Nerve root	Dermatome afferent (sensory)	Myotome efferent (motor)	Reflexes	Functional application
Cervical plexus	C1	Touch: Vertex of skull	Upper neck muscles	None	None
	C2	Touch: Temple, forehead, occiput	Upper neck muscles	None	None
	C3	Touch: Entire neck, posterior cheek, temporal area, under mandible	Trapezius, splenius, capitis	None	Scapula retraction, neck extension Sensation to cheek and side of neck
	C4	Touch: Shoulder area, clavicular area, upper scapular area	Trapezius, levator scapulae	None	Scapula retraction & elevation Sensation to clavicle and upper scapula
Brachial plexus	C5	Touch: Deltoid area, anterior aspect of entire arm to base of thumb	Supraspinatus, infraspinatus, deltoid, biceps brachii	Biceps brachii	Shoulder abduction Sensation to lateral side of arm & elbow
	C6	Touch: Anterior arm, radial side of hand to thumb and index finger	Biceps, supinator, wrist extensors	Biceps brachii, brachioradialis	Elbow flexion, wrist extension Sensation to lateral side of forearm including thumb & index fingers
	C7	Touch: Lateral arm and forearm to index, long, and ring fingers	Triceps brachii, wrist flexors	Triceps brachii	Elbow extension, wrist flexion Sensation to middle of anterior forearm and long finger
	C8	Touch: Medial side of forearm to ring and little fingers	Ulnar deviators, thumb extensors, thumb adductors (rarely triceps)	None	Wrist ulnar deviation, thumb extension Sensation to posterior elbow & medial forearm to little fingers
	T1	Touch: Medial arm and forearm to wrist	Intrinsic muscles of the hand except for opponens pollicis and abductor pollicis brevis	None	Abduction and adduction of fingers Sensation medial arm & elbow

(continued)

	Nerve root	Dermatome afferent (sensory)	Myotome efferent (motor)	Reflexes	Functional application
	T2	Touch: Medial side of upper arm to medial elbow, pectoral and midscapular areas	Intercostal muscles	None	Sensation to medial upper arm, upper chest, and midscapular area
	T3–T12	Touch: T3–T6, upper thorax; T5–T7, coastal margin; T8–T12, abdomen and lumbar region	Intercostal muscles, abdominal muscles	None	Sensation to chest, abdomen, and low back
Lumbosacral plexus	L1	Touch: lower abdomen, groin, lumbar region from 2nd to 4th vertebrae, upper & outer aspect of buttocks	Quadratus Lumborum	None	Sensation to low back, over trochanter and groin
	L2	Touch: lower lumbar region, upper buttock, anterior aspect of thigh	Iliopsoas, quadriceps	None	Hip flexion Sensation to back, front of thigh to knee
	L3	Touch: medial aspect of thigh to knee, anterior aspect of lower 1/3 of the thigh to just below patella	Psoas, quadriceps	Patella or knee extensors	Hip flexion and knee extension Sensation to back, upper buttock, anterior thigh and knee, medial lower leg
	L4	Touch: medial aspect of lower leg & foot, inner border of foot, great toe	Tibialis anterior, extensor hallucis and digitorum longus, peroneals	Patella or knee extensors	Ankle dorsiflexion, transverse tarsal/subtalar inversion Sensation to medial buttock, lateral thigh, medial leg, dorsum of foot, big toe
	L5	Touch: lateral border of leg, anterior surface of the lower leg, top of foot to middle three toes	Extensor hallucis and digitorum longus, peroneals, gluteus maximus and medius, and dorsiflexors	None	Great toe extension, transverse talar/subtalar eversion Sensation to upper lateral leg, anterior surface of the lower leg, middle three toes
	S1	Touch: posterior aspect of the lower 1/4 of the leg, posterior aspect of the foot, including the heel, lateral border of the foot & sole	Gastrocnemius, soleus, gluteus maximus and medius, hamstrings, peroneals	Achilles reflex	Ankle plantarflexion, knee flexion, transverse talar/subtalar eversion Sensation to lateral leg, lateral foot, lateral two toes, plantar aspect of foot
	S2	Touch: posterior central strip of the leg from below the gluteal fold to 3/4 of the way down the leg	Gastrocnemius, soleus, gluteus maximus, hamstrings	None	Ankle plantarflexion and toe flexion Sensation to posterior thigh and upper posterior leg
	S3	Touch: Groin, medial thigh to knee	Intrinsic foot muscles	None	Sensation to groin and adductor region
	S4	Touch: Perineum, genitals, lower sacrum	Bladder, rectum	None	Urinary and bowel control Sensation to saddle area, genitals, anus

Proprioception and kinesthesis

The performance of various activities is significantly dependent upon neurological feedback from the body. Very simply, we use the various senses to determine a response to our environment, as when we use sight to know when to lift our hand to catch a fly ball. We are all familiar with the senses of smell, touch, sight, hearing, and taste. We are also aware of other sensations, such as pain, pressure, heat, and cold, but we often take for granted the sensations associated with neuromuscular activity through *proprioception*. Proprioceptors are internal receptors located in the skin, joints, muscles, and tendons which provide us feedback relative to the tension, length, and contraction state of muscle, the position of the body and limbs, and movements of the joints. These proprioceptors in combination with the other sense organs of the body are vital in *kinesthesis*, which is the awareness of the position and movement of the body in space. Proprioceptors specific to the muscles are muscle spindles and Golgi tendon organs (GTO), whereas Meissner's corpuscles, Ruffini's corpuscles, Pacinian corpuscles, and Krause's end-bulbs are proprioceptors specific to the joints and skin.

Muscle spindles, concentrated primarily in the muscle belly between the fibers, are sensitive to stretch and rate of stretch. As a result, when stretch occurs an impulse is sent to the CNS. The CNS then activates the motor neurons of the muscle and causes it to contract. The knee jerk or patella tendon reflex can be used as an example. When the reflex hammer strikes the patella tendon, it causes a quick stretch to the musculotendinous unit of the quadriceps. In response, the quadriceps fires and the knee extends. To an extent, the more sudden the tap of the hammer, the more significant the reflexive contraction. The stretch reflex provided by the muscle spindle may be utilized to facilitate a greater response, as in the case of a quick short squat before attempting a jump. The quick stretch placed upon the muscles in the squat enables the same muscles to generate more force in subsequently jumping off the floor.

The Golgi tendon organ, found in the tendon close to the muscle-tendon junction, is sensitive to both muscle tension and active contraction. The GTO is much less sensitive to stretch than muscle spindles are, and requires a greater stretch to be activiated. Tension in tendons and consequently in the GTO increases as the muscle contracts, which in turn activates the GTO. When the GTO stretch threshold is reached, an impulse is sent to the CNS, which in turn causes the muscle to relax and facilitates activation of the antagonists as a protective mechanism. That is, the GTO protects us from an excessive contraction by causing it to relax.

Pacinian corpuscles, concentrated around joint capsules, ligaments, and tendon sheaths and beneath the skin, are activated by rapid changes in the joint angle and by pressure changes affecting the capsule. This activation lasts only briefly and is not effective in detecting constant pressure. Pacinian corpuscles are helpful in providing feedback regarding the location of a body part in space following quick movements such as running or jumping.

Ruffini's corpuscles, located in deep layers of the skin and the joint capsule, are activated by strong and sudden joint movements as well as pressure changes. Unlike Pacinian corpuscles, their reaction to pressure changes are slower to develop, but their activation is continued as long as pressure is maintained. They are essential in detecting even minute joint position changes and providing information as to the exact joint angle.

Meissner's corpuscles and Krause's end-bulbs are located in the skin and in subcutaneous tissues. While they are important in receiving stimuli from touch, they are not so relevant to our discussion of kinesthesis. See Table 2.3 for further comparisons of sensory receptors.

The quality of movement and how we react to position change is significantly dependent upon the proprioceptive feedback from the muscles and joints. Like the other factors involving body movement, proprioception may be enhanced through specific training.

TABLE 2.3 • **Sensory receptors**

Receptors	Sensitivity	Location
Muscle spindles	Subconscious muscle sense	Skeletal muscles
Golgi tendon organs	Subconscious muscle sense	In tendons, near muscle-tendon junction
Pacinian corpuscles	Pressure, vibration	Subcutaneous, submucosa & subserous tissues around joints & external genitals, mammary glands
Ruffini's corpuscles	Touch, pressure	Skin & subcutaneous tissue of fingers, collagenous fibers of the joint capsule
Meissner's corpuscles	Fine touch, vibration	In skin
Krause's end-bulbs	Touch, thermal changes	Skin, subcutaneous tissue, lip & eyelid mucosa, external genitals

Neuromuscular concepts

All or none principle

When a particular muscle contracts, the contraction actually occurs at the muscle fiber level within a particular motor unit. In a typical muscle contraction, the number of muscle fibers contracting within the muscle may vary significantly, from relatively few to virtually all of the muscle fibers, depending on the number of muscle fibers within each activated motor unit and the number of motor units activated. Regardless of the number involved, the individual muscle fibers within a given motor unit will fire and contract either maximally or not at all. This is referred to as the "all or none principle." The difference between a particular muscle contracting to lift a minimal resistance versus the same muscle contracting to lift a maximal resistance is the number of muscle fibers recruited. The number of muscle fibers recruited may be increased by activating those motor units containing a greater number of muscle fibers, by activating more motor units, or by increasing the frequency of motor unit activation.

Muscle length–tension relationship

The maximal ability of a muscle to develop tension and exert force varies depending upon the length of the muscle during contraction. Generally, depending upon the particular muscle involved, the greatest amount of tension can be developed when a muscle is stretched between 100% and 130% of its resting length. As a muscle is stretched beyond this point, the amount of force it can exert significantly decreases. Likewise, a proportional decrease in the ability to develop tension occurs as a muscle is shortened. When a muscle is shortened to around 50% to 60% of resting length, its ability to develop contractile tension is essentially reduced to zero. This principle may be seen at work when we squat slightly to stretch the calf, hamstrings, and quadriceps before contracting them concentrically to jump. When attempting to isolate a muscle, we may take advantage of this principle to effectively reduce the contribution of other muscles in the group. For example, in hip extension, we may isolate the work of the gluteus maximus by maximally shortening the hamstrings with flexion of the knee to reduce their ability to act as hip extensors. See Fig. 2.7.

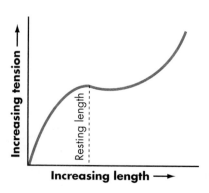

FIG. 2.7 • Muscle length–tension relationship.

Muscle force–velocity relationship

When the muscle is either concentrically or eccentrically contracting, the rate of length change is significantly related to the amount of force potential. When contracting concentrically against a light resistance, the muscle is able to contract at a high velocity. As the resistance increases, the maximal velocity at which the muscle is able to contract decreases. Eventually, as the load increases, the velocity decreases to zero; this results in an isometric contraction.

As the load increases even further beyond that which the muscle can maintain with an isometric contraction, the muscle begins to lengthen, resulting in an eccentric contraction or action. A slight increase in the load will result in relatively low velocity of lengthening. As the load increases even further, the velocity of lengthening will increase as well. Eventually, the load may increase to the point where the muscle can no longer resist. This will result in uncontrollable lengthening, or more likely, dropping of the load.

From this explanation you can see that there is an inverse relationship between concentric velocity and force production. As the force needed to cause movement of an object increases, the velocity of concentric contraction decreases. Furthermore, there is a somewhat proportional relationship between eccentric velocity and force production. As the force needed to control the movement of an object increases, the velocity of eccentric lengthening increases, at least until the point at which control is lost. This is illustrated in Fig. 2.8.

Angle of pull

Another factor of considerable importance in using the leverage system is the angle of pull of the muscles on the bone. The angle of pull may be defined as the angle between the line of pull of the muscle and the bone on which it inserts. For the sake of clarity and consistency, we need to specify that the actual angle referred to is the angle of attachment facing away from the joint as opposed to the angle on the side of the joint. With every degree of joint motion, the angle of pull changes. Joint movements and insertion angles involve mostly small angles of pull. The angle of pull decreases as the bone moves away from its anatomical position through the contraction of the local muscle group. This range of movement depends on the type of joint and bony structure.

Most muscles work at a small angle of pull, generally less than 50 degrees. The amount of muscular force needed to cause joint movement is affected by the angle of pull. Three components of muscular force are involved. The *rotary component,* also referred to as the vertical component, is the component of muscular force that acts perpendicular to the long axis of the bone (lever). When the to line of muscular force is at 90 degrees to the bone on which it attaches, all of the muscular force is rotary force; therefore, 100% of the force is contributing to the movement. That is, all of the force is being used to rotate the lever about its axis. The closer the angle of pull to 90 degrees, the greater the rotary component. At all other degrees of the angle of pull, one of the other two components of force is operating in addition to the rotary component. The same rotary component is continuing, although with less force, to rotate the lever about its axis. The second force component is the horizontal or *nonrotary component* and is either a *stabilizing component* or a *dislocating component,* depending on whether the angle of pull is less than or greater than 90 degrees. If the angle is less than 90 degrees, the force is a stabilizing force, because its

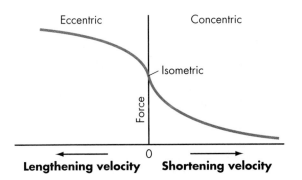

FIG. 2.8 ● Muscle force–velocity relationship.

pull directs the bone toward the joint axis. If the angle is greater than 90 degrees, the force is dislocating, because its pull directs the bone away from the joint axis (Fig. 2.9).

In some activities, it is desirable to have a person begin a movement when the angle of pull is at 90 degrees. Many boys and girls are unable to do a chin-up (pull-up) unless they start with the elbow in a position to allow the elbow flexor muscle group to approximate a 90-degree angle with the forearm.

This angle makes the chin-up easier because of the more advantageous angle of pull. The application of this fact can compensate for lack of sufficient strength. In its range of motion, a muscle pulls a lever through a range characteristic of itself, but it is most effective when approaching and going beyond 90 degrees. An increase in strength is the only solution for muscles that operate at disadvantageous angles of pull and require a greater force to operate efficiently.

Biarticular or multiarticular muscles

Biarticular muscles are those that cross, and act on two different joints. Depending on a variety of factors, a biarticular muscle may contract and cause motion at either one or both of its joints. Biarticular muscles have two advantages over uniarticular muscles. They can cause and/or control motion at more than one joint, and they may be able to maintain a relatively constant length due to "shortening" at one joint and "lengthening" at another joint. The muscle does not actually shorten at one joint and lengthen at the other; instead, the concentric shortening of the muscle to move one joint is offset by motion of the other joint, which moves its attachment of the muscle farther away. This maintenance of a relatively constant length results in the muscle ability to continue its exertion of force.

The biarticular muscles of the hip and knee provide excellent examples of two different patterns of action. An example of a *concurrent* movement pattern occurs when both the knee and the hip extend at the same time. If only the knee were to extend, the rectus femoris would shorten and lose tension as do the other quadriceps muscles, but its relative length and subsequent tension may be maintained due to its relative lengthening at the hip joint during extension. When a ball is kicked, an example of a *countercurrent* movement pattern may be observed.

FIG. 2.9 ● **A** to **C,** Components of force due to the angle of pull.

Modified from Hall SJ: *Basic biomechanics,* St. Louis, 1991, Mosby.

40   www.mhhe.com/floyd15e

During the forward movement phase of the lower extremity, the rectus femoris is concentrically contracted to both flex the hip and extend the knee. These two movements, when combined, increase the tension or stretch on the hamstring muscles at both the knee and the hip.

Multiarticular muscles act on three or more joints due to the line of pull between their origin and insertion crossing multiple joints. The principles discussed relative to biarticular muscles apply in a similar fashion to multiarticular muscles.

Reciprocal inhibition or innervation

As stated earlier, antagonist muscle groups must relax and lengthen when the agonist muscle group contracts. This effect, reciprocal innervation, occurs through reciprocal inhibition of the antagonists. Activation of the motor units of the agonists causes a reciprocal neural inhibition of the motor units of the antagonists. This reduction in neural activity of the antagonists allows them to subsequently lengthen under less tension. This may be demonstrated by comparing the ease at which one can stretch the hamstrings when simultaneously contracting the quadriceps versus attempting to stretch the hamstrings without the quadriceps contracted.

Active and passive insufficiency

As a muscle shortens, its ability to exert force diminishes, as discussed earlier. When the muscle becomes shortened to the point at which it cannot generate or maintain active tension, *active insufficiency* is reached. If the opposing muscle becomes stretched to the point at which it can no longer lengthen and allow movement, *passive insufficiency* is reached. These principles are most easily observed in either biarticular or multiarticular muscles when the full range of motion is attempted in all of the joints crossed by the muscle.

An example occurs when the rectus femoris contracts concentrically to both flex the hip and extend the knee. It may completely perform either action one at a time, but is actively insufficient to obtain full range at both joints simultaneously. Likewise, the hamstrings will not usually stretch enough to allow both maximal hip flexion and maximal knee extension; hence, they are passively insufficient. As a result of these phenomena, it is virtually impossible to actively extend the knee fully when beginning with the hip fully flexed, or vice versa.

Web sites

Neurologic Exam: An anatomical approach

http://.medlib.med.utah.edu/neurologicexam/ home_exam.html

A very thorough site regarding neurological exam including numerous movies with both normal & pathological results.

Cranial Nerves: Review info

www.gwc.maricopa.edu/class/bio201/cn/ cranial.htm

A good resource on the cranial nerves.

University of Arkansas for Medical Sciences Nerve tables

http://anatomy.uams.edu/HTMLpages/ anatomyhtml/nerves.html

Numerous tables of all nerves throughout the body.

A Cyberanatomy Tutorial of the Brachial Plexus and its Associated Injuries

http://anatome.ncl.ac.uk/tutorials/brachial1/text/

A hands on guide to the Brachial Plexus.

Dermatomes

www.meddean.luc.edu/lumen/MedEd/ GrossAnatomy/learnem/dermat/main_der.htm

An interactive review of the body's dermatomes.

Loyola University Medical Education Network Master Muscle List

www.meddean.luc.edu/lumen/MedEd/ GrossAnatomy/dissector/mml/

An interactive and graphical review of the muscles indexed alphabetically and by region.

Spinal Cord and Nervous System

www.driesen.com/spine_and_spinal_cord.htm

A review of the spinal cord and nervous system.

Proprioception Exercises Can Improve Balance

http://sportsmedicine.about.com/library/weekly/ aa062200.htm

Proprioception

Meds 1 Neurophysiology 2003

www.med.uwo.ca/physiology/courses/medsweb/

A site with Flash animations regarding neurophysiology.

Muscles

**http://users.rcn.com/jkimball.ma.ultranet/
BiologyPages/M/Muscles.html**

A review of the science behind muscle contractions.

An introduction to the mechanism of muscle contraction

www.ebsa.org/npbsn41/intro_muscle.html

A graphical review of muscle contraction physiology.

Laboratory and review exercises

1. Observe on a fellow student some of the muscles found in Figs. 2.1 and 2.2.
2. With a partner, choose a diarthrodial joint on the body and carry out each of the following exercises:
   a. Familiarize yourself with all of the joint's various movements and list them.
   b. Determine which muscle or muscle groups are responsible for each of the movements you listed in 2a.
   c. For the muscles or muscle groups you listed for each movement in 2b, determine the type of contraction occurring.
   d. Determine how to change the parameters of gravity and/or resistance so that the opposite muscles contract to control the same movements in 2c. Name the type of contraction occurring.
   e. Determine how to change the parameters of movement, gravity, and/or resistance so that the same muscles listed in 2c contract differently to control the opposite movement.
3. With the wrist in neutral, extend the fingers maximally and attempt to maintain the position and then extend the wrist maximally. What happens to the fingers and why?
4. Sit up very straight on a table with the knees flexed 90 degrees and the feet hanging free. Maintain this position while then flexing the right hip and attempting to cross your legs to place the right leg across the left knee. Is this difficult? What tends to happen to the low back and trunk? How can you modify this activity to make it easier?
5. Request a partner to stand with eyes closed while you position his/her arms in an odd position at the shoulders, elbows, and wrists. Ask your partner to describe the exact position of each joint while keeping the eyes closed. Then have your partner begin in the anatomical position, close the eyes, and subsequently reassume the position in which you had previously placed them. Explain the neuromechanisms involved in your partner's being able to both sense the joint position you placed them in and then reassume the same position.
6. Determine your one-repetition maximum for a biceps curl beginning in full extension and ending in full flexion. Carry out each of the following exercises with adequate periods for recovery in between.
   a. Begin with your elbow flexed 45 degrees and have a partner hand you a weight slightly heavier than your one-repetition maximum (approximately 5 pounds). Attempt to lift this through the remaining range of flexion. Can you reach full flexion? Explain your results.
   b. Begin with your elbow in 90 degrees of flexion. Have your partner hand you an even slightly heavier weight than in 6a. Attempt to hold the elbow flexed in this position for 10 seconds. Can you do so? Explain.
   c. Begin with your elbow in full flexion. Have your partner hand you an even slightly heavier weight than in 6b. Attempt to slowly lower the weight under control till you reach full extension. Can you do this? Explain.

References

Hamilton N, Luttgens K: *Kinesiology: scientific basis of human motion,* ed 10, Boston, 2002, McGraw-Hill.

Kreighbaum E, Barthels KM: *Biomechanics: a qualitative approach for studying human movement,* ed 4, Boston, 1996, Allyn & Bacon.

Lindsay DT: *Functional human anatomy,* St. Louis, 1996, Mosby.

Logan GA, McKinney WC: *Anatomic kinesiology,* ed 3, Dubuque, IA, 1982, Wm. C. Brown.

National Strength and Conditioning Association; Baechle TR, Earle RW: *Essentials of strength training and conditioning,* ed 2, Champaign, IL, 2000, Human Kinetics.

Neumann DA: *Kinesiology of the musculoskeletal system: foundations for physical rehabilitation,* St. Louis, 2002, Mosby.

Norkin CC, Levangie PK: *Joint structure and function—a comprehensive analysis,* Philadelphia, 1983, Davis.

Rasch PJ: *Kinesiology and applied anatomy,* ed 7, 1989, Philadelphia, Lea & Febiger.

Van De Graaff KM: *Human anatomy,* ed 4, Dubuque, IA, 1995, Wm. C. Brown.

Van De Graaf KM, Fox SI, LaFleur KM: *Synopsis of human anatomy & physiology,* Dubuque, IA, 1997, Wm. C. Brown.

Chapter 3

Basic Biomechanical Factors and Concepts

Objectives

- To know and understand how knowledge of levers can help improve physical performance

- To know and understand how the musculoskeletal system functions as a series of simple machines

- To know and understand how knowledge of torque and lever arm lengths can help improve physical performance

- To know and understand how knowledge of Newton's laws of motion can help improve physical performance

- To know and understand how knowledge of balance, equilibrium, and stability can help improve physical performance

- To know and understand how knowledge of force and momentum can help improve physical performance

- To know and understand the basic effects of mechanical loading on the tissues of the body

---

Online Learning Center Resources

Visit *Manual of Structural Kinesiology's* Online Learning Center at **www.mhhe.com/floyd15e** for additional information and study material for this chapter, including:

- *Self-grading quizzes*
- *Anatomy flashcards*
- *Animations*

Many students in kinesiology classes have some knowledge, from a college or high school physics or physical science course, of the physical laws that affect motion. They need to review these facts and principles as they learn to apply them to motion in the human body. This area, the study of mechanics as it relates to the functional and anatomical analysis of biological systems and especially humans, is known as *biomechanics.* We can understand movements of the human body more completely by studying its mechanical characteristics and principles.

A brief discussion of some of these biomechanical characteristics and principles is included in this chapter.

Mechanics, the study of physical actions of forces, can be subdivided into *statics* and *dynamics.* Statics involves the study of systems that are in a constant state of motion, whether at rest with no motion or moving at a constant velocity without acceleration. Statics involves all forces acting on the body being in balance, resulting in the body being in equilibrium. Dynamics involves the study of systems in motion with acceleration. A system in acceleration is unbalanced due to unequal forces acting on the body. Additional components of biomechanical study include *kinematics* and *kinetics.* Kinematics is concerned with the description of motion and includes consideration of time, displacement, velocity, acceleration, and space factors of a system's motion. Kinetics is the study of forces associated with the motion of a body.

Types of machines found in the body

In studying the movements associated with various physical activities, the musculoskeletal system may be thought of as a series of simple machines. Machines are used to increase mechanical advantage. The mechanical aspect of each component should be considered in analysis with respect to the components' machine-like function.

Machines function in four ways:

1. to balance multiple forces
2. to enhance force in an attempt to reduce the total force needed to overcome a resistance
3. to enhance range of motion and speed of movement so that resistance may be moved farther or faster than the applied force
4. to alter the resulting direction of the applied force. The arrangement of the musculoskeletal system provides for three types of machines in producing movement: levers, wheel axles, and pulleys. Of these, the lever is the most common.

Levers

It is difficult for a person to visualize his or her body as a system of levers. The topic may seem academic to some, but this is far from true. A person moves through the use of his or her system of levers. The anatomical levers of the body cannot be changed, but, when the system is properly understood, it can be used more efficiently to maximize the muscular efforts of the body.

A lever is defined as a rigid bar that turns about an *axis* of rotation, or fulcrum. The axis is the point of rotation about which the lever moves.

The lever rotates about the axis as a result of *force* (sometimes referred to as effort, *E*) being applied to it to cause its movement against a *resistance* or weight. In the body, the bones represent the bars, the joints are the axes, and the

muscles contract to apply the force. The amount of resistance can vary from maximal to minimal. In fact, the bones themselves or weight of the body segment may be the only resistance applied. All lever systems have each of these three components in one of three possible arrangements.

The arrangement or location of these three points in relation to one another determines the type of lever and the kind of motion for which they are best suited. These points are the axis, the point of force application (usually the muscle insertion), and the point of resistance application (sometimes the center of gravity of the lever and sometimes the location of an external resistance). When the axis (*A*) is placed between the force (*F*) and the resistance (*R*), a first-class lever is produced (Figs. 3.1 and 3.2). In second-class levers, the resistance is between the axis and the force (Figs. 3.1 and 3.3). If the force is placed between the axis and the resistance, a third-class lever is created (Figs. 3.1 and 3.4). Table 3.1 provides a summary of the three classes of levers and the characteristics of each.

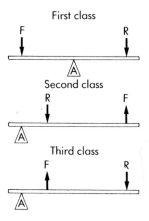

FIG. 3.1 ● Classification of levers.

Modified from Hall SJ: *Basic biomechanics,* ed 4, 2003, McGraw-Hill.

FIG. 3.2 ● **A** and **B**, First-class levers.

A modified from Booher JM, Thibodeau GA: *Athletic injury assessment,* ed 4, 2000, McGraw-Hill;
B modified from Hall SJ: *Basic biomechanics,* ed 4, 2003, McGraw-Hill.

First-class levers

Typical examples of a first-class lever are the crowbar, the seesaw, and the triceps in elbow extension. An example of this type of lever in the body is seen with the triceps applying the force to the olecranon (*F*) in extending the nonsupported forearm (*R*) at the elbow (*A*). Other examples of this type of lever may be seen in the body when the agonist and antagonist muscle groups on either side of a joint axis are contracting simultaneously, with the agonist producing force and the antagonist supplying the resistance. A first-class lever (Fig. 3.2) is designed basically to produce balanced movements when the axis is midway between the force and the resistance (e.g., a seesaw). When the axis is close to the force, the lever produces speed and range of motion (e.g., the triceps in elbow extension). When the axis is close to the resistance, the lever produces force motion (e.g., a crowbar).

In applying the principle of levers to the body, it is important to remember that the force is ap-plied where the muscle inserts in the bone, not in the belly of the muscle. For example, in elbow extension with the shoulder fully flexed and the arm beside the ear, the triceps applies the force to the olecranon of the ulna behind the axis of the elbow joint. As the applied force exceeds the amount of forearm resistance, the elbow extends.

The type of lever may be changed for a given joint and muscle, depending on whether the body segment is in contact with a surface such as a floor or wall. For example, we have demonstrated that the triceps in elbow extension is a first-class lever with the hand free in space where the arm is pushed away from the body. By placing the hand in contact with the floor, as in performing a push-up to push the body away from the floor, the same muscle action at this joint now changes the lever to second class, because the axis is at the hand and the resistance is the body weight at the elbow joint.

TABLE 3.1 • Classification of levers and characteristics of each

Class	Arrangement	Arm movement	Functional design	Relationship to axis	Practical example	Human example
1st	**F–A–R** Axis between force and resistance	Resistance arm and force arm move in opposite directions	Balanced movements	Axis near middle	Seesaw	Erector spinae extending the head on cervical spine
			Speed and range of motion	Axis near force	Scissors	Triceps brachii in extending the elbow
			Force motion	Axis near resistance	Crow bar	
2nd	**A–R–F** Resistance between axis and force	Resistance arm and force arm move in the same direction	Force motion (large resistance can be moved with relatively small force)	Axis near resistance	Wheel barrow, nutcracker	Gastrocnemius and soleus in plantar flexing the foot to raise the body on the toes
3rd	**A–F–R** Force between axis and resistance	Resistance arm and force arm move in the same direction	Speed and range of motion (requires large force to move a relatively small resistance)	Axis near force	Shoveling dirt, catapult	Biceps brachii and brachialis in flexing the elbow

FIG. 3.3 • **A** and **B,** Second-class levers.

A modified from Booher JM, Thibodeau GA: *Athletic injury assessment,* ed 4, 2000, McGraw-Hill;
B modified from Hall SJ: *Basic biomechanics,* ed 4, 2003, McGraw-Hill.

Second-class levers

A second-class lever (Fig. 3.3) is designed to produce force movements, since a large resistance can be moved by a relatively small force. An example of a second-class lever is a wheelbarrow. Besides the example given previously of the tri-

ceps extending the elbow in a push-up, a similar example of a second-class lever in the body is plantar flexion of the foot to raise the body up on the toes. The ball (*A*) of the foot serves as the axis of rotation as the ankle plantar flexors apply force to the calcaneus (*F*) to lift the resistance of the

Speed and range of motion

FIG. 3.4 • **A** and **B,** Third-class levers.

A modified from Booher JM, Thibodeau GA: *Athletic injury assessment,* ed 4, 2000, McGraw-Hill;
B modified from Hall SJ: *Basic biomechanics,* ed 4, 2003, McGraw-Hill.

body at the tibial articulation (*R*) with the foot. Opening the mouth against resistance provides another example of a second-class lever. There are relatively few other occurrences of second-class levers in the body.

Third-class levers

Third-class levers (Fig. 3.4), with the force being applied between the axis and the resistance, are designed to produce speed and range-of-motion movements. Most of the levers in the human body are of this type, which require a great deal of force to move even a small resistance. Examples include a screen door operated by a short spring and application of lifting force to a shovel handle with the lower hand while the upper hand on the shovel handle serves as the axis of rotation.

The biceps brachii is a typical example in the body. Using the elbow joint (*A*) as the axis, the biceps brachii applies force at its insertion on the radial tuberosity (*F*) to rotate the forearm up, with its center of gravity (*R*) serving as the point of resistance application.

The brachialis is an example of true third-class leverage. It pulls on the ulna just below the elbow, and, since the ulna cannot rotate, the pull is direct and true. The biceps brachii, on the other hand, supinates the forearm as it flexes, so that the third-class leverage applies to flexion only.

Other examples include the hamstrings contracting to flex the leg at the knee while in a standing position and the iliopsoas when it is used to flex the thigh at the hip.

Factors in use of anatomical levers

Our anatomical leverage system can be used to gain a mechanical advantage that will improve simple or complex physical movements. Some individuals unconsciously develop habits of using human levers properly, but frequently this is not true.

Torque and length of lever arms

To understand the leverage system, the concept of torque must be understood. *Torque,* or movement of force, is the turning effect of an eccentric force. *Eccentric force* is a force that is applied in a direction not in line with the center of rotation of an object with a fixed axis. In objects without a fixed axis, it is an applied force that is not in line with the object's center of gravity. For rotation to occur, an eccentric force must be applied. In the human body, the contracting muscle applies an eccentric force (not to be confused with eccentric contraction) to the bone on which it attaches and causes the bone to rotate about an axis at the joint. The amount of torque can be determined by multiplying the amount of force (*force magnitude*) by the *force arm.* The perpendicular distance between the location of force application and the axis is known as the force arm, moment arm, or torque arm. The force arm may be best understood as the shortest distance from the axis of rotation to the line of action of the force. The greater the distance of the force arm, the more torque produced by the force. A frequent practical application of torque and levers occurs when we purposely increase the force arm length in order to increase the torque so that we can more easily move a relatively large resistance. This is commonly referred to as increasing our leverage.

It is also important to note the *resistance arm,* which may be defined as the distance between the axis and the point of resistance application. In discussing the application of levers, it is necessary to understand the length relationship between the two lever arms. There is an inverse relationship between force and the force arm, just as there is between resistance and the resistance arm. The longer the force arm, the less force required to move the lever if the resistance and resistance arm remain constant. In addition, if the force and force arm remain constant, a greater resistance may be moved by shortening the resistance arm.

Also, there is a proportional relationship between the force components and the resistance components. That is, for movement to occur when either of the resistance components increases, there must be an increase in one or both of the force components. See Fig. 3.5 for an illustration of these relationships. Even slight variations in the location of the force and the resistance are important in determining the effective force of the muscle. This point can be illustrated in the following simple formula, using the biceps brachii muscle in each example:

$$F \times FA = R \times RA$$
(Force) × (Force arm) = (Resistance) × (Resistance arm)

FIG. 3.5 ● Relationship between force, force arms, resistance, and resistance arms.
A, If the force arm and resistance arm are equal in length, a force equal to the resistance is required to balance it; **B,** As the force arm becomes shorter an increasing amount of force is required to move a relatively smaller resistance; **C,** As the force arm becomes longer, a decreasing amount of force is required to move a relatively larger resistance.

Initial example

$$F \times 0.1 \text{ meter} = 45 \text{ Newtons} \times 0.25 \text{ meter}$$
$$0.1 \times F = 11.25 \text{ Newton-meters}$$
$$F = 112.5 \text{ Newton-meters}$$

Example A

Increase the (FA) by changing the insertion 0.05 meters:

$$F \times 0.15 \text{ meter} = 45 \text{ Newtons} \times 0.25 \text{ meter}$$
$$0.15 \times F = 11.25 \text{ Newton-meters}$$
$$F = 75 \text{ Newton-meters}$$

A change of 0.05 meters in the insertion can make a considerable difference in the force necessary to move the lever.

Example B

Reduce the (RA) by changing the point of resistance application 0.05 meters:

$$F \times 0.1 \text{ meter} = 45 \text{ Newtons} \times 0.2 \text{ meter}$$
$$0.1 \times F = 9 \text{ Newton-meters}$$
$$F = 90 \text{ Newton-meters}$$

Shortening the resistance arm can decrease the amount of force necessary to move the lever.

Example C

Change the (R) amount by reducing the resistance 1 Newton:

$$F \times 0.1 \text{ meter} = 44 \text{ Newtons} \times 0.25 \text{ meter}$$
$$0.1 \times F = 11 \text{ Newton-meters}$$
$$F = 110 \text{ Newton-meters}$$

Obviously, decreasing the amount of resistance can decrease the amount of force needed to move the lever.

The system of leverage in the human body is built for speed and range of movement at the expense of force. Short force arms and long resistance arms require great muscular strength to produce movement. In the forearm, the attachments of the biceps and triceps muscles clearly illustrate this point, since the force arm of the biceps is 1 to 2 inches and that of the triceps less than 1 inch. Many other similar examples are found all over the body. From a practical point of view, this means that the muscular system should be strong to supply the necessary force for body movements, especially in strenuous sports activities.

When we speak of human leverage in relation to sport skills, we are generally referring to several levers. For example, in throwing a ball, there are levers at the shoulder, elbow, and wrist joints.

In fact, it can be said that there is one long lever from the feet to the hand.

The longer the lever, the more effective it is in imparting velocity. A tennis player can hit a tennis ball harder with a straight-arm drive than with a bent elbow because the lever (including the racket) is longer and moves at a faster speed.

Fig. 3.6 indicates that a longer lever (Z') travels faster than a shorter lever (S') in traveling the same number of degrees. In sports activities in which it is possible to increase the length of a lever with a racket or bat, the same principle applies.

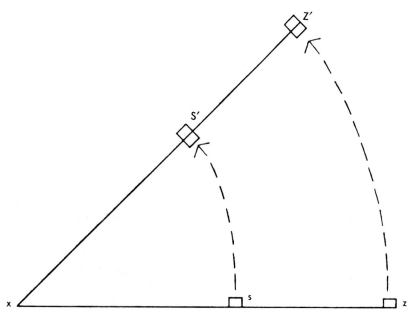

FIG. 3.6 ● Length of levers.

In baseball, hockey, golf, field hockey, and other sports, long levers similarly produce more linear force and thus better performance. For quickness of movement, it is sometimes desirable to have a short lever arm, such as when a baseball catcher brings the hand back to the ear to secure a quick throw or when a sprinter shortens the knee lever through flexion so much that the sprinter almost catches his or her spikes in his or her gluteal muscles.

Wheels and axles

Wheels and axles are used primarily to enhance range of motion and speed of movement in the musculoskeletal system. A wheel and an axle essentially function as a form of lever. When either the wheel or the axle turns, the other must turn as well. Both complete one turn at the same time. The center of the wheel and the axle both correspond to the fulcrum. Both the radius of the wheel and the radius of the axle correspond to the force arms. If the radius of the wheel is greater than the radius of the axle, then, due to the longer force arm, the wheel has a mechanical advantage over the axle. That is, a relatively smaller force may be applied to the wheel to move a relatively greater resistance applied to the axle. Very simply, if the radius of the wheel is three times the radius of the axle, then the wheel has a 3 to 1 mechanical advantage over the axle, as in Fig. 3.7. The mechanical advantage of a wheel and axle for this scenario may be calculated by considering the radius of the wheel over that of the axle.

$$\text{Mechanical advantage} = \frac{\text{radius of the wheel}}{\text{radius of the axle}}$$

If the application of force is reversed so that it is applied to the axle, then the mechanical advantage results from the wheel's turning a greater distance and speed. Using the same example, if the wheel radius is three times greater than the radius of the

axle, the outside of the wheel will turn at a speed three times that of the axle. Additionally, the distance that the outside of the wheel turns will be three times that of the outside of the axle. The mechanical advantage of a wheel and axle for this scenario may be calculated by considering the radius of the wheel over the axle.

$$\text{Mechanical advantage} = \frac{\text{force on the axle}}{\text{force on the wheel}}$$

An example of the muscles applying force to the axle to result in greater range of motion and speed may be seen in the upper extremity, in the case of the internal rotators attaching to the humerus. The humerus acts as the axle. The hand and wrist are located at the outside of the wheel when the elbow is flexed approximately 90 degrees. With a relatively small amount of humerus rotation, the hand and wrist travel a great distance. Using the wheel and axle in this manner allows us to significantly increase the speed at which we can throw objects.

Pulleys

Single pulleys function to change the effective direction of force application. Numerous weight machines utilize pulleys to alter the direction of the resistive force. In the human body, an excellent example is provided by the lateral malleolus, acting as a pulley around which the tendon of the peroneus longus runs. As these muscles contract they pull toward their bellies, which is toward the knee. Due to their use of the lateral malleolus as a pulley (Fig. 3.8), the force is

FIG. 3.8 ● Pulley. The lateral malleolus serving as a pulley for the peroneus longus tendon.

From Hamilton N, Luttgens K: *Kinesiology: scientific basis of human motion,* ed 10, McGraw-Hill, 2002.

FIG. 3.7 ● Wheel and axle.

transmitted to the plantar aspect of the foot; this results in downward and outward movement of the foot.

Laws of motion and physical activities

Motion is fundamental in physical education and sports activity. Body motion is generally produced, or at least started, by some action of the muscular system. Motion cannot occur without a force, and the muscular system is the source of force in the human body. Thus, development of the muscular system is indispensable to movement.

Basically, there are two types of motion: *linear motion* and *angular motion.* Linear motion, also referred to as translatory motion, is motion along a line. If the motion is along a straight line, it is *rectilinear* motion, whereas motion along a curved line is known as *curvilinear* motion. Angular motion, also known as rotary motion, involves rotation around an axis. In the human body, the axis of rotation is provided by the various joints. In a sense, these two types of motion are related, since angular motion of the joints can produce the linear motion of walking.

For example, in many sports activities, the cumulative angular motion of the joints of the body imparts linear motion to a thrown object (ball, shot) or to an object struck with an instrument (bat, racket).

Displacement refers to a change in position or location of an object from its original point of reference, whereas *distance*, or the path of movement, refers to the actual sum length of measurement traveled. An object may have traveled a distance of 10 meters along a linear path in two or more directions but be displaced from its original reference point by only 6 meters. *Angular displacement* refers to the change in location of a rotating body. *Linear displacement* is the distance that a system moves in a straight line.

We are sometimes concerned about the time it takes for displacement to occur. *Speed* is how fast an object is moving, or the distance an object travels in a specific amount of time. *Velocity* includes the direction and describes the rate of displacement.

A brief review of Newton's laws of motion will indicate the many applications of these laws to physical education activities and sports. Newton's laws explain all the characteristics of motion, and they are fundamental to understanding human movement.

Law of inertia

A body in motion tends to remain in motion at the same speed in a straight line unless acted on by a force; a body at rest tends to remain at rest unless acted on by a force.

Inertia may be described as the resistance to action or change. In terms of human movement, *inertia* refers to resistance to acceleration or deceleration. Inertia is the tendency for the current state of motion to be maintained, regardless of whether the body segment is moving at a particular velocity or is motionless.

Muscles produce the force necessary to start motion, stop motion, accelerate motion, decelerate motion, or change the direction of motion. Put another way, inertia is the reluctance to change status; only force can do it. The greater the mass of an object, the greater its inertia. Therefore, the greater the mass, the more force needed to significantly change an object's inertia. Numerous examples of this law are found in physical education activities. A sprinter in the starting blocks must apply considerable force to overcome resting inertia. A runner on an indoor track must apply considerable force to overcome moving inertia and stop before hitting the wall. Fig. 3.9 provides an example of how a skier in motion remains in motion, even though airborne after skiing off a hill. Balls and other objects that are thrown or struck require force to stop them. Starting, stopping, and changing direction—a part of many physical activities—provide many other examples of the law of inertia applied to body motion.

FIG. 3.9 ● An example of Newton's first law of motion.

From Hamilton N, Luttgens K: *Kinesiology: scientific basis of human motion,* ed 10, McGraw-Hill, 2002.

Since force is required to change inertia, it is obvious that any activity that is carried out at a steady pace in a consistent direction will conserve energy, and that any irregularly paced or directed activity will be very costly to energy reserves. This explains in part why activities such as handball and basketball are so much more fatiguing than jogging or dancing.

Law of acceleration

A change in the acceleration of a body occurs in the same direction as the force that caused it. The change in acceleration is directly proportional to the force causing it and inversely proportional to the mass of the body.

Acceleration may be defined as the rate of change in velocity. To attain speed in moving the body, a strong muscular force is generally necessary. *Mass*, the amount of matter in a body, affects the speed and acceleration in physical movements. A much greater force is required from the muscles to accelerate an 80-kilogram man than to accelerate a 58-kilogram man to the same running speed. Also, it is possible to accelerate a baseball faster than a shot because of the difference in weight. The force required to run at half speed is less than the force required to run at top speed. To impart speed to a ball or an object, it is necessary to rapidly accelerate the part of the body holding the object. Football, basketball, track, and field hockey are a few sports that demand speed and acceleration.

Law of reaction

For every action there is an opposite and equal reaction.

As we place force on a supporting surface by walking over it, the surface provides an equal resistance back in the opposite direction to the soles of our feet. Our feet push down and back, while the surface pushes up and forward. The force of the surface reacting to the force we place on it is referred to as *ground reaction force*. We provide the action force, while the surface provides the reaction force. It is easier to run on a hard track than on a sandy beach because of the difference in the ground reaction forces of the two surfaces. The track resists the runner's propulsion force, and the reaction drives the runner ahead. The sand dissipates the runner's force, and the reaction force is correspondingly reduced, with the apparent loss in forward force and speed (Fig. 3.10). A sprinter applies a force in excess of 1335 Newtons on the starting blocks, which resist with an equal force. When a body is in flight, as it is in jumping,

FIG. 3.10 ● An example of Newton's third law of motion. To accelerate forward, a walker must push backward. Notice how the front part of the footprint in the sand is more deeply depressed than the rear.

From Hamilton N, Luttgens K: *Kinesiology: scientific basis of human motion*, ed 10, McGraw-Hill, 2002.

movement of one part of the body produces a reaction in another part. This occurs because there is no resistive surface to supply a reaction force.

Friction

Friction is the force that results from the resistance between the surfaces of two objects moving upon one another. Depending upon the activity involved, we may desire increased or decreased friction. In running, we depend upon friction forces between our feet and the ground so that we may exert force against the ground and propel ourselves forward. When friction is reduced due to a slick ground or shoe surface, we are more likely to slip. In skating, we desire decreased friction so that we may slide across the ice with less resistance. Friction may be further characterized as either static friction or kinetic friction. *Static friction* refers to the amount of friction between two objects that have not yet begun to move, whereas *kinetic friction* is the friction occurring between two objects that are sliding upon one another. Static friction is always greater than kinetic friction. As a result, it is always more difficult to initiate dragging an object across a surface than it is to continue. Static friction may be increased by increasing the normal or perpendicular forces pressing the two objects together, as in adding more weight to one object sitting on the other object. To determine the amount of friction forces, we must consider both the forces pressing the two objects together and the *coefficient of friction,* which depends upon the hardness and roughness of the surface textures. The coefficient of friction is the ratio between the force needed to overcome the friction over the force holding the surfaces together. *Rolling friction* is the resistance to an object rolling across a surface, such as a ball rolling across a court or a tire rolling across the ground. Rolling friction is always much less than static or kinetic friction.

Balance, equilibrium, and stability

Balance is the ability to control equilibrium, either static or dynamic. In relation to human movement, *equilibrium* refers to a state of zero acceleration where there is no change in the speed or direction of the body. Equilibrium may be either static or dynamic. If the body is at rest or completely motionless, it is in *static equilibrium. Dynamic equilibrium* occurs when all of the applied and inertial forces acting on the moving body are in balance, resulting in movement with unchanging speed or direction. For us to control equilibrium and, hence, achieve balance, we need to maximize *stability.* Stability is the resistance to a change in the body's acceleration or, more appropriately, the resistance to a disturbance of the body's equilibrium. Stability may be enhanced by determining the body's *center of gravity* and changing it appropriately. The center of gravity is the point at which all of the body's mass and weight is equally balanced or equally distributed in all directions.

Balance is important for the resting body, as well as for the moving body. Generally, balance is to be desired, but there are circumstances in which movement is improved when the body tends to be unbalanced. Following are certain general factors that apply toward enhancing equilibrium, maximizing stability, and ultimately achieving balance:

1. A person has balance when the center of gravity falls within the base of support.

2. A person has balance in direct proportion to the size of the base. The larger the base of support, the more balance.

3. A person has balance depending on the weight (mass). The greater the weight, the more balance.

4. A person has balance depending on the height of the center of gravity. The lower the center of gravity, the more balance.

5. A person has balance depending on where the center of gravity is in relation to the base of support. The balance is less if the center of gravity is near the edge of the base. However, when anticipating an oncoming force, stability may be improved by placing the center of gravity nearer the side of the base of support expected to receive the force.

6. In anticipation of an oncoming force, stability may be increased by enlarging the size of the base of support in the direction of the anticipated force.

7. Equilibrium may be enhanced by increasing the friction between the body and the surfaces it contacts.

8. Rotation about an axis aids balance. A moving bike is easier to balance than a stationary bike.

9. Kinesthetic physiological functions contribute to balance. The semicircular canals of the inner ear, vision, touch (pressure), and kinesthetic sense all provide balance information to the performer. Balance and its components of equilibrium and stability are essential in all movements. They are all affected by the constant force of gravity, as well as by inertia. Walking has been described as an activity in which a person throws the body in and out of balance with each step. In rapid running movements in which moving inertia is high, the individual has to lower the center of gravity to maintain balance when stopping or changing direction. On the other hand, jumping activities attempt to raise the center of gravity as high as possible.

Force

Muscles are the main source of force that produces or changes movement of a body segment, the entire body, or an object thrown, struck, or stopped. Strong muscles are able to produce more force than weak muscles. This refers to both maximum and sustained exertion over a period of time.

Forces either push or pull on an object in an attempt to affect motion or shape. Without forces acting on an object, there is no motion. Force is the product of mass times acceleration. The mass of a body segment or the entire body times the speed of acceleration determines the force. Obviously, in football this is very important, yet it is just as important in other activities that use only a part of the human body. When one throws a ball, the force applied to the ball is equal to the mass of the arm times the arm's speed of acceleration. Also, as previously discussed, leverage is important.

$$\text{Force} = \text{mass} \times \text{acceleration}$$
$$F = m \times a$$

The quantity of motion or, more scientifically stated, the *momentum,* which is equal to mass times velocity, is important in skill activities. The greater the momentum, the greater the resistance to change in the inertia or state of motion.

It is not necessary to apply maximum force and thus increase the momentum of a ball or an object being struck in all situations. In skillful performance, regulation of the amount of force is necessary. Judgment as to the amount of force required to throw a softball a given distance, hit a golf ball 200 yards, or hit a tennis ball across the net and into the court is important.

In activities involving movement of various joints, as in throwing a ball or putting a shot, there should be a summation of forces from the beginning of movement in the lower segment of the body to the twisting of the trunk and movement at the shoulder, elbow, and wrist joints. The speed at which a golf club strikes the ball is the result of a summation of forces of the trunk, shoulders, arms, and wrists. Shot-putting and discus and javelin throwing are other good examples that show that summation of forces is essential.

Mechanical loading basics

As we utilize the musculoskeletal system to exert force on the body to move and to interact with the ground and other objects or people, significant mechanical loads are generated and absorbed by the tissues of the body. The forces causing these loads may be internal or external. Only muscles can actively generate internal force, but tension in tendons, connective tissues, ligaments, and joints capsules may generate passive internal forces. External forces are produced from outside the body and originate from gravity, inertia, or direct contact. All tissues, in varying degrees, resist changes in their shape. Obviously, tissue deformation may result from external forces, but it must be realized that we also have the ability to generate internal forces large enough to fracture bones, dislocate joints, and disrupt muscles and connective tissues. To prevent injury or damage from tissue deformation, we must use the body to

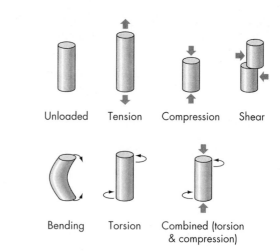

FIG. 3.11 ● Mechanical loading forces.

absorb energy from both internal and external forces. Along this line, it is to our advantage to absorb this force over larger aspects of our body rather than smaller ones, and to spread the absorption rate over a greater period of time. Additionally, the stronger and healthier we are, the more likely we are able to withstand excessive mechanical loading and the resultant excessive tissue deformation. Tension (stretching or strain), compression, shear, bending, and torsion (twisting) are all forces that act individually or in combination to provide mechanical loading that could result in excessive tissue deformation. Fig. 3.11 illustrates the mechanical forces that act on tissues of the body.

Throwing

In the performance of various sport skills, many applications of the laws of leverage, motion, and balance may be found. A skill common to many activities is throwing. The object thrown may be some type of ball, but it is frequently an object of another size or shape, such as a rock, beanbag, Frisbee, discus, or javelin. A brief analysis of some of the basic mechanical principles involved in the skill of throwing will help indicate the importance of understanding the applications of these principles. Many activities involve these and sometimes other mechanical principles. Motion is basic to throwing when the angular motion (p. 40) of the levers (bones) of the body (trunk, shoulder, elbow, and wrist) is used to give linear motion to the ball when it is released.

Newton's laws of motion apply in throwing because the individual's inertia and the ball's inertia

(p. 51) must be overcome by the application of force. The muscles of the body provide the force to move the body parts and the ball held in the hand. The *law of acceleration* (Newton's second law) comes into operation with the muscular force necessary to accelerate the arm, wrist, and hand. The greater the force (mass times acceleration) that a person can produce, the faster the arm will move and, thus, the greater the speed that will be imparted to the ball. The reaction of the feet against the surface on which the person stands indicates the application of the *law of reaction.*

The leverage factor is very important in throwing a ball or an object. The longer the lever, the greater the speed that can be imparted to the ball. For all practical purposes, the body from the feet to the fingers can be considered as one long lever. The longer the lever, either from natural body length or from the movements of the body to the extended backward position (as in throwing a softball, with extension of the shoulder and the elbow joints), the greater will be the arc through which it accelerates, and thus the greater the speed imparted to the thrown object.

In certain circumstances, when the ball is to be thrown only a short distance, as in baseball when it is thrown by the catcher to the bases, the short lever is advantageous because it takes less total time to release the ball.

Balance, or equilibrium, is a factor in throwing when the body is rotated to the rear in the beginning of the throw. This motion moves the body nearly out of balance to the rear, and then balance changes again in the body with the forward movement. Balance is again established with the follow-through, when the feet are spread and the knees and trunk are flexed to lower the center of gravity.

Summary

The preceding discussion has been a brief overview of some of the factors affecting motion. Analysis of human motion in light of the laws of physics poses a problem: how comprehensive is the analysis to be? It can become very complex, particularly when body motion is combined with the manipulation of an object in the hand involved in throwing, kicking, striking, or catching.

These factors become involved when an analysis is attempted of the activities common to our physical education program—football, baseball, basketball, track and field, field hockey, and swimming, to mention a few. However, a physical educator who is to have a complete view of which factors control human movement must have a working knowledge of both the physiological and the biomechanical principles of kinesiology.

It is beyond the scope of this book to make a detailed analysis of other activities. Some sources that consider these problems in detail are listed in the references.

Web sites

Biomechanics World Wide:

www.per.ualberta.ca/biomechanics

This site enables the reader to search the biomechanics journals for recent information regarding mechanism of injury.

Biomechanics: The Magazine of Body Movement and Medicine:

www.biomech.com/

International Society of Biomechanics:

www.isbweb.org/

Software, data, information, resources, yellow pages, conferences.

University of Arkansas Medical School Gross Anatomy for Medical Students:

http://anatomy.uams.edu/htmlpages/ anatomyhtml/gross.html

Dissections, anatomy tables, atlas images, links, etc.

Sports Coach—Levers

www.brianmac.demon.co.uk/levers.htm

A basic review of levers with excellent links to the study of muscle training & function.

Physics Concepts—Simple Machines

www.ceeo.tufts.edu/curriculum/classroom/ simple_machines.htm

An overview of physics concepts involved in the study of biomechanics.

Design and Technology—Mechanism

http://fp.keystage3dt.f9.co.uk/mechanisms.htm

A graphical overview with animations detailing the mechanisms of changing an input force and movement into an output force and movement.

Worksheet exercises

1. Develop special projects and class reports by individual or small groups of students on the mechanical analysis of all the skills involved in the following:
   a. Basketball
   b. Baseball
   c. Dancing
   d. Diving
   e. Football
   f. Field hockey
   g. Golf
   h. Gymnastics
   i. Soccer
   j. Swimming
   k. Tennis
   l. Wrestling

2. Develop term projects and special class reports by individual or small groups of students about the following factors in motion:
   a. Balance
   b. Force
   c. Gravity
   d. Motion
   e. Torque
   f. Leverage
   g. Projectiles
   h. Friction
   i. Buoyancy
   j. Aerodynamics
   k. Hydrodynamics
   l. Restitution
   m. Spin
   n. Rebound angle
   o. Momentum
   p. Center of gravity
   q. Equilibrium
   r. Stability
   s. Base of support
   t. Inertia
   u. Linear displacement
   v. Angular displacement
   w. Speed
   x. Velocity

3. Develop demonstrations, term projects, or special reports by individuals or small groups of students on the following activities:
   a. Lifting
   b. Throwing
   c. Standing
   d. Walking
   e. Running
   f. Jumping
   g. Falling
   h. Sitting
   i. Pushing and pulling
   j. Striking

References

Adrian MJ, Cooper JM: *The biomechanics of human movement,* Indianapolis, IN, 1989, Benchmark Press.

American Academy of Orthopaedic Surgeons: *Athletic training and sports medicine,* ed 2, Park Ridge, IL, 1991, American Academy of Orthopaedic Surgeons.

Barham JN: *Mechanical kinesiology,* St. Louis, 1978, Mosby.

Broer MR: *An introduction to kinesiology,* Englewood Cliffs, NJ, 1968, Prentice-Hall.

Broer MR, Zernicke RF: *Efficiency of human movement,* ed 3, Philadelphia, 1979, Saunders.

Bunn JW: *Scientific principles of coaching,* ed 2, Englewood Cliffs, NJ, 1972, Prentice-Hall.

Cooper JM, Adrian M, Glassow RB: *Kinesiology,* ed 5, St. Louis, 1982, Mosby.

Donatelli R, Wolf SL: *The biomechanics of the foot and ankle,* Philadelphia, 1990, Davis.

Hall SJ: *Basic biomechanics,* ed 4, New York, 2000, McGraw-Hill Companies, Inc.

Hinson M: *Kinesiology,* ed 4, New York, 1981, McGraw-Hill Companies, Inc.

Kegerreis S, Jenkins WL, Malone TR: Throwing injuries, *Sports Injury Management* 2:4, 1989.

Kelley DL: *Kinesiology: fundamentals of motion description,* Englewood Cliffs, NJ, 1971, Prentice-Hall.

Kreighbaum E, Barthels KM: *Biomechanics: a qualitative approach for studying human movement,* ed 3, New York, 1990, Macmillan.

Logan GA, McKinney WC: *Anatomic kinesiology,* ed 3, New York, 1982, McGraw-Hill Companies, Inc.

Luttgens K, Hamilton N: *Kinesiology: scientific basis of human motion,* ed 10, New York, 2002, McGraw-Hill.

Neumann, DA: *Kinesiology of the musculoskeletal system: foundations for physical rehabilitation,* St. Louis, 2002, Mosby.

Nordin M, Frankel VH: *Basic biomechanics of the musculoskeletal system,* ed 2, Philadelphia, 1989, Lea & Febiger.

Norkin CC, Levangie PK: *Joint structure and function: a comprehensive analysis,* Philadelphia, 1983, Davis.

Northrip JW, Logan GA, McKinney WC: *Analysis of sport motion: anatomic and biomechanic perspectives,* ed 3, New York, 1983, McGraw-Hill Companies, Inc.

Piscopo J, Baley J: *Kinesiology: the science of movement,* New York, 1981, John Wiley & Sons.

Prentice WE: *Arheim's principles of athletic training,* ed 11, New York, 2003, McGraw-Hill.

Rasch PJ: *Kinesiology and applied anatomy,* ed 7, Philadelphia, 1989, Lea & Febiger.

Scott MG: *Analysis of human motion,* ed 2, New York, 1963, Appleton-Century-Crofts.

Weineck J: *Functional anatomy in sports,* ed 2, St. Louis, 1990, Mosby.

Wirhed R: *Athletic ability and the anatomy of motion,* London, 1984, Wolfe.

Chapter 4

The Shoulder Girdle

Objectives

- To identify on the skeleton important bony features of the shoulder girdle

- To label on a skeletal chart the important bony features of the shoulder girdle

- To draw on a skeletal chart the muscles of the shoulder girdle and indicate shoulder girdle movements using arrows

- To demonstrate, using a human subject, all of the movements of the shoulder girdle and list their respective planes of movement and axes of rotation

- To palpate the muscles of the shoulder girdle on a human subject and list their antagonists

- To palpate the joints of the shoulder girdle on a human subject during each movement through the full range of motion

---

Online Learning Center Resources

Visit *Manual of Structural Kinesiology's* Online Learning Center at **www.mhhe.com/floyd15e** for additional information and study material for this chapter, including:

- *Self-grading quizzes*
- *Anatomy flashcards*
- *Animations*

Brief descriptions of the most important bones in the shoulder region will help you understand the skeletal structure and its relationship to the muscular system.

Bones

Two bones are primarily involved in movements of the shoulder girdle (Figs. 4.1 and 4.2). They are the scapula and clavicle, which generally move as a unit. Their only bony link to the axial skeleton is provided by the clavicle's articulation with the sternum. Key bony landmarks for studying the shoulder girdle are the manubrium, clavicle, coracoid process, acromion process, glenoid fossa, lateral border, inferior angle, medial border, superior angle, and spine of the scapula (Figs. 4.1, 4.2, 4.3).

Joints

When analyzing shoulder girdle (scapulothoracic) movements, it is important to realize that the scapula moves on the rib cage because the joint motion actually occurs at the sternoclavicular joint and to a lesser amount at the acromioclavicular joint (see Figs. 4.1 and 4.2).

Sternoclavicular (SC)

This is classified as a (multiaxial) arthrodial joint. It moves anteriorly 15 degrees with protraction and posteriorly 15 degrees with retraction. It moves superiorly 45 degrees with elevation and inferiorly 5 degrees with depression. Some rotation of the clavicle along its axis during various movements of the shoulder girdle result in slight

Know for test

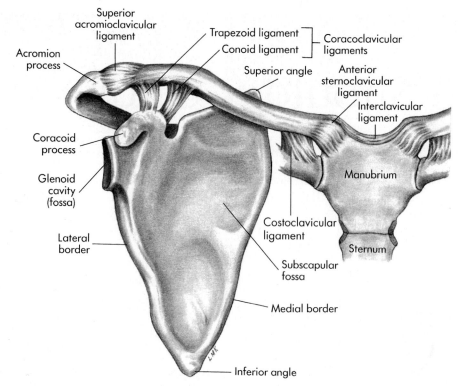

FIG. 4.1 ● Right shoulder girdle, anterior view.

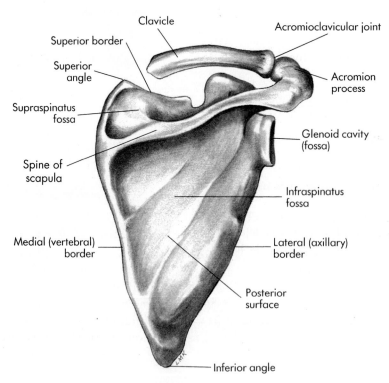

FIG. 4.2 ● Right scapula, posterior view.

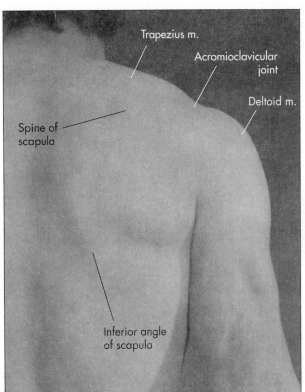

FIG. 4.3 ● Right shoulder girdle surface anatomy, anterior and posterior views.

rotary gliding movement at the sternoclavicular joint. It is supported anteriorly by the anterior sternoclavicular ligament and posteriorly by the posterior ligament. Additionally, the costoclavicular and interclavicular ligaments provide stability against superior displacement.

Acromioclavicular (AC)

This is classified as an arthrodial joint. It has a 20- to 30-degree total gliding and rotational motion accompanying other shoulder girdle and shoulder joint motions. In addition to the strong support provided by the coracoclavicular ligaments (trapezoid and conoid), the superior and inferior acromioclavicular ligaments provide stability to this often injured joint. The coracoclavicular joint, classified as a syndesmotic-type joint, functions through its ligaments to greatly increase the stability of the acromioclavicular joint.

Scapulothoracic

This is not a true synovial joint, due to its not having regular synovial features and due to the fact that its movement is totally dependent on the sternoclavicular and acromioclavicular joints. Even though scapula movement occurs as a result of motion at the SC and AC joints, the scapula can be described as having a total range of 25-degree abduction-adduction movement, 60-degree upward-downward rotation, and 55-degree elevation-depression. The scapulothoracic joint is supported dynamically by its muscles and lacks ligamentous support, since it has no synovial features.

Movements FIG. 4.4 & FIG. 4.5

In analyzing shoulder girdle movements, it is often helpful to focus on a specific scapular bony landmark, such as the inferior angle (posteriorly), the glenoid fossa (laterally), and the acromion process (anteriorly). All of these movements have their pivotal point where the clavicle joins the sternum at the sternoclavicular joint.

Movements of the shoulder girdle can be described as movements of the scapula. See Figs. 4.4 and 4.5 for movements of the shoulder girdle.

Abduction (protraction)

Movement of the scapula laterally away from the spinal column, as in reaching for an object in front of the body.

know for test

Abduction
(protraction)

A

Adduction
(retraction)

B

Elevation

C

Depression

D

Upward rotation

E

Downward rotation

F

FIG. 4.4 ● Movements of the shoulder girdle.

— elevation

adduction

Rhomboids
Trapezius
Levator scapulae

Rhomboids
Trapezius
Levator
scapulae

Serratus
Anterior
Pectoralis
minor

— abduction

Trapezius
Serratus anterior

Rhomboids
Pectoralis minor
Levator scapulae

Trapezius
Pectoralis minor

DepRession

FIG. 4.5 ● Actions of the scapular muscles.

Adduction (retraction)

Movement of the scapula medially toward the spinal column, as in pinching the shoulder blades together.

Upward rotation

Turning the glenoid fossa upward and moving the inferior angle superiorly and laterally away from the spinal column

Downward rotation

Returning the inferior angle medially and inferiorly toward the spinal column and the glenoid fossa to its normal position. (Once the scapula has returned to its anatomical position, further downward rotation actually results in the superior angle moving slightly superomedial.)

Elevation

Upward or superior movement, as in shrugging the shoulders

Depression

Downward or inferior movement, as in returning to normal position

To accomplish some of the previously listed shoulder girdle movements, the scapula must rotate or tilt on its axis. While these are not primary movements of the shoulder girdle, they are necessary for the scapula to move normally throughout its range of motion during shoulder girdle movements.

Lateral tilt

Consequential movement during abduction in which the scapula rotates about its vertical axis, resulting in posterior movement of the medial border and anterior movement of the lateral border

Medial tilt

Return from lateral tilt; consequential movement during extreme adduction in which the scapula rotates about its vertical axis, resulting in anterior movement of the medial border and posterior movement of the lateral border

Chapter
4

Upward tilt (anterior tilt)

Consequential rotational movement of the scapula about the frontal axis occurring during hyperextension of the glenohumeral joint, resulting in the superior border moving anteroinferiorly and the inferior angle moving posterosuperiorly

Downward tilt (posterior tilt)

Consequential rotational movement of the scapula about the frontal axis occurring during hyperflexion of the glenohumeral joint, resulting in the superior border moving posteroinferiorly and the inferior angle moving anterosuperiorly

The shoulder joint and shoulder girdle work together in carrying out upper extremity activities. It is critical to understand that movement of the shoulder girdle is not dependent on the shoulder joint and its muscles. However, the muscles of the shoulder girdle are essential in providing a scapula-stabilizing effect, so that the muscles of the shoulder joint will have a stable base from which to exert force for powerful movement involving the humerus. Consequently, the shoulder girdle muscles contract to maintain the scapula in a relatively static position during many shoulder joint actions. As the shoulder joint goes through more extreme ranges of motion, the scapular muscles contract to move the shoulder girdle as well to enhance movement of the entire upper extremity. The shoulder girdle movements that usually accompany shoulder joint movements are addressed in Table 5.1 in Chapter 5.

Muscles

There are five muscles primarily involved in shoulder girdle movements. To avoid confusion, it is helpful to group muscles of the shoulder girdle

separately from those of the shoulder joint. The subclavius muscle is also included in this group, but it is not regarded as a primary mover in any actions of the shoulder girdle. All five shoulder girdle muscles have their origin on the axial skeleton, with their insertion located on the scapula and/or the clavicle. Shoulder girdle muscles do not attach to the humerus, nor do they cause actions of the shoulder joint. The pectoralis minor, serratus anterior, and subclavius are located anteriorly, and the trapezius, rhomboid, and levator scapula are posterior.

The shoulder girdle muscles are essential in providing dynamic stability of the scapula, so that it can serve as a relative base of support for shoulder joint activities such as throwing, batting, and blocking.

Shoulder girdle muscles—location

Anterior
Primarily abduction and depression
- Pectoralis minor
- Serratus anterior
- Subclavius

Posterior
Primarily adduction and elevation
- Trapezius
- Rhomboid
- Levator scapula

It is important to understand that muscles may not necessarily be active throughout the absolute full range of motion for which they are noted as being agonists.

Table 4.1 provides a detailed breakdown of the muscles responsible for primary movements of the shoulder girdle.

TABLE 4.1 • Agonist muscles of the shoulder girdle

	Muscle	Origin	Insertion	Action	Plane of Motion	Palpation	Innervation
Anterior muscles	Pectoralis minor	Anterior surfaces of the 3rd to 5th ribs	Coracoid process of the scapula	Abduction	Transverse	Difficult to palpate, but can be palpated under the pectoralis major muscle in the pit of the shoulder during powerful downward movement	Medial pectoral nerve (C8 & T1)
				Downward rotation	Frontal		
				Depression	Frontal		
	Serratus anterior	Surface of the upper 9 ribs at the side of the chest	Anterior aspect of the whole length of the medial border of the scapula	Abduction	Transverse	Front and lateral side of the chest below the 5th and 6th ribs just proximal to their origin during abduction	Long thoracic nerve (C5–C7)
				Upward rotation	Frontal		
Posterior muscles	Trapezius upper fibers	Base of skull, occipital protuberance, and posterior ligaments of neck	Posterior aspect of the lateral 3rd of the clavicle	Elevation	Frontal	Halfway between occipital protuberance to C6 and laterally to acromion, particularly during elevation	Spinal accessory nerve and branches of C3 & C4
				Extension of head at neck	Sagittal		
	Trapezius middle fibers	Spinous process of 7th cervical and upper 3 thoracic vertebrae	Medial border of the acromion process and upper border of the scapular spine	Elevation	Frontal	From C7 to T3 and laterally to acromion process and scapula spine, particularly during adduction	
				Adduction	Transverse		
				Upward rotation	Frontal		
	Trapezius lower fibers	Spinous process of 4th–12th thoracic vertebrae	Triangular space at the base of the scapular spine	Adduction	Transverse	From T4 to T12 and medial aspect of scapula spine, particularly during depression and adduction	
				Depression	Frontal		
				Upward rotation	Frontal		
	Rhomboids	Spinous processes of the last cervical and the first 5 thoracic vertebrae	Medial border of the scapula, below the scapula spine	Adduction	Transverse	Difficult to palpate due to being deep to trapezius, but may be palpated through the trapezius during adduction	Dorsal scapula nerve (C5)
				Downward rotation	Frontal		
				Elevation	Frontal		
	Levator Scapulae	Transverse processes of the upper 4 cervical vertebrae	Medial border of the scapula	Elevation	Frontal	Difficult to palpate due to being deep to trapezius; best palpated at insertion just medial to the superior angle of scapula, particularly during slight elevation	Dorsal scapula nerve C5 and branches of C3 & C4

Chapter 4

Note: The subclavius is not listed since it is not a prime mover in shoulder girdle movements.

Nerves

The muscles of the shoulder girdle are innervated primarily from the nerves of the cervical plexus and brachial plexus as illustrated in Figs. 4.6 and 4.7. The trapezius is innervated by the spinal accessory nerve and from branches of C3 and C4. In addition to supplying the trapezius, C3 and C4 also innervate the levator scapula. The levator scapula receives further innervation from the dorsal scapula nerve originating from C5. The dorsal scapula nerve also innervates the rhomboid. The long thoracic nerve originates from C5, C6, and C7 and innervates the serratus anterior. The medial pectoral nerve arises from C8 and T1 to innervate the pectoralis minor.

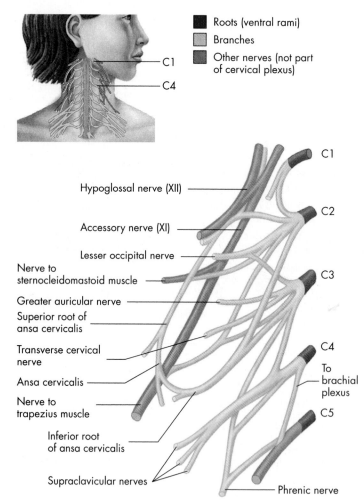

FIG. 4.6 • Cervical plexus, anterior view. The roots of the plexus are formed by the ventral rami of the spinal nerves C1–C4.

From Seeley RR, Stephens TD, Tate P: *Anatomy & physiology,* ed 6, Dubuque, IA, 2003, McGraw-Hill.

Roots: C5, C6, C7, C8, T1
Trunks: upper, middle, lower
Anterior divisions
Posterior divisions
Cords: posterior, lateral, medial
Branches: Axillary nerve
Radial nerve
Musculocutaneous nerve
Median nerve
Ulnar nerve

C5
T1

C4

C5

Dorsal scapular nerve
Suprascapular nerve
Subclavian nerve
Lateral cord
Posterior cord
Axillary nerve
Radial nerve
Musculo-cutaneous nerve
Medial and lateral pectoral nerves
Median nerve
Ulnar nerve
Medial brachial cutaneous nerve

Upper trunk
C6
Middle trunk
C7
Long thoracic nerve
C8
Lower trunk
T1
Medial cord

FIG. 4.7 ● Brachial plexus, anterior view. The roots of the plexus are formed by the ventral rami of the spinal nerves C5–T1 and join to form an upper, middle, and lower trunk. Each trunk divides into anterior and posterior divisions. The divisions join together to form the posterior, lateral, and medial cords from which the major brachial plexus nerves arise.

From Seeley RR, Stephens TD, Tate P: *Anatomy & physiology,* ed 6, Dubuque, IA, 2003, McGraw-Hill.

✱ Trapezius muscle   FIG. 4.8

(tra-peˊzi-us)

✱ Origin

Upper fibers: base of skull, occipital protuberance, and posterior ligaments of neck
Middle fibers: spinous processes of seventh cervical and upper three thoracic vertebrae
Lower fibers: spinous processes of fourth through twelfth thoracic vertebrae

✱ Insertion

Upper fibers: posterior aspect of the lateral third of the clavicle
Middle fibers: medial border of the acromion process and upper border of the scapular spine
Lower fibers: triangular space at the base of the scapular spine

✱ Action

Upper fibers: elevation of the scapula; extension of the head at the neck
Middle fibers: elevation, upward rotation, and adduction of the scapula
Lower fibers: depression, adduction, and upward rotation of the scapula

Palpation

Upper fibers: halfway between occipital protuberance to C6 and laterally to acromion, particularly during elevation
Middle fibers: from C7 to T3 and laterally to acromion process and scapula spine, particularly during adduction
Lower fibers: from T4 to T12 and medial aspect of scapula spine, particularly during depression and adduction

Origin - moves the least

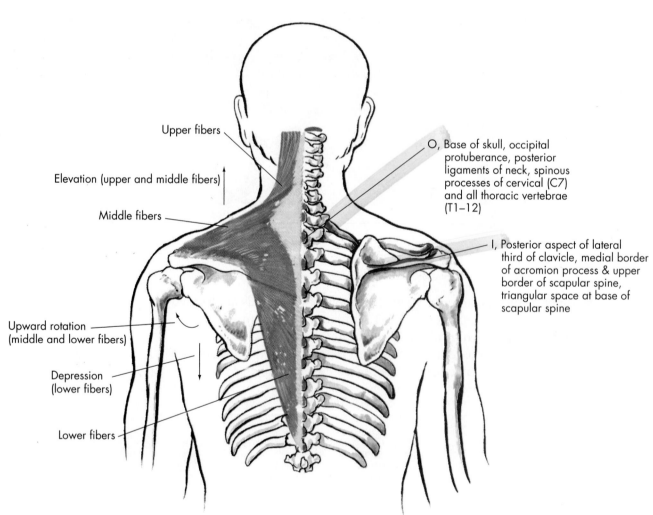

FIG. 4.8 ● Trapezius muscle. *O*, Origin; *I*, insertion; posterior view.

Innervation

Spinal accessory nerve (cranial nerve XI) and
branches of C3, C4

Application, strengthening, and flexibility

The upper fibers are a thin and relatively weak part of the muscle. They provide some elevation of the clavicle. Due to their origin on the base of the skull, they assist in extension of the head.

The middle fibers are stronger and thicker and provide strong elevation, upward rotation, and adduction (retraction) of the scapula.

The lower fibers assist in adduction (retraction) and rotate the scapula upward.

When all the parts of the trapezius are working together, they tend to pull upward and adduct at the same time. Typical action of the trapezius muscle is fixation of the scapula for deltoid action. Continuous action in upward rotation of the scapula permits the arms to be raised over the head. The muscle is always used in preventing the glenoid fossae from being pulled down during the lifting of objects with the arms. It is also typically seen in action during the holding of an object overhead. Holding the arm at the side horizontally shows typical fixation of the scapula by the trapezius muscle, while the deltoid muscle holds the arm in that position. The muscle is used strenuously when lifting with the hands, as in picking up a heavy wheelbarrow. The trapezius must prevent the scapula from being pulled downward. Carrying objects on the tip of the shoulder also calls this muscle into play. Strengthening of the upper and middle fibers can be accomplished through shoulder-shrugging exercises. The middle and lower fibers can be strengthened through bent rowing from a prone position and side arm shoulder joint abduction exercises.

To stretch the trapezius, each portion needs to be specifically addressed. The upper fibers may be stretched by using one hand to pull the head and neck forward into flexion or slight lateral flexion to the opposite side while the ipsilateral hand is hooked under a table edge to maintain the scapula in depression. The middle fibers are stretched to some extent with the procedure used for the upper fibers, but they may be stretched further by using a partner to passively pull the scapula into full protraction. The lower fibers are perhaps best stretched with the subject in a side-lying position while a partner grasps the lateral border and inferior angle of the scapula and moves it passively into maximal elevation and protraction.

Levator scapulae muscle   FIG. 4.9

(le-va´tor scap´u-lae)

Origin

Transverse processes of the upper four cervical vertebrae

Insertion

Medial border of the scapula above the base of the scapular spine

Action

Elevates the medial margin of the scapula

Palpation

Difficult to palpate due to being deep to trapezius; best palpated at insertion just medial to the superior angle of scapula, particularly during slight elevation

Innervation

Dorsal scapula nerve C5 and branches of C3 and C4

Application, strengthening, and flexibility

Shrugging the shoulders calls the levator scapulae muscle into play, along with the upper trapezius muscle. Fixation of the scapula by the pectoralis minor muscle allows the levator scapulae muscles on both sides to extend the neck or to flex laterally if used on one side only.

The levator scapula is perhaps best stretched by rotating the head approximately 45 degrees to the opposite side and flexing the cervical spine actively while maintaining the scapula in a relaxed, depressed position.

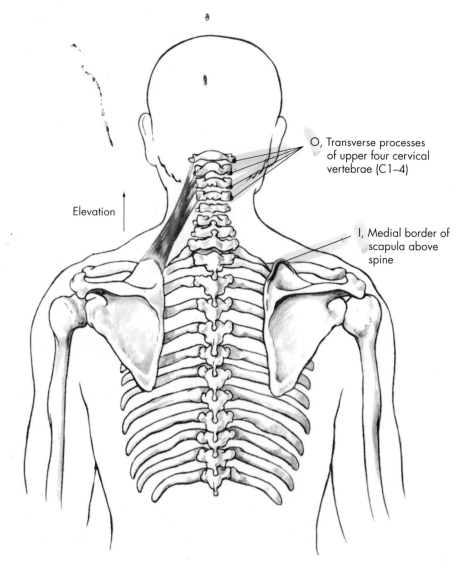

Elevation

O, Transverse processes of upper four cervical vertebrae (C1–4)

I, Medial border of scapula above spine

FIG. 4.9 ● Levator scapulae muscle. *O,* Origin; *I,* insertion; posterior view.

Rhomboid muscles—major and minor   FIG. 4.10

(rom´boyd)

✗ ### Origin

Spinous processes of the last cervical and the first five thoracic vertebrae

✗ ### Insertion

Medial border of the scapula, below the spine of the scapula

✗ ### Action

The rhomboid major and minor muscles work together

Adduction (retraction): draw the scapula toward the spinal column

Downward rotation: from the upward rotated position; they draw the scapula into downward rotation

Elevation: slight upward movement accompanying adduction

Palpation

Difficult to palpate due to being deep to trapezius, but may be palpated through the trapezius during adduction

Innervation

Dorsal scapula nerve (C5)

Application, strengthening, and flexibility

The rhomboid muscles fix the scapula in adduction (retraction) when the muscles of the shoulder joint adduct or extend the arm. These muscles are used powerfully in chinning. As one hangs from the horizontal bar, suspended by the hands, the scapula tends to be pulled away from the top of the chest. When the chinning movement begins, it is the rhomboid muscles that rotate the medial border of the scapula down and back toward the spinal column. Note their favorable position to do this.

The trapezius and rhomboid muscles working together produce adduction with slight elevation of the scapula. To prevent this elevation, the latissimus dorsi muscle is called into play.

Chin-ups and dips are excellent exercises for developing strength in this muscle. The rhomboids may be stretched by passively moving the scapula into full protraction while maintaining depression. Upward rotation may assist in this stretch as well.

FIG. 4.10 ● Rhomboid muscles (major and minor). *O*, Origin; *I*, insertion; posterior view.

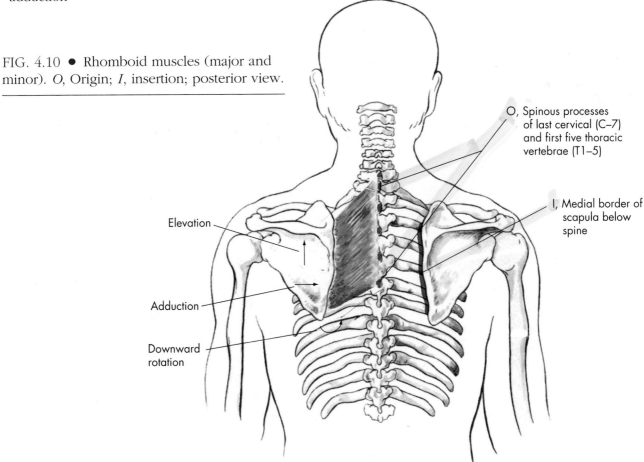

O, Spinous processes of last cervical (C–7) and first five thoracic vertebrae (T1–5)

I, Medial border of scapula below spine

Elevation

Adduction

Downward rotation

Serratus anterior muscle   FIG. 4.11

(ser-a'tus an-tir'e-or)

Origin

Surface of the upper nine ribs at the side of the chest

Insertion

Anterior aspect of the whole length of the medial
border of the scapula

Action

Abduction (protraction): draws the medial border of
the scapula away from the vertebrae

Upward rotation: longer, lower fibers tend to draw
the inferior angle of the scapula farther away from
the vertebrae, thus rotating the scapula upward
slightly

Palpation

Front and lateral side of the chest below the fifth
and sixth ribs just proximal to their origin during
abduction

Innervation

Long thoracic nerve (C5–C7)

Application, strengthening, and flexibility

The serratus anterior muscle is used commonly in
movements drawing the scapula forward with
slight upward rotation, such as throwing a baseball, shooting and guarding in basketball, and tackling in football. It works along with the pectoralis
major muscle in typical action, such as throwing a
baseball. Additionally, the serratus anterior prevents winging of the scapula.

The serratus anterior muscle is used strongly in
doing push-ups, especially in the last 5 to 10 degrees of motion. The bench press and overhead
press are good exercises for this muscle. A winged
scapula condition indicates a definite weakness of
the serratus anterior, which may result from an injury to the long thoracic nerve.

The serratus anterior can be stretched by standing, facing a corner and placing each hand at
shoulder level on the two walls. As you lean in
and attempt to place your nose in the corner, both
scapula are pushed into an adducted position,
which stretches the serratus anterior.

Chapter
4

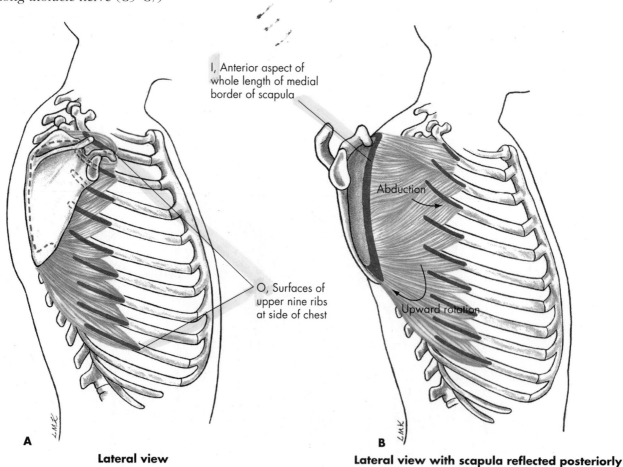

FIG. 4.11 ● Serratus anterior muscle. *O*, Origin; *I*, insertion; lateral view.

Pectoralis minor muscle   FIG. 4.12

(pek-to-ra´lis mi´nor)

Origin
Anterior surfaces of the third to fifth ribs

Insertion
Coracoid process of the scapula

Action
Abduction (protraction): draws the scapula forward and tends to tilt the lower border away from the ribs

Downward rotation: as it abducts, it draws the scapula downward

Depression: when the scapula is rotated upward, it assists in depression

Palpation
Difficult to palpate, but can be palpated under the pectoralis major muscle in the pit of the shoulder during powerful downward movement

Innervation
Medial pectoral nerve (C8–T1)

Application, strengthening, and flexibility

The pectoralis minor muscle is used, along with the serratus anterior muscle, in true abduction (protraction) without rotation. This is seen particularly in movements such as push-ups. True abduction of the scapula is necessary. Therefore, the serratus anterior draws the scapula forward with a tendency toward upward rotation, the pectoralis minor pulls forward with a tendency toward downward rotation, and the two pulling together give true abduction, which is necessary in push-ups. These muscles will be seen working together in most movements of pushing with the hands.

The pectoralis minor is most used in depressing and rotating the scapula downward from an upwardly rotated position, as in pushing the body upward on dip bars.

The wall push-up in the corner, as used for the serratus anterior, is helpful for improving flexibility in the pectoralis minor. Additionally, lying supine with a rolled towel directly under the thoracic spine while a partner pushes each scapula into retraction places this muscle on stretch.

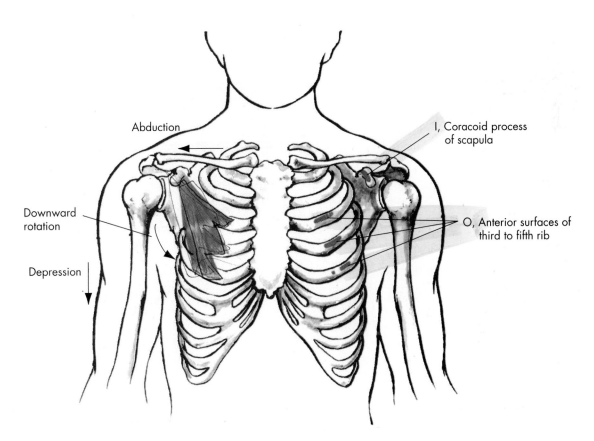

FIG. 4.12 ● Pectoralis minor muscle. *O*, Origin; *I*, insertion; anterior view.

Subclavius muscle FIG. 4.13

(sub-klá-ve-us)

 Origin

Superior aspect of first rib at its junction with its costal cartilage

 Insertion

Inferior groove in the midportion of the clavicle

 Action

Stabilization and protection of the sternoclavicular joint

Depression

Palpation

Cannot be palpated

Innervation

Nerve fibers from C5 and C6

Application, strengthening, and flexibility

The subclavius pulls the clavicle inferiorly toward the sternum. In addition to assisting in depressing the clavicle and the shoulder girdle, it has a significant role in protecting and stabilizing the sternoclavicular joint during upper extremity movements. It may be strengthened during activities in which there is active depression, such as dips. Extreme elevation of the shoulder girdle provides a stretch to the subclavius.

FIG. 4.13 ● Subclavius muscle. *O,* Origin; *I,* insertion; anterior view.

Chapter 4

Web sites

Anatomy & Physiology Tutorials:

www.gwc.maricopa.edu/class/bio201/index.htm

Radiologic Anatomy Browser:

http://radlinux1.usuf1.usuhs.mil/rad/iong/index.html

This site has numerous radiological views of the musculoskeletal system.

University of Arkansas Medical School Gross Anatomy for Medical Students:

http://anatomy.uams.edu/htmlpages/anatomyhtml/gross.html

Dissections, anatomy tables, atlas images, links, etc.

Loyola University Medical Center: Structure of the Human Body:

www.meddean.luc.edu/lumen/MedEd/GrossAnatomy/GA.html

An excellent site with many slides, dissections, tutorials, etc., for the study of human anatomy

Wheeless' Textbook of Orthopaedics:

www.ortho-u.net/

This site has an extensive index of links to the fractures, joints, muscles, nerves, trauma, medications, medical topics, lab tests, and links to orthopedic journals and other orthopedic and medical news.

Premiere Medical Search Engine:

www.medsite.com

This site allows the reader to enter any medical condition and it will search the net to find relevant articles.

Virtual Hospital:

www.vh.org

Numerous slides, patient information, etc.

Dynamic Human version 2.0 CD-ROM: The Visual Guide to Anatomy & Physiology:

www.mhhe.com/biosci/ap/dynamichuman2/

Web site that accompanies the CD-ROM

Worksheet exercises

As an aid to learning, for in-class or out-of-class assignments, or for testing, tear-out worksheets are found at the end of the text (pp. 324 and 325).

Skeletal worksheet (no. 1)

Draw and label on the worksheet the following muscles:
a. Trapezius
b. Rhomboid major and minor
c. Serratus anterior
d. Levator scapulae
e. Pectoralis minor
f. Subclavius

Human figure worksheet (no. 2)

Label the circles next to the arrows with the appropriate letter that corresponds to the movements of the shoulder girdle indicated by the arrow:
a. Adduction (retraction)
b. Abduction (protraction)
c. Rotation upward
d. Rotation downward
e. Elevation
f. Depression

Laboratory and review exercises

1. Locate the following prominent skeletal features on a human skeleton and on a subject:
   a. Scapula
      1. Medial border
      2. Inferior angle
      3. Superior angle
      4. Coracoid process
      5. Spine of scapula
      6. Glenoid cavity
      7. Acromion process
      8. Supraspinatus fossa
      9. Infraspinatus fossa
   b. Clavicle
      1. Sternal end
      2. Acromial end
   c. Joints
      1. Sternoclavicular joint
      2. Acromioclavicular joint

2. How and where do you palpate the following muscles on a human subject?
   a. Serratus anterior
   b. Trapezius
   c. Rhomboid major and minor
   d. Levator scapulae
   e. Pectoralis minor
      NOTE: "How" means palpating during active contraction and possibly resisting a primary movement of the muscle. Some muscles have several primary movements, such as the trapezius with rotation upward and adduction. "Where" refers to the location on the body where the muscle can be felt.

3. Palpate the sternoclavicular and acromioclavicular joint movements and the muscles primarily involved while demonstrating the following shoulder girdle movements.
   a. Adduction
   b. Abduction
   c. Rotation upward
   d. Rotation downward
   e. Elevation
   f. Depression

4. List the planes in which each of the following shoulder girdle movements occur. List the respective axis of rotation for each movement in each plane.
   a. Adduction
   b. Abduction
   c. Rotation upward
   d. Rotation downward
   e. Elevation
   f. Depression

5. Fill in the muscle analysis chart below by listing the muscles primarily involved in each movement.

6. Fill in the antagonistic muscle action chart on p. 75 by listing the muscle(s) or parts of muscles that are antagonist in their actions to the muscles in the left column.

Muscle analysis chart • Shoulder girdle

Shoulder girdle	
Abduction	Adduction
Elevation	Depression
Upward rotation	Downward

Antagonistic muscle action chart • Shoulder girdle

Agonist	Antagonist
Serratus anterior	
Trapezius (upper fibers)	
Trapezius (middle fibers)	
Trapezius (lower fibers)	
Rhomboid	
Levator scapulae	
Pectoralis minor	

Chapter

4

References

Andrews JR, Wilk KE: *The athlete's shoulder,* New York, 1994, Churchill Livingstone.

Andrews JR, Zarins B, Wilk KE: *Injuries in baseball,* Philadelphia, 1998, Lippincott-Raven.

Field D: *Anatomy: palpation and surface markings,* ed 3, Oxford, 2001, Butterworth-Heinemann.

Hislop HJ, Montgomery J: *Daniels and Worthingham's muscle testing: techniques of manual examination,* ed 6, Philadelphia, 1995, Saunders.

McMurtrie H, Rikel JK: *The coloring review guide to human anatomy,* 1991, McGraw-Hill Companies, Inc., New York.

Neumann, DA: *Kinesiology of the musculoskeletal system: foundations for physical rehabilitation,* St. Louis, 2002, Mosby.

Norkin CC, Levangie PK: *Joint structure and functional comprehensive analysis,* Philadelphia, 1983, Davis.

Rasch PJ: *Kinesiology and applied anatomy,* ed 7, Philadelphia, 1989, Lea & Febiger.

Seeley RR, Stephens TD, Tate P: *Anatomy & physiology,* ed 6, Dubuque, IA, 2003, McGraw-Hill.

Smith LK, Weiss EL, Lehmkuhl LD: *Brunnstrom's clinical kinesiology,* ed 5, Philadelphia, 1996, Davis.

Sobush DC, et al: The Lennie test for measuring scapula position in healthy young adult females: a reliability and validity study, *Journal of Orthopedic and Sports Physical Therapy* 23:39, January 1996.

Soderburg GL: *Kinesiology—application to pathological motion,* Baltimore, 1986, Williams & Wilkins.

Van de Graaff KM: *Human anatomy,* ed 6, Dubuque, IA. 2002, McGraw Hill.

The Shoulder Joint

Objectives

- To identify on a human skeleton or human subject selected bony structures of the shoulder joint

- To label on a skeletal chart selected bony structures of the shoulder joint

- To draw on a skeletal chart the muscles of the shoulder joint and indicate, using arrows, shoulder joint movements

- To demonstrate with a fellow student all of the movements of the shoulder joints and list their respective planes and axes of rotation

- To learn and understand how movements of the scapula accompany movements of the humerus in achieving movement of the entire shoulder complex

- To determine and list the muscles of the shoulder joint and their antagonists

- To organize and list the muscles that produce the movements of the shoulder girdle and the shoulder joint

---

Online Learning Center Resources

Visit *Manual of Structural Kinesiology's* Online Learning Center at **www.mhhe.com/floyd15e** for additional information and study material for this chapter, including:

- *Self-grading quizzes*
- *Anatomy flashcards*
- *Animations*

The only attachment of the shoulder joint to the axial skeleton is with the clavicle at the sternoclavicular joint. Movements of the shoulder joint are many and varied. It is unusual to have movement of the humerus without scapula movement. When the humerus is flexed above shoulder level, the scapula is elevated, rotated upward, and abducted. With glenohumeral abduction above shoulder level, the scapula is rotated upward and elevated. Adduction of the humerus results in rotation downward and depression, whereas extension of the humerus results in depression, rotation downward, and adduction of the scapula. The scapula abducts with humeral internal rotation and horizontal adduction. Scapula adduction accompanies external rotation and horizontal abduction of the humerus. For a summary of these movements, refer to Table 5.1.

Because the shoulder joint has such a wide range of motion in so many different planes, it also has a significant amount of laxity, which often results in instability problems such as rotator cuff impingement, subluxations, and dislocations. The price of mobility is reduced stability. The concept that the more mobile a joint is, the less stable it is and that the more stable it is, the less mobile it is applies generally throughout the body, but particularly in the shoulder joint.

Bones

The scapula, clavicle, and humerus serve as attachments for most of the muscles of the shoulder joint. Learning the specific location and importance of certain bony landmarks is critical to understanding the functions of the shoulder complex. Some of these scapular landmarks are the supraspinatus fossa, infraspinatus fossa, subscapular fossa, spine

TABLE 5.1 • Pairing of shoulder girdle and shoulder joint movements (When the muscles of the shoulder joint perform the actions in the left column through any substantial range of motion, the muscles of the shoulder girdle work in concert by performing the actions in the right column)

Shoulder joint	Shoulder girdle
Abduction	Upward rotation
Adduction	Downward rotation
Flexion	Elevation/upward rotation
Extension	Depression/downward rotation
Internal rotation	Abduction (protraction)
External rotation	Adduction (retraction)
Horizontal abduction	Adduction (retraction)
Horizontal adduction	Abduction (protraction)
Diagonal abduction (overhand activities)	Adduction (retraction)/upward rotation/elevation
Diagonal abduction (overhand activities)	Abduction (protraction)/depression/downward rotation

of the scapula, glenoid cavity, coracoid process, acromion process, and inferior angle. Humeral landmarks are the head, greater tubercle, lesser tubercle, intertubercular groove, and deltoid tuberosity (review Figs. 4.1, 4.2 and see Fig. 5.1).

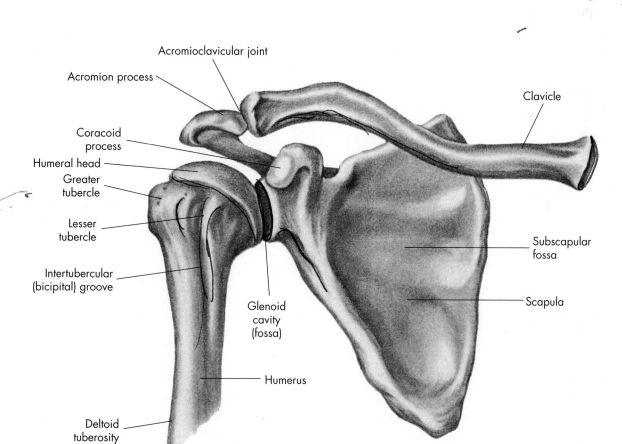

FIG. 5.1 • Right glenohumeral joint, anterior view.

Joint

The shoulder joint, specifically known as the glenohumeral joint, is a multiaxial ball-and-socket joint classified as enarthrodial (Fig. 5.1). Its stability is enhanced slightly by the glenoid labrum, a cartilaginous ring that surrounds the glenoid fossa just inside its periphery. It is further stabilized by the glenohumeral ligaments, especially anteriorly and inferiorly. The anterior glenohumeral ligaments become taut as external rotation, extension, abduction, and horizontal abduction occur, whereas the very thin posterior capsular ligaments become taut in internal rotation, flexion, and horizontal adduction. In recent years the importance of the inferior glenohumeral ligament in providing both anterior and posterior stability has come to light (see Figs. 5.2 and 5.3). It is, however, important to note that, due to the wide range of motion involved in the glenohumeral joint, the ligaments are quite lax until the extreme ranges of motion are reached. Stability is sacrificed to gain mobility.

Movement of the humerus from the side position is common in throwing, tackling, and striking activities. Flexion and extension of the shoulder joint are performed frequently when supporting body weight in a hanging position or in a movement from a prone position on the ground.

Determining the exact range of each movement for the glenohumeral joint is difficult because of the accompanying shoulder girdle movement. However, if the shoulder girdle is prevented from moving, then the glenohumeral joint movements are generally thought to be in the following ranges: 90 to 95 degrees abduction, 0 degrees adduction (prevented by the trunk) or 75 degrees anterior to the trunk, 40 to 60 degrees of extension, 90 to 100 degrees of flexion, 70 to 90 degrees of internal and external rotation, 45 degrees of horizontal abduction, and 135 degrees of horizontal adduction. If the shoulder girdle is free to move, then the total range of the combined joints is 170 to 180 degrees of abduction and 170 to 180 degrees of flexion.

The shoulder joint is frequently injured because of its anatomical design. A number of factors contribute to its injury rate, including the shallowness of the glenoid fossa, the laxity of the ligamentous structures necessary to accommodate its wide range of motion, and the lack of strength and endurance in the muscles, which are essential in providing dynamic stability to the joint. As a result, anterior or anteroinferior glenohumeral subluxations and dislocations are quite common with physical activity. Although posterior dislocations are fairly rare in occurrence, problems about the shoulder due to posterior instability are somewhat commonplace.

Another frequent injury is to the rotator cuff. The subscapularis, supraspinatus, infraspinatus, and teres minor muscles make up the rotator cuff. They are small muscles whose tendons cross the front, top, and rear of the head of the humerus to attach on the lesser and greater tuberosities, respectively. Their point of insertion enables them to rotate the humerus, an essential movement in this freely movable joint. Most important, how-

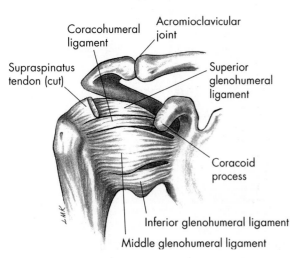

FIG. 5.2 ● Glenohumeral ligaments, anterior view.

FIG. 5.3 ● Glenohumeral joint, lateral view with humerus removed.

ever, is the vital role that the rotator cuff muscles play in maintaining the humeral head in correct approximation within the glenoid fossa while the more powerful muscles of the joint move the humerus through its wide range of motion.

Movements   FIGS. 5.4 and 5.5

Flexion

Movement of the humerus straight anteriorly.

Extension

Movement of the humerus straight posteriorly, sometimes referred to as hyperextension.

Abduction

Upward lateral movement of the humerus out to the side, away from the body.

Adduction:

Downward movement of the humerus medially toward the body from abduction.

External rotation

Movement of the humerus laterally around its long axis away from the midline.

Internal rotation

Movement of the humerus medially around its long axis toward the midline.

Horizontal adduction (flexion)

Movement of the humerus in a horizontal or transverse plane toward and across the chest.

Horizontal abduction (extension)

Movement of the humerus in a horizontal or transverse plane away from the chest.

Diagonal abduction

Movement of the humerus in a diagonal plane away from the midline of the body.

Diagonal adduction

Movement of the humerus in a diagonal plane toward the midline of the body.

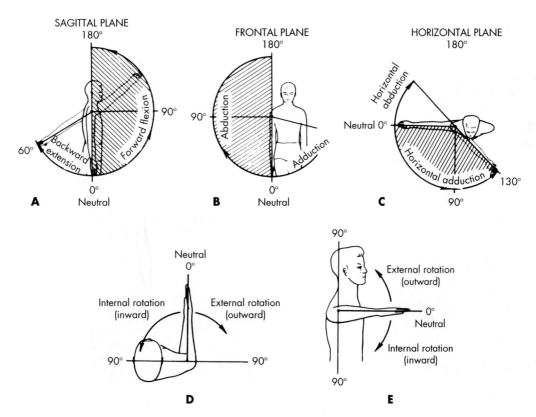

FIG. 5.4 ● Range of motion of the shoulder. **A,** Flexion and extension; **B,** abduction and adduction; **C,** horizontal abduction and adduction; **D,** internal and external rotation with the arm at the side of the body; and **E,** internal and external rotation with the arm abducted to 90°.

Flexion   A

Extension   B

Abduction   C

Adduction   D

Internal rotation   E

External rotation   F

FIG. 5.5 ● Movements of the shoulder joint.

Horizontal abduction G

Horizontal adduction H

Diagonal abduction I

Diagonal adduction J

FIG. 5.5 continued ● Movements of the shoulder joint.

Chapter
5

Muscles

When attempting to learn and understand the muscles of the glenohumeral joint, it may be helpful to group them according to their location and function. All of the muscles that originate on the scapula and clavicle may be thought of as intrinsic glenohumeral muscles. The intrinsic muscles include the deltoid, the coracobrachialis, the teres major, and the rotator cuff group, which is composed of the subscapularis, the supraspinatus, the infraspinatus, and the teres minor. Extrinsic glenohumeral muscles are the latissimus dorsi and pectoralis major. It may also be helpful to organize the muscles according to their general location. The pectoralis major, coracobrachialis, and subscapularis are anterior muscles. Located superiorly are the deltoid and supraspinatus. The latissimus dorsi, teres major, infraspinatus, and teres minor are located posteriorly.

The biceps brachii and triceps brachii (long head) are also involved in glenohumeral movements. Primarily, the biceps brachii assists in flexing and horizontally adducting the shoulder, whereas the long head of the triceps brachii assists in extension and horizontal abduction. Further discussion of these muscles appears in Chapter 6.

Shoulder joint muscles—location

Anterior
   Pectoralis major
   Coracobrachialis
   Subscapularis
Superior
   Deltoid
   Supraspinatus
Posterior
   Latissimus dorsi
   Teres major
   Infraspinatus
   Teres minor

Muscle identification

In Figs. 5.6 and 5.8, identify the anterior and posterior muscles of the shoulder joint and shoulder girdle. Compare Fig. 5.6 with Fig. 5.7 and Fig. 5.8 with Fig. 5.9, and refer to Table 5.2 for a detailed breakdown of the agonist muscles for the glenohumeral joint.

FIG. 5.6 ● Anterior shoulder joint and shoulder girdle muscles.

FIG. 5.7 ● Anterior muscles.

From Booher JA, Thibodeau GA: *Athletic injury assessment,* ed 2, St. Louis, 1989, Mosby.

Trapezius m. Biceps brachii m.

Deltoid m.

Triceps
brachii m.

Teres major m.

Latissimus
dorsi m.

FIG. 5.8 ● Posterior shoulder joint and shoulder
girdle muscles.

Splenius capitis m.

Levator scapulae m.
Trapezius m.
Supraspinatus m.

Spine of scapula

Trapezius m.

Rhomboideus major m.

Deltoid m.

Infraspinatus m.

Teres minor m.

Teres major m.

Fascia over infraspinatus

Latissimus dorsi m. (cut)
Erector spinae m.

Triceps brachii m.

Rib

Latissimus dorsi m.

Serratus posterior inferior m.

Exterior abdominal oblique m.

Lumbodorsal fascia

FIG. 5.9 ● Posterior muscles.

TABLE 5.2 • Agonist muscles of the glenohumeral joint

	Muscle	Origin	Insertion	Action	Plane of motion	Palpation	Innervation
Anterior muscles	Pectoralis major upper fibers	Medial half of anterior surface of clavicle	Flat tendon 2 or 3 inches wide to lateral lip of intertubercular groove of humerus	Internal rotation	Transverse	From medial end of clavicle to the intertubercular groove of the humerus, during flexion	Lateral pectoral nerve (C5, C6, C7)
				Horizontal adduction			
				Diagonal adduction	Diagonal		
				Flexion	Sagittal		
				Abduction	Frontal		
	Pectoralis major lower fibers	Anterior surface of costal cartilages of first six ribs, and adjoining portion of sternum	Flat tendon 2 or 3 inches wide to lateral lip of intertubercular groove of humerus	Internal rotation	Transverse	From the lower ribs and sternum to the intertubercular groove of the humerus, during resisted extension from a flexed position	Medial pectoral nerve (C8, T1)
				Horizontal adduction			
				Diagonal adduction	Diagonal		
				Extension	Sagittal		
				Adduction	Frontal		
	Subscapularis	Entire anterior surface of subscapular fossa	Lesser tubercle of humerus	Internal rotation	Transverse	Cannot be palpated due to being deep to the pectoralis major	Upper and lower subscapular nerve (C5, C6)
	Coracobrachialis	Coracoid process of scapula	Middle of medial border of humeral shaft	Horizontal adduction	Transverse	The belly may be palpated high up on the medial arm and towards the coracoid process, particularly with resisted adduction	Musculotaneous nerve (C5, C6, C7)
				Diagonal adduction	Diagonal		
Superior muscles	Deltoid anterior fibers	Anterior lateral third of clavicle	Deltoid tuberosity on the lateral humerus	Abduction	Frontal	From the clavicle toward the anterior humerus during resisted flexion	Axillary nerve (C5, C6)
				Flexion	Sagittal		
				Horizontal adduction	Transverse		
				Diagonal adduction	Diagonal		
	Deltoid middle fibers	Lateral aspect of acromion	Deltoid tuberosity on lateral humerus	Abduction	Frontal	From the lateral border of the acromion down towards the deltoid tuberosity during resisted abduction	
				Horizontal abduction	Transverse		
	Deltoid posterior fibers	Inferior edge of spine of scapula	Deltoid tuberosity on lateral humerus	Abduction	Frontal	From the lower lip of the spine of the scapula toward the posterior humerus during resisted extension	
				Horizontal abduction	Transverse		
				Diagonal abduction	Diagonal		
	Supraspinatus	Medial two-thirds of supraspinatus fossa	Superiorly on greater tubercle of humerus	Abduction	Frontal	Above the spine of the scapula during initial abduction in the scapula plane	Suprascapula nerve (C5)

(continued)

TABLE 5.2 (continued) • Agonist muscles of the glenohumeral joint

	Muscle	Origin	Insertion	Action	Plane of motion	Palpation	Innervation
Posterior muscles	Latissimus dorsi	Posterior crest of ilium, back of sacrum and spinous processes of lumbar and lower six thoracic vertebrae, slips from lower three ribs	Medial side of intertubercular groove of humerus	Extension	Sagittal	The tendon may be palpated as it passes under the teres major at the posterior wall of the axilla, particularly during resisted extension and internal rotation. The muscle can be palpated in the upper lumbar/lower thoracic area during extension from a flexed position	Thoracodorsal (C6, C7, C8)
				Adduction	Frontal		
				Internal rotation	Transverse		
	Teres major	Posteriorly on inferior third of lateral border of scapula and just superior to inferior angle	Medial lip of intertubercular groove of humerus	Extension	Sagittal	Just above the latissimus dorsi on the posterior scapula surface, moving diagonally upward and laterally from the inferior angle of the scapula during resisted internal rotation	Lower subscapular nerve (C5, C6)
				Adduction	Frontal		
				Internal rotation	Transverse		
	Infraspinatus	Medial aspect of infraspinatus fossa just below spine of scapula	Posteriorly on greater tubercle of humerus	External rotation	Transverse	Just below the spine of the scapula passing upwards and laterally to the humerus during resisted external rotation	Suprascapula nerve (C5, C6)
				Horizontal abduction			
				Diagonal abduction	Diagonal		
	Teres minor	Posteriorly on upper and middle aspect of lateral border of scapula	Posteriorly on greater tubercle of humerus	External rotation	Transverse	Just above the teres minor on the posterior scapula surface, moving diagonally upward and laterally from the inferior angle of the scapula during resisted external rotation	Axillary nerve (C5, C6)
				Horizontal abduction			
				Diagonal abduction	Diagonal		

Note: The biceps brachii assists in flexion, horizontal adduction, and diagonal adduction, while the long head of the triceps brachii assists in extension, adduction, horizontal abduction, and diagonal abduction. Due to their coverage in Chapter 6, neither is listed above.

Chapter 5

Nerves FIGS. 5.10, 5.11

The muscles of the shoulder joint are all innervated from the nerves of the brachial plexus. The pectoralis major is innervated by the pectoral nerves. Specifically, the lateral pectoral nerve arising from C5, C6, and C7 innervates the clavicular head, while the medial pectoral nerve arising from C8 and T1 innervates the sternal head. The thoracodorsal nerve, arising from C6, C7, and C8, supplies the latissimus dorsi. The axillary nerve (Fig. 5.10), branching from C5 and C6, innervates the deltoid and teres minor. A lateral patch of skin over the deltoid region of the arm is provided sensation by the axillary nerve. Both the upper and lower subscapular nerves arising from C5 and C6 innervate the subscapularis, while only the lower subscapular nerve supplies the teres major. The supraspinatus and infraspinatus are innervated by the suprascapula nerve, which originates from C5 and C6. The musculocutaneous nerve, as seen in Fig. 5.11, branches from C5, C6, and C7 and innervates the coracobrachialis. It supplies sensation to the radial aspect of the forearm.

FIG. 5.10 • Muscular and cutaneous distribution of the axillary nerve.

FIG. 5.11 • Muscular and cutaneous distribution of the musculocutaneous nerve.

Deltoid muscle FIG. 5.12

(del-toyd´)

Origin

Anterior fibers: anterior lateral third of the clavicle
Middle fibers: lateral aspect of the acromion
Posterior fibers: inferior edge of the spine of the scapula

Insertion

Deltoid tuberosity on the lateral humerus

Action

Anterior fibers: abduction, flexion, horizontal adduction, and internal rotation of the glenohumeral joint
Middle fibers: abduction of the glenohumeral joint
Posterior fibers: abduction, extension, horizontal abduction, and external rotation of the glenohumeral joint

Palpation

Anterior fibers: from the clavicle toward the anterior humerus during resisted flexion
Middle fibers: from the lateral border of the acromion down toward the deltoid tuberosity during resisted abduction
Posterior fibers: from the lower lip of the spine of the scapula toward the posterior humerus during resisted extension

Innervation

Axillary nerve (C5, C6)

Application, strengthening, and flexibility

The deltoid muscle is used commonly in any lifting movement. The trapezius muscle stabilizes the scapula as the deltoid pulls on the humerus. The anterior fibers of the deltoid muscle flex and internally rotate the humerus. The posterior fibers extend and externally rotate the humerus. The anterior fibers also horizontally adduct the humerus while the posterior fibers horizontally abduct it. This muscle is used in all lifting movements. Any movement of the humerus on the scapula will involve part or all of the deltoid muscle.

Lifting the humerus from the side to the position of abduction is a typical action of the deltoid. Side-arm dumbbell raises are excellent for strengthening the deltoid, especially the middle fibers. By abducting the arm in a slightly horizontally adducted (30 degrees) position, the anterior deltoid fibers can be emphasized. The posterior fibers can be strengthened better by abducting the arm in a slightly horizontally abducted (30 degrees) position.

Stretching the deltoid requires varying positions, depending on the fibers to be stretched. The anterior deltoid is stretched by taking the humerus into extreme horizontal abduction or by extreme extension and adduction. The middle deltoid is stretched by taking the humerus into extreme adduction behind the back. Extreme horizontal adduction stretches the posterior deltoid.

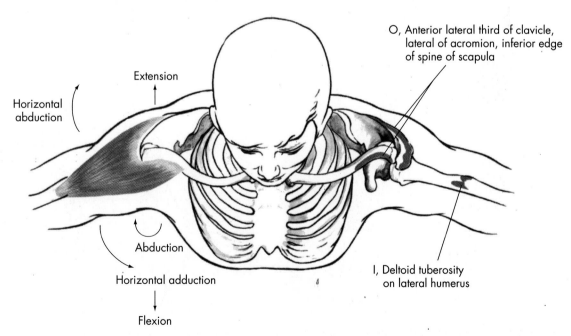

FIG. 5.12 ● Deltoid muscle, superior view. *O*, Origin; *I*, insertion.

Pectoralis major muscle   FIG. 5.13

(pek-to-ra´lis ma´jor)

Origin

Upper fibers (clavicular head): medial half of the anterior surface of the clavicle

Lower fibers (sternal head): anterior surfaces of the costal cartilage of the first six ribs, and adjacent portion of the sternum

Insertion

Flat tendon 2 or 3 inches wide to the outer lip of the intertubercular groove of the humerus

Action

Upper fibers (clavicular head): internal rotation, horizontal adduction, flexion, abduction (once the arm is abducted 90 degrees, the upper fibers assist in further abduction), and adduction (with the arm below 90 degrees of abduction) of the glenohumeral joint

Lower fibers (sternal head): internal rotation, horizontal adduction, extension, and adduction of the glenohumeral joint

Palpation

Upper fibers: from the medial end of the clavicle to the intertubercular groove of the humerus, during flexion

Lower fibers: from the lower ribs and sternum to the intertubercular groove of the humerus, during resisted extension from a flexed position

Innervation

Upper fibers: lateral pectoral nerve (C5–C7)
Lower fibers: medial pectoral nerve (C8, T1)

Application, strengthening, and flexibility

The pectoralis major muscle aids the serratus anterior muscle in drawing the scapula forward as it moves the humerus in flexion and internal rotation. Even though the pectoralis major is not attached to the scapula, it is effective in this scapula protraction because of its anterior pull on the humerus, which joins to the scapula at the glenohumeral joint. Typical action is shown in throwing a baseball. As the glenohumeral joint is flexed, the humerus is internally rotated and the scapula is drawn forward with upward rotation. It also works as a helper of the latissimus dorsi muscle when extending and adducting the humerus from a raised position.

The pectoralis major and the anterior deltoid work closely together. The pectoralis major is used powerfully in push-ups, pull-ups, throwing, and tennis serves. With a barbell, the subject takes a supine position on a bench with the arms at the side and moves the arms to a horizontally adducted position. This exercise, known as bench pressing, is widely used for pectoralis major development.

Externally rotating the shoulder stretches the entire pectoralis major. It is also stretched when the shoulder is horizontally abducted. Extending the shoulder fully provides stretching to the upper pectoralis major, while full abduction stretches the lower pectoralis major.

FIG. 5.13 ● Pectoralis major muscle. *O,* Origin; *I,* insertion.

Adduction

Internal rotation

O, Medial half of anterior surface of clavicle, anterior surface of costal cartilages of first six ribs, adjoining portion of sternum

I, Flat tendon 2 or 3 inches wide to outer lip of intertubercular groove of humerus

Latissimus dorsi muscle   FIG. 5.13

(lat-is´i-mus dor´si)

Origin

Posterior crest of the ilium, back of the sacrum and spinous processes of the lumbar and lower six thoracic vertebrae (T6–T12); slips from the lower three ribs

Insertion

Medial lip of the intertubercular groove of the humerus

Action

Adduction of the glenohumeral joint
Extension of the glenohumeral joint
Internal rotation of the glenohumeral joint
Horizontal abduction of the glenohumeral joint

Palpation

The tendon may be palpated as it passes under the teres major at the posterior wall of the axilla, particularly during resisted extension and internal rotation. The muscle can be palpated in the upper lumbar/lower thoracic area during extension from a flexed position.

Innervation

Thoracodorsal nerve (C6–C8)

Application, strengthening, and flexibility

The latissimus dorsi muscle has strong action in adduction of the humerus. Due to the upward rotation of the scapula that accompanies glenohumeral abduction, the latissimus effectively downwardly rotates the scapula by way of its action in pulling the entire shoulder girdle downward in active glenohumeral adduction. It is one of the most important extensor muscles of the humerus and contracts powerfully in chinning.

Exercises in which the arms are pulled down bring the latissimus dorsi muscle into powerful contraction. Chinning, rope climbing, dips on parallel bars, and other uprise movements on the horizontal bar are good examples. In barbell exercises, the basic rowing and pullover exercises are good for developing the "lats." Pulling the bar of an overhead pulley system down toward the shoulders, known as "lat pulls," is a common exercise for this muscle.

The latissimus dorsi is stretched with the teres major when the shoulder is externally rotated while in a 90-degree abducted position. This stretch may be accentuated further by abducting the shoulder fully while maintaining external rotation and then laterally flexing and rotating the trunk to the opposite side.

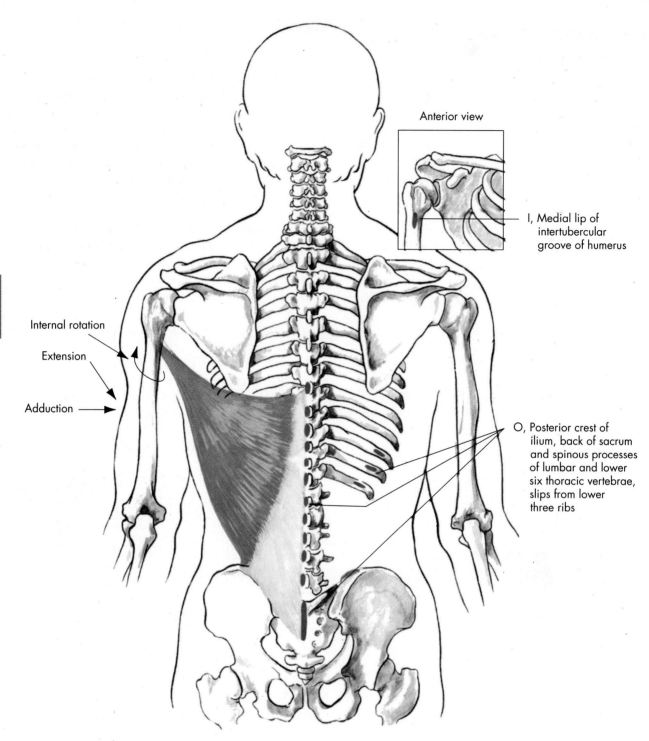

Anterior view

I, Medial lip of
intertubercular
groove of humerus

Internal rotation

Extension

Adduction

O, Posterior crest of
ilium, back of sacrum
and spinous processes
of lumbar and lower
six thoracic vertebrae,
slips from lower
three ribs

FIG. 5.14 ● Latissimus dorsi muscle. *O*, Origin; *I*, insertion.

Coracobrachialis muscle   FIG. 5.15
(kor-a-ko-bra´ki-a´lis)

Origin
Coracoid process of the scapula

Insertion
Middle of the medial border of the humeral shaft

Action
Flexion of the glenohumeral joint
Adduction of the glenohumeral joint
Horizontal adduction of the glenohumeral joint

Palpation
The belly may be palpated high up on the medial
  arm and towards the coracoid process, particularly
  with resisted adduction

Innervation
Musculocutaneous nerve (C5–C7)

Application, strengthening, and flexibility
The coracobrachialis is not a powerful muscle,
but it does assist in flexion and adduction and is
most functional in moving the arm horizontally
toward and across the chest. It is best strengthened by horizontally adducting the arm against
resistance, as in bench pressing. It may also be
strengthened by performing lat pulls, which are
defined on page 89.

The coracobrachialis is best stretched in extreme horizontal abduction, although extreme extension also stretches this muscle.

Chapter

5

FIG. 5.15 ● Coracobrachialis muscle, anterior view. *O*, Origin; *I*, insertion.

Rotator cuff muscles

Figs. 5.16 and 5.17 illustrate the rotator cuff muscle group, which, as previously mentioned, is most important in maintaining the humeral head in its proper location within the glenoid cavity. The acronym **SITS** may be used in learning the names of the supraspinatus, infraspinatus, teres minor, and subscapularis. These muscles, which are not very large in comparison with the deltoid and pectoralis major, must possess not only adequate strength but also a significant amount of muscular endurance to ensure their proper functioning, particularly in repetitive overhead activities such as throwing, swimming, and pitching. Quite often when these types of activities are conducted with poor technique, muscle fatigue, or inadequate warm-up and conditioning, the rotator cuff muscle group, particularly the supraspinatus, fails to dynamically stabilize the humeral head in the glenoid cavity, leading to further rotator cuff problems such as tendinitis and rotator cuff impingement within the subacromial space.

FIG. 5.16 ● Rotator cuff muscles, superior view.

FIG. 5.17 ● Rotator cuff muscles, anterolateral view.

Subscapularis muscle FIG. 5.18

(sub-skap-u-la´ris)

Origin

Entire anterior surface of the subscapular fossa

Insertion

Lesser tubercle of the humerus

Action

Internal rotation of the glenohumeral joint
Adduction of the glenohumeral joint
Extension of the glenohumeral joint
Stabilization of the humeral head in the glenoid
  fossa

Palpation

Cannot be palpated due to being deep to the
  pectoralis major

Innervation

Upper and lower subscapular nerve (C5, C6)

Application, strengthening, and flexibility

The subscapularis muscle, another rotator cuff muscle, holds the head of the humerus in the glenoid fossa from in front and below. It acts with the latissimus dorsi and teres major muscles in its typical movement but is less powerful in its action because of its proximity to the joint. The muscle also requires the help of the rhomboid in stabilizing the scapula to make it effective in the movements described. The subscapularis is relatively hidden behind the rib cage in its location on the anterior aspect of the scapula in the subscapular fossa. It may be strengthened with exercises similar to those used for the latissimus dorsi and teres major, such as rope climbing and lat pulls. A specific exercise for its development is done by internally rotating the arm against resistance in the beside-the-body position at 0 degrees of glenohumeral abduction.

External rotation with the arm adducted by the side stretches the subscapularis.

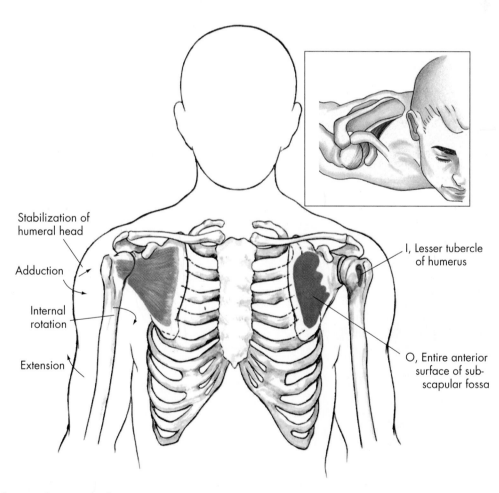

FIG. 5.18 ● Subscapularis muscle, anterior view. *O*, Origin; *I*, insertion.

Supraspinatus muscle FIG. 5.19

(su´pra-spi-na´tus)

Origin

Medial two-thirds of the supraspinatus fossa

Insertion

Superiorly on the greater tubercle of the humerus

Action

Weak abduction

Stabilization of the humeral head in the glenoid
fossa

Palpation

Above the spine of the scapula during initial abduction in the scapula plane

Innervation

Suprascapular nerve (C5)

Application, strengthening, and flexibility

The supraspinatus muscle holds the head of the
humerus in the glenoid fossa. In throwing movements, it provides important dynamic stability by
maintaining the proper relationship between the
humeral head and the glenoid fossa. In the cocking phase of throwing, there is a tendency for
the humeral head to subluxate anteriorly. In the
follow-through phase, the humeral head tends to
move posteriorly.

The supraspinatus, along with the other rotator
cuff muscles, must have excellent strength and
endurance to prevent abnormal and excessive
movement of the humeral head in the fossa.

The supraspinatus is the most often injured rotator cuff muscle. Acute severe injuries may occur
with trauma to the shoulder. However, mild to
moderate strains or tears often occur with athletic
activity, particularly if the activity involves repeti-
tious overhead movements, such as throwing or
swimming.

Injury or weakness in the supraspinatus may be
detected when the athlete attempts to substitute
the scapula elevators and upward rotators to obtain humeral abduction. An inability to smoothly
abduct the arm against resistance is indicative of
possible rotator cuff injury.

The supraspinatus muscle may be called into
play whenever the middle fibers of the deltoid
muscle are used. An "empty-can exercise" may be
used to emphasize supraspinatus action. This is
performed by internally rotating the humerus, followed by abducting the arm to 90 degrees in a 30-
to 45-degree horizontally adducted position, as if
one were emptying a can.

Adducting the arm behind the back with the
shoulder internally rotated and extended stretches
the supraspinatus.

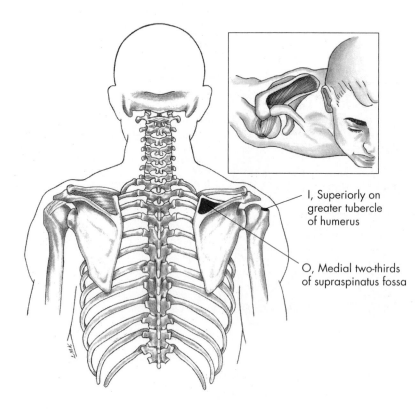

I, Superiorly on
greater tubercle
of humerus

O, Medial two-thirds
of supraspinatus fossa

FIG. 5.19 ● Supraspinatus muscle,
posterior view. *O*, Origin; *I*, insertion.

Infraspinatus muscle   FIG. 5.20

(in´fra-spi-na´tus)

Origin

Medial aspect of the infraspinatus fossa just below the spine of the scapula

Insertion

Posteriorly on the greater tubercle of the humerus

Action ·

External rotation of the glenohumeral joint
Horizontal abduction of the glenohumeral joint
Extension of the glenohumeral joint
Stabilization of the humeral head in the glenoid fossa

Palpation

Just below the spine of the scapula passing upwards and laterally to the humerus during resisted external rotation

Innervation

Suprascapular nerve (C5, C6)

Application, strengthening, and flexibility

The infraspinatus and teres minor muscles are effective when the rhomboid muscles stabilize the scapula. When the humerus is rotated outward, the rhomboid muscles flatten the scapula to the back and fixate it so that the humerus may be rotated.

The infraspinatus is vital to maintaining the posterior stability of the glenohumeral joint. It is the most powerful of the external rotators and is the second most commonly injured rotator cuff muscle.

Both the infraspinatus and the teres minor can best be strengthened by externally rotating the arm against resistance in the 15- to 20-degree abducted position and the 90-degree abducted position.

Stretching of the infraspinatus is accomplished with internal rotation and extreme horizontal adduction.

Chapter
5

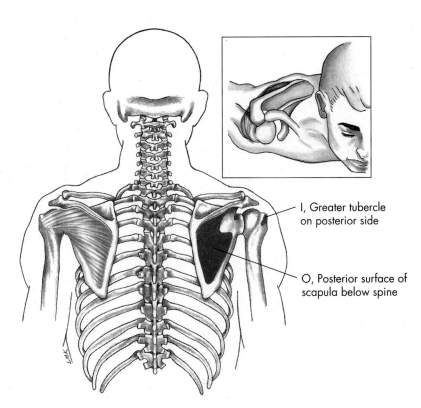

I, Greater tubercle on posterior side

O, Posterior surface of scapula below spine

FIG. 5.20 ● Infraspinatus muscle, posterior view. *O*, Origin; *I*, insertion.

Teres minor muscle   FIG. 5.21

(teʹrez miʹnor)

Origin

Posteriorly on the upper and middle aspect of the lateral border of the scapula

Insertion

Posteriorly on the greater tubercle of the humerus

Action

External rotation of the glenohumeral joint
Horizontal abduction of the glenohumeral joint
Extension of the glenohumeral joint
Stabilization of the humeral head in the glenoid fossa

Palpation

Just above the teres minor on the posterior scapula surface, moving diagonally upward and laterally from the inferior angle of the scapula during resisted external rotation

Innervation

Axillary nerve (C5, C6)

Application, strengthening, and flexibility

The teres minor functions very similarly to the infraspinatus in providing dynamic posterior stability to the glenohumeral joint. Both of these muscles perform the same actions together. The teres minor is strengthened with the same exercises that are used in strengthening the infraspinatus.

The teres minor is stretched similarly to the infraspinatus by internally rotating the shoulder while moving into extreme horizontal adduction.

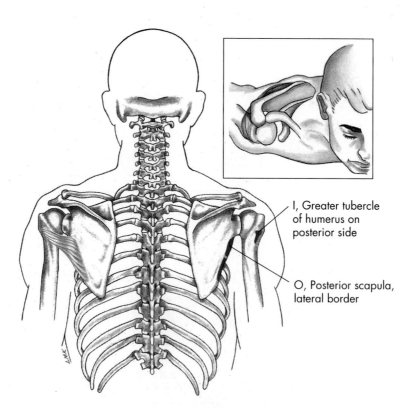

I, Greater tubercle of humerus on posterior side

O, Posterior scapula, lateral border

FIG. 5.21 ● Teres minor muscle, posterior view. *O,* Origin; *I,* insertion.

Teres major muscle   FIG. 5.22

(te´rez ma´jor)

Origin

Posteriorly on the inferior third of the lateral border of the scapula and just superior to the inferior angle

Insertion

Medial lip of the intertubercular groove of the humerus

Action

Extension of the glenohumeral joint, particularly from the flexed position to the posteriorly extended position

Internal rotation of the glenohumeral joint

Adduction of the glenohumeral joint, particularly from the abducted position down to the side and toward the midline of the body

Palpation

Just above the latissimus dorsi on the posterior scapula surface, moving diagonally upward and laterally from the inferior angle of the scapula during resisted internal rotation

Innervation

Lower subscapular nerve (C5, C6)

Application, strengthening, and flexibility

The teres major muscle is effective only when the rhomboid muscles stabilize the scapula or move the scapula in downward rotation. Otherwise, the scapula would move forward to meet the arm.

This muscle works effectively with the latissimus dorsi. It assists the latissimus dorsi, pectoralis major, and subscapularis in adducting, internally rotating, and extending the humerus. It is said to be the latissimus dorsi's "little helper." It may be strengthened by lat pulls, rope climbing, and internal rotation exercises against resistance.

Externally rotating the shoulder in a 90-degree abducted position stretches the teres major.

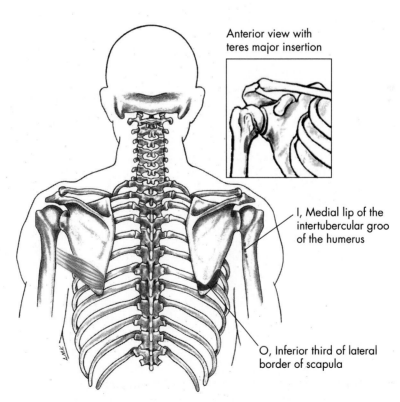

Anterior view with teres major insertion

I, Medial lip of the intertubercular groo of the humerus

O, Inferior third of lateral border of scapula

FIG. 5.22 ● Teres major muscle, posterior view. *O*, Origin; *I*, insertion.

Web sites

Anatomy & Physiology Tutorials:

www.gwc.maricopa.edu/class/bio201/index.htm

Radiologic Anatomy Browser:

http://radlinux1.usuf1.usuhs.mil/rad/iong/index.html

This site has numerous radiological views of the musculoskeletal system.

University of Arkansas Medical School Gross Anatomy for Medical Students:

http://anatomy.uams.edu/htmlpages/anatomyhtml/gross.html

Dissections, anatomy tables, atlas images, links, etc.

Loyola University Medical Center: Structure of the Human Body:

www.meddean.luc.edu/lumen/MedEd/GrossAnatomy/GA.html

An excellent site with many slides, dissections, tutorials, etc., for the study of human anatomy.

Wheelless' Textbook of Orthopaedics:

www.ortho-u.net/

This site has an extensive index of links to the fractures, joints, muscles, nerves, trauma, medications, medical topics, and lab tests, as well as links to orthopedic journals and other orthopedic and medical news.

Premiere Medical Search Engine:

www.medsite.com

This site allows the reader to enter any medical condition and it will search the net to find relevant articles.

Arthroscopy.Com.:

www.arthroscopy.com/sports.htm

Patient information on various musculoskeletal problems of the upper and lower extremity

Virtual Hospital:

www.vh.org

Numerous slides, patient information, etc.

Dynamic Human version 2.0 CD-ROM: The Visual Guide to Anatomy & Physiology:

www.mhhe.com/biosci/ap/dynamichuman2/

Web site that accompanies this CD-ROM

Worksheet exercises

As an aid to learning, for in-class or out-of-class assignments, or for testing, tear-out worksheets are found at the end of the text (pp. 326 and 327).

Skeletal worksheet (no. 1)

Draw and label on the worksheet the following muscles:
a. Deltoid
b. Supraspinatus
c. Subscapularis
d. Teres major
e. Infraspinatus
f. Teres minor
g. Latissimus dorsi
h. Pectoralis major
i. Coracobrachialis

Human figure worksheet (no. 2)

Label and indicate with arrows the following movements of the shoulder joint:
a. Abduction
b. Adduction
c. Flexion
d. Extension
e. Horizontal adduction
f. Horizontal abduction
g. Internal rotation
h. External rotation

Laboratory and review exercises

1. Locate the following parts of the humerus and scapula on a human skeleton and on a subject:
   a. Greater tubercle
   b. Lesser tubercle
   c. Neck
   d. Shaft
   e. Intertubercular groove
   f. Medial epicondyle
   g. Lateral epicondyle
   h. Trochlea
   i. Capitulum
   j. Supraspinatus fossa
   k. Infraspinatus fossa
   l. Spine of the scapula
2. How and where can the following muscles be palpated on a human subject?
   a. Deltoid
   b. Teres major
   c. Infraspinatus
   d. Teres minor

e. Latissimus dorsi

f. Pectoralis major (upper and lower)

   NOTE: Using the pectoralis major muscle, indicate how various actions allow muscle palpation.

3. Demonstrate and locate on a human subject the muscles that are primarily used in the following shoulder joint movements:
   a. Abduction
   b. Adduction
   c. Flexion
   d. Extension
   e. Horizontal adduction
   f. Horizontal abduction
   g. External rotation
   h. Internal rotation

4. List the planes in which each of the following glenohumeral joint movements occur. List the respective axis of rotation for each movement in each plane.
   a. Abduction
   b. Adduction
   c. Flexion
   d. Extension
   e. Horizontal adduction
   f. Horizontal abduction
   g. External rotation
   h. Internal rotation

5. Why is it essential that both anterior and posterior muscles of the shoulder joint be properly developed? What are some activities or sports that would cause unequal development? equal development?

6. Using an articulated skeleton, compare the relationship of the greater tubercle to the undersurface of the acromion in each of the following situations:
   a. Flexion with the humerus internally rotated versus externally rotated
   b. Abduction with the humerus internally versus externally rotated
   c. Horizontal adduction with the humerus internally versus externally rotated

7. What practical application do the activities or sports in question #5 support if
   a. The rotator cuff muscles are not functioning properly due to fatigue or lack of appropriate strength and endurance?
   b. The scapula stabilizers are not functioning properly due to fatigue or lack of strength and endurance?

8. Pair up with a partner with the back exposed. Use your hand to grasp your partner's right scapula along the lateral border to prevent scapula movement. Have your partner slowly abduct the glenohumeral joint as much as possible. Note the difference in total abduction possible normally versus when you restrict movement of the scapula. Repeat the same exercise, except hold the inferior angle of the scapula tightly against the chest wall while you have your partner internally rotate the humerus. Note the difference in total internal rotation possible normally versus when you restrict movement of the scapula.

9. Analyze movements and muscles in both the shoulder girdle and shoulder joint when the following activities are performed:
   a. Chinning (actual pull)
   b. Throwing a baseball (throw only)
   c. Batting a baseball (striking ball)
   d. Performing a push-up (actual push)

10. Fill in the antagonistic muscle action chart (p. 100) by listing the muscle(s) or parts of muscles that are antagonist in their actions to the muscles in the left column.

11. Fill in the muscle analysis chart (p. 101) by listing the muscles primarily involved in each joint movement.

Antagonistic muscle action chart • Glenohumeral joint

Agonist	Antagonist
Deltoid (anterior fibers)	
Deltoid (middle fibers)	
Deltoid (posterior fibers)	
Supraspinatus	
Subscapularis	
Teres major	
Infraspinatus/teres minor	
Latissimus dorsi	
Pectoralis major (upper fibers)	
Pectoralis major (lower fibers)	
Coracobrachialis	

Muscle analysis chart • Shoulder girdle and shoulder joint

Shoulder Girdle	Shoulder Joint
Adduction	Extension
Abduction	Flexion
Elevation	Horizontal adduction
Depression	Horizontal abduction
Upward rotation	Abduction
Downward rotation	Adduction
	External rotation
	Internal rotation
	Diagonal abduction (overhand activities)
	Diagonal adduction (overhand activities)

References

Andrews JR, Wilk KE: *The athlete's shoulder,* New York, 1994, Churchill Livingstone.

Andrews JR, Zarins B, Wilk KE: *Injuries in baseball,* Philadelphia, 1988, Lippincott-Raven.

Field D: *Anatomy: palpation and surface markings,* ed 3, Oxford, 2001, Butterworth-Heinemann.

Garth WP, et al: Occult anterior subluxations of the shoulder in noncontact sports, *American Journal of Sports Medicine* 15:579, November–December 1987.

Hislop HJ, Montgomery J: *Daniels and Worthingham's muscle testing: techniques of manual examination,* ed 6, Philadelphia, 1995, Saunders.

Perry JF, Rohe DA, Garcia AO: *The kinesiology workbook,* Philadelphia, 1992, Davis.

Rasch PJ: *Kinesiology and applied anatomy,* ed 7, Philadelphia, 1989, Lea & Febiger.

Sieg KW, Adams SP: *Illustrated essentials of musculoskeletal anatomy,* ed 2, Gainesville, FL, 1985, Megabooks.

Smith LK, Weiss EL, Lehmkuhl LD: *Brunnstrom's clinical kinesiology,* ed 5, Philadelphia, 1996, Davis.

Stacey E: Pitching injuries to the shoulder, *Athletic Journal* 65:44, January 1984.

Chapter
5

Chapter 6

The Elbow and Radioulnar Joints

Objectives

- To identify on a human skeleton selected bony features of the elbow and radioulnar joints

- To label selected bony features on a skeletal chart

- To draw and label the muscles on a skeletal chart

- To palpate the muscles on a human subject and list their antagonists

- To list the planes of motion and their respective axes of rotation

- To organize and list the muscles that produce the primary movements of the elbow joint and the radioulnar joint

---

Online Learning Center Resources

Visit *Manual of Structural Kinesiology's* Online Learning Center at **www.mhhe.com/floyd15e** for additional information and study material for this chapter, including:

- *Self-grading quizzes*
- *Anatomy flashcards*
- *Animations*

Almost any movement of the upper extremity will involve the elbow and radioulnar joints. Quite often, these joints are grouped together because of their close anatomical relationship. For this reason, novice students may confuse motions of the elbow with those of the radioulnar joint. In addition, radioulnar joint motion may be incorrectly attributed to the wrist joint because it appears to occur there. However, with close inspection, movements of the elbow joint can be clearly distinguished from those of the radioulnar joints, just as the radioulnar movements can be distinguished from those of the wrist.

Bones

The ulna is much larger proximally than the radius (Fig. 6.1), but distally the radius is much larger than the ulna (see Fig. 7.1 in Chapter 7). The scapula and humerus serve as the proximal attachments for the muscles that flex and extend the elbow. The ulna and radius serve as the distal attachments for the same muscles. The scapula, humerus, and ulna serve as proximal attachments for the muscles that pronate and supinate the radioulnar joints. The distal attachments of the radioulnar joint muscles are located on the radius.

The medial condyloid ridge, olecranon process, coranoid process, and radial tuberosity are important bony landmarks for these muscles. Additionally, the medial epicondyle, lateral epicondyle, and lateral supracondylar ridge are key bony landmarks for the muscles of the wrist and hand, discussed in Chapter 7.

A

B

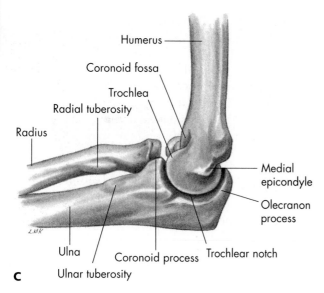

C

FIG. 6.1 ● Right Elbow joint. **A,** anterior view; **B,** lateral view; **C,** medial view.

Joints

The elbow joint is classified as a ginglymus or hinge-type joint that allows only flexion and extension (Fig. 6.1). The elbow may actually be thought of as two interrelated joints, the humeroulnar and the radiohumeral joints. Elbow motions primarily involve movement between the articular surfaces of the humerus and ulna—specifically, the humeral trochlear fitting into the trochlear notch of the ulna. The head of the radius has a relatively small amount of contact with the capitulum of the humerus. As the elbow reaches full extension, the olecranon process of the ulna is received by the olecranon fossa of the humerus. This arrangement provides increased joint stability when the elbow is fully extended.

As the elbow flexes approximately 20 degrees or more, its bony stability is somewhat unlocked, allowing for more side-to-side laxity. The stability of the elbow in flexion is more dependent on the collateral ligaments, such as the lateral or radial collateral ligament and especially the medial or ulnar collateral ligament (Fig. 6.2). The ulnar collateral ligament is critical to providing medial support to prevent the elbow from abducting (not a normal movement of the elbow) when stressed in physical activity. Many contact sports, particularly sports with throwing activities, place stress on the medial aspect of the joint, resulting in injury. The radial collateral ligament on the opposite side provides lateral stability and is rarely injured. Additionally, the annular ligament is located laterally, providing a sling effect around the radial head to secure its stability.

A **Lateral view**

Articular capsule
Radial collateral ligament
Annular ligament

Joint capsule
Annular ligament
Medial epicondyle of humerus
Tendon of biceps brachii m. (cut)
Coronoid process of ulna
Ulnar collateral ligament

Medial view **B**

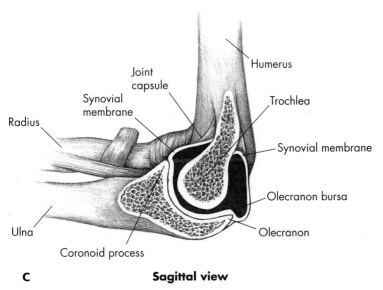

Radius
Synovial membrane
Joint capsule
Humerus
Trochlea
Synovial membrane
Olecranon bursa
Ulna
Olecranon
Coronoid process

C **Sagittal view**

FIG. 6.2 ● Right Elbow joint with ligaments detailed. **A,** Lateral view; **B,** medial view; **C,** sagittal cut view.

The elbow is capable of moving from 0 degrees of extension to approximately 145 to 150 degrees of flexion, as detailed in Fig. 6.3.

The radioulnar joint is classified as a trochoid or pivot-type joint. The radial head rotates around in its location at the proximal ulna. This rotary movement is accompanied by the distal radius rotating around the distal ulna. The radial head is maintained in its joint by the annular ligament.

The radioulnar joint can supinate approximately 80 to 90 degrees from the neutral position. Pronation varies from 70 to 90 degrees (Fig. 6.4).

Due to the radius and ulna being held tightly together between the proximal and distal articulations by an interosseus membrane, the joint between the shafts of these bones is often referred to as syndesmosis type of joint. There is substantial rotary motion between the bones despite this classification.

A   **B**

FIG. 6.3 ● ROM of the elbow: flexion, extension, and hyperextension. **A,** Flexion and hyperextension. *Flexion:* zero to 150°. *Extension:* 150° to zero. *Hyperextension:* measured in degrees beyond the zero starting point. This motion is not present in all persons. When it is present, it may vary from 5° to 15°; **B,** Measurement of limited motion. (The unshaded area indicates the limited ROM). Limited motion may be expressed in the following ways: (1) the elbow flexes from 30° to 90° (30°–90°); (2) the elbow has a flexion deformity of 30° with further flexion to 90°.

A   **B**

FIG. 6.4 ● ROM of the forearm: pronation and supination. **A,** Pronation and supination. *Pronation:* zero to 80° or 90°. *Supination:* zero to 80° or 90°. *Total forearm motion:* 160° to 180°. Persons may vary in the range of supination and pronation. Some may reach the 90° arc, and others may have only 70° plus; **B,** Limited motion. *Supination:* 45° (0–45°). *Total joint motion:* 105°.

Movements FIGS. 6.3, 6.4, 6.5

Elbow movements

Flexion

Movement of the forearm to the shoulder by bending the elbow to decrease its angle

Extension

Movement of the forearm away from the shoulder by straightening the elbow to increase its angle

Radioulnar joint movements

Pronation

Internal rotary movement of the radius on the ulna that results in the hand moving from the palm-up to the palm-down position

Supination

external rotary movement of the radius on the ulna that results in the hand moving from the palm-down to the palm-up position

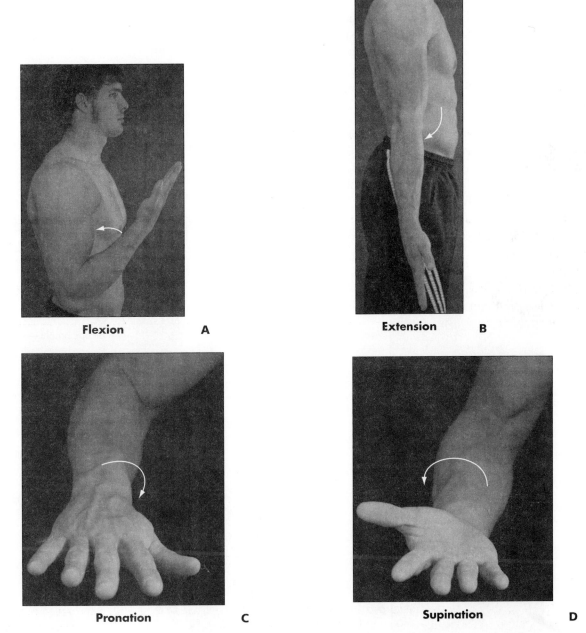

FIG. 6.5 • Movements of the elbow and radioulnar joint. **A,** Elbow flexion; **B,** elbow extension; **C,** radioulnar pronation; **D,** radioulnar supination.

Muscles

The muscles of the elbow and radioulnar joints may be more clearly understood when separated by function. The elbow flexors, located anteriorly, are the biceps brachii, the brachialis, and the brachioradialis, with some weak assistance from the pronator teres (Figs. 6.6, 6.7 & 6.10).

The triceps brachii, located posteriorly, is the primary elbow extensor, with assistance provided by the anconeus (Figs. 6.8, 6.9 & 6.10). The pronator group, located anteriorly, consists of the pronator teres, the pronator quadratus, and the brachioradialis. The brachioradialis also assists with supination, which is controlled mainly by the supinator muscle and the biceps brachii. The supinator muscle is located posteriorly. See Table 6.1.

A common problem associated with the muscles of the elbow is "tennis elbow," which usually involves the extensor digitorum muscle near its origin on the lateral epicondyle. This condition, known technically as *lateral epicondylitis,* is quite frequently associated with gripping and lifting activities. Medial epicondylitis, a somewhat less common problem frequently referred to as "golfer's elbow," is associated with the wrist flexor and pronator group near their origin on the medial epicondyle. Both of these conditions involve muscles which cross the elbow but act primarily on the wrist and hand. These muscles will be addressed in Chapter 7.

Elbow and radioulnar joint muscles—location

Anterior
- Primarily flexion and pronation
  - Biceps brachii
  - Brachialis
  - Brachioradialis
  - Pronator teres
  - Pronator quadratus

Posterior
- Primarily extension and supination
  - Triceps brachii
  - Anconeus
  - Supinator

FIG. 6.6 ● Anterior upper extremity muscles.

FIG. 6.7 ● Anterior upper extremity muscles.

FIG. 6.8 ● Posterior upper extremity muscles.

Trapezius m.

Acromion process of scapula

Deltoid m.

Triceps brachii m.

Brachioradialis m.

Ulnar nerve

Extensor carpi radialis longus m.

Anconeus

Extensor carpi radialis brevis m.

Flexor carpi ulnaris m.

Extensor carpi ulnaris m.

Extensor digitorum m.

Extensor digiti minimi m.

Extensor retinaculum

FIG. 6.9 ● Posterior upper extremity muscles.

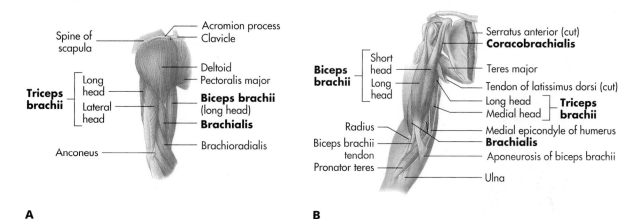

Spine of scapula

Acromion process

Clavicle

Triceps brachii

Long head

Lateral head

Deltoid

Pectoralis major

Biceps brachii
(long head)

Brachialis

Brachioradialis

Anconeus

A

Biceps brachii

Short head

Long head

Serratus anterior (cut)

Coracobrachialis

Teres major

Tendon of latissimus dorsi (cut)

Long head

Medial head

Triceps brachii

Radius

Biceps brachii tendon

Pronator teres

Medial epicondyle of humerus

Brachialis

Aponeurosis of biceps brachii

Ulna

B

FIG. 6.10 ● Muscles of the arm. **A,** Lateral view of the right shoulder and arm; **B,** Anterior view of the right shoulder and arm (deep). Deltoid, pectoralis major, and pectoralis minor muscle removed to reveal deeper structures.

Radioulnar joint

TABLE 6.1 • Agonist muscles of the elbow and radioulnar joints

Muscle	Origin	Insertion	Action	Plane of motion	Palpation	Innervation
Biceps brachii long head	Supraglenoid tubercle above the superior lip of the glenoid fossa	Tuberosity of the radius and bicipital aponeurosis	Supination of the forearm	Transverse	Easily palpated on the anterior humerus. The long head and short head tendons may be palpated in the inter-tubercular groove and just inferior to the coracoid process, respectively. Distally, the biceps tendon is palpated just antero-medial to the elbow joint during supination and flexion.	Musculo-cutaneous nerve (C5, C6)
			Flexion of the elbow	Sagittal		
			Weak flexion of the shoulder joint			
Biceps brachii short head	Coracoid process of the scapula and upper lip of the glenoid fossa		Supination of the forearm	Transverse		
			Flexion of the elbow	Sagittal		
			Weak flexion of the shoulder joint			
Brachialis	Distal half of the anterior portion of the humerus	Coranoid process of the ulna	Flexion of the elbow	Sagittal	Deep on either side of the biceps tendon during flexion/extension	Musculo-cutaneous nerve (C5, C6)
Brachio-radialis	Distal 2/3 of the lateral condyloid (supracondylar) ridge of the humerus	Lateral surface of the distal end of the radius at the styloid process	Flexion of the elbow	Sagittal	Anterolaterally on the proximal forearm during resisted elbow flexion with the radioulnar joint positioned in neutral	Radial nerve (C5, C6)
			Pronation from supination to neutral	Transverse		
			Supination from pronation to neutral			
Pronator teres	Distal part of the medial condyloid ridge of the humerus and medial side of the proximal ulna	Middle 1/3 of the lateral surface of the radius	Pronation of the forearm	Transverse	Anteromedial surface of the proximal forearm during resisted pronation	Median nerve (C6, C7)
			Weak flexion of the elbow	Sagittal		
Pronator quadratus	Distal 1/4 of the anterior side of the ulna	Distal 1/4 of the anterior side of the radius	Pronation of the forearm	Transverse	Cannot be palpated	Median nerve (C6, C7)

Anterior muscles (primarily flexors and pronators)

TABLE 6.1 (continued) • **Agonist muscles of the elbow and radioulnar joints**

	Muscle	Origin	Insertion	Action	Plane of motion	Palpation	Innervation
Posterior muscles (primarily extensors and supinators)	Triceps brachii long head	Infraglenoid tubercle below inferior lip of glenoid fossa of the scapula	Olecranon process of the ulna	Extension of the elbow joint	Sagittal	Proximally as a tendon on the postero-medial arm to underneath the posterior deltoid during resisted shoulder extension/ adduction	Radial nerve (C7, C8)
				Extension of the shoulder joint			
				Adduction of the shoulder joint	Frontal		
	Triceps brachii lateral head	Upper half of the posterior surface of the humerus		Extension of the elbow joint	Sagittal	Posterior arm during resisted extension from a flexed position (lateral head is higher and lateral, medial head is lower and medial). Distally, the tendon may be felt just proximal to the olecranon process.	
	Triceps brachii medial head	Distal 2/3 of the posterior surface of the humerus		Extension of the elbow joint			
	Supinator	Lateral epicondyle of the humerus and neighboring posterior part of the ulna	Lateral surface of the proximal radius just below the head	Supination of the forearm	Transverse	Cannot be palpated	Radial nerve (C6)
	Anconeus	Posterior surface of the lateral condyle of the humerus	Posterior surface of the olecranon process of the ulna	Extension of the elbow	Sagittal	Posterolateral aspect of the proximal ulna to the olecranon process during resisted extension	Radial nerve (C7, C8)

Note: The flexor carpi radialis, palmaris longus, flexor carpi ulnaris, and flexor digitorum superficialis assist in weak flexion of the elbow, while the extensor carpi ulnaris, extensor carpi radialis brevis, extensor carpi radialis longus, and extensor digitorum assist in weak extension of the elbow. Due to their coverage in Chapter 7, they are not listed above.

Chapter

6

Nerves   FIGS. 5.11, 6.11, 6.12

The muscles of the elbow and radioulnar joints are all innervated from the median, musculocutaneous, and radial nerves of the brachial plexus. The radial nerve, originating from C5, C6, C7, and C8, provides innervation for the triceps brachii, brachioradialis, supinator, and anconeus (Fig. 6.11). More specifically, the posterior interosseous nerve, derived from the radial nerve, supplies the supinator. The radial nerve also provides sensation to the posterolateral arm, forearm, and hand. The median nerve, illustrated in Fig. 6.12, innervates the pronator teres and further branches to become the anterior interosseus nerve, which supplies the pronator quadratus. The median nerve's most important related derivations are from C6 and C7. It provides sensation to the palmar aspect of the hand and first three phalanages. The palmar aspect of the radial side of the fourth finger is also provided sensation, along with the dorsal aspect of the index and long fingers. The musculocutaneous nerve, shown in Fig. 5.11, branches from C5 and C6 and supplies the biceps brachii and brachialis.

Posterior cord of brachial plexus

Medial cord of brachial plexus

Lateral cord of brachial plexus

Radial nerve

Long head of triceps brachii m.

Lateral head of triceps brachii m.

Medial head of triceps brachii m.

Anconeus m.

Supinator m.

Extensor carpi ulnaris m.

Extensor digiti minimi m.

Extensor digitorum m.

Brachioradialis m.

Extensor carpi radialis longus m.

Extensor carpi radialis brevis m.

Abductor pollicis longus m.

Extensor pollicis longus and brevis mm.

Extensor indicis m.

Creek

FIG. 6.11 ● Muscular and cutaneous distribution of the radial nerve.

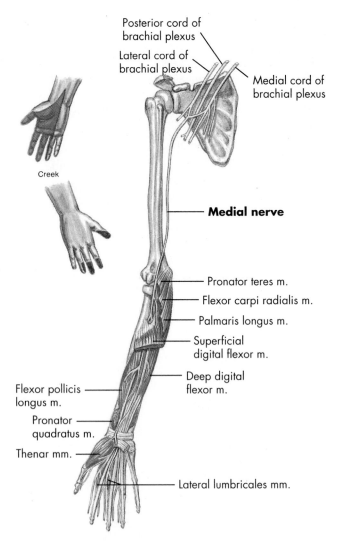

Posterior cord of brachial plexus

Lateral cord of brachial plexus

Medial cord of brachial plexus

Creek

Medial nerve

Pronator teres m.

Flexor carpi radialis m.

Palmaris longus m.

Superficial digital flexor m.

Deep digital flexor m.

Flexor pollicis longus m.

Pronator quadratus m.

Thenar mm.

Lateral lumbricales mm.

FIG. 6.12 ● Muscular and cutaneous distribution of the median nerve.

Biceps brachii muscle   FIG. 6.13

(bi´seps bra´ki-i)

Origin

Long head: supraglenoid tubercle above the superior lip of the glenoid fossa

Short head: coracoid process of the scapula and upper lip of the glenoid fossa

Insertion

Tuberosity of the radius and bicipital aponeurosis

Action

Flexion of the elbow
Supination of the forearm
Weak flexion of the shoulder joint

Palpation

Easily palpated on the anterior humerus. The long head and short head tendons may be palpated in the intertubercular groove and just inferior to the coracoid process, respectively. Distally, the biceps tendon is palpated just anteromedial to the elbow joint during supination and flexion.

Innervation

Musculocutaneous nerve (C5, C6)

Application, strengthening, and flexibility

The biceps is commonly known as a two-joint (shoulder and elbow), or biarticular, muscle. However, technically it should be considered a three-joint (multiarticular) muscle—shoulder, elbow, and radioulnar. It is weak in actions of the shoulder joint, although it does assist in providing dynamic anterior stability to maintain the humeral head in the glenoid fossa. It is more powerful in flexing the elbow when the radioulnar joint is supinated. It is also a strong supinator, particularly if the elbow is flexed. Palms away from the face (pronation) decrease the effectiveness of the biceps, partly as a result of the disadvantageous pull of the muscle as the radius rotates. The same muscles are used in elbow joint flexion, regardless of forearm pronation or supination.

Flexion of the forearm with a barbell in the hands, known as "curling," is an excellent exercise to develop the biceps brachii. This movement can be performed one arm at a time with dumbbells or both arms simultaneously with a barbell. Other activities in which there is powerful flexion of the forearm are chinning and rope climbing.

Due to the multiarticular orientation of the biceps, all three joints must be positioned appropriately to achieve optimal stretching. The elbow must be extended maximally with the shoulder in full extension. The biceps may also be stretched by beginning with full elbow extension and progressing into full horizontal abduction at approximately 70 to 110 degrees of shoulder abduction. In all cases, the forearm should be fully pronated to achieve maximal lengthening of the biceps brachii.

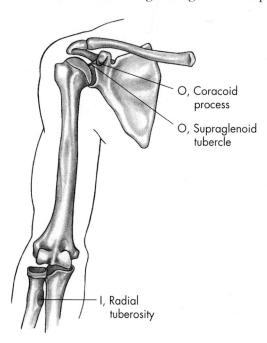

FIG. 6.13 ● Biceps brachii muscle, anterior view. *O*, Origin; *I*, insertion.

Brachialis muscle   FIG. 6.14

(bra´ki-a´lis)

Origin
Distal half of the anterior portion of the humerus

Insertion
Coronoid process of the ulna

Action
True flexion of the elbow

Palpation
Deep on either side of the biceps tendon during flexion/extension

Innervation
Musculocutaneous nerve and sometimes branches from radial and median nerves (C5, C6)

Application, strengthening, and flexibility
The brachialis muscle is used along with other flexor muscles, whether in pronation or supination.

It pulls on the ulna, which does not rotate, thus making this muscle the only pure flexor of this joint.

The brachialis muscle is called into action whenever the elbow flexes. It is exercised along with elbow curling exercises, as described for the biceps brachii, pronator teres, and brachioradialis muscles. Elbow flexion activities that occur with the forearm pronated isolate the brachialis to some extent by reducing the effectiveness of the biceps brachii. Since the brachialis is a pure flexor of the elbow, it can be stretched maximally only by extending the elbow with the shoulder relaxed and flexed. Forearm positioning should not affect the stretch on the brachialis unless the forearm musculature itself limits elbow extension, in which case the forearm is probably best positioned in neutral.

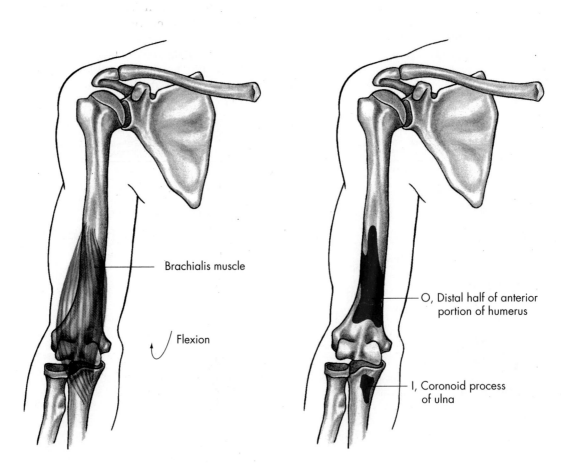

Brachialis muscle

Flexion

O, Distal half of anterior portion of humerus

I, Coronoid process of ulna

FIG. 6.14 ● Brachialis muscle, anterior view. *O*, Origin; *I*, insertion.

Brachioradialis muscle   FIG. 6.15
(bra´ki-o-ra´di-a´lis)

Origin
Distal two-thirds of the lateral condyloid (supracondylar) ridge of the humerus

Insertion
Lateral surface of the distal end of the radius at the
styloid process

Action
Flexion of the elbow
Pronation from supinated position to neutral
Supination from pronated position to neutral

Palpation
Anterolaterally on the proximal forearm during resisted elbow flexion with the radioulnar joint positioned in neutral

Innervation
Radial nerve (C5, C6)

Application, strengthening, and flexibility
The brachioradialis muscle acts as a flexor best
in a midposition or neutral position between
pronation and supination. In a supinated position
of the forearm, it tends to pronate as it flexes. In a
pronated position, it tends to supinate as it flexes.
This muscle is favored in its action of flexion
when the neutral position between pronation and
supination is assumed, as previously suggested.
Its insertion at the end of the radius makes it a
strong elbow flexor. Its ability as a supinator decreases as the radioulnar joint moves toward neutral. Similarly, its ability to pronate decreases as
the forearm reaches neutral. As you will see in
Chapter 7, nearly all of the muscles originating off
the lateral epicondyle have some action as weak
elbow extensors. This is not the case with the
brachioradialis, due to its line of pull being anterior to the elbow's axis of rotation.

The brachioradialis may be strengthened by
performing elbow curls against resistance, particularly with the radioulnar joint in the neutral
position. In addition, the brachioradialis may be
developed by performing pronation and supination movements through the full range of motion
against resistance.

The brachioradialis is stretched by maximally
extending the elbow with the shoulder in flexion
and the forearm in either maximal pronation or
maximal supination.

FIG. 6.15 ● Brachioradialis muscle, lateral view. *O*, Origin; *I*, insertion.

Triceps brachii muscle   FIG. 6.16

(tri´seps bra´ki-i)

Origin

Long head: infraglenoid tubercle below inferior lip
of glenoid fossa of the scapula

Lateral head: upper half of the posterior surface of
the humerus

Medial head: distal two-thirds of the posterior
surface of the humerus

Insertion

Olecranon process of the ulna

Action

All heads: extension of the elbow

Long head: extension of the shoulder joint

Adduction of the shoulder joint

Palpation

Posterior arm during resisted extension from a
flexed position (lateral head is higher and lateral,
medial head is lower and medial). Distally, the
tendon may be felt just proximal to the olecranon
process.

Proximally as a tendon on the posteromedial arm to
underneath the posterior deltoid during resisted
shoulder extension/adduction

Innervation

Radial nerve (C7, C8)

Application, strengthening, and flexibility

Typical action of the triceps brachii is shown in
push-ups when there is powerful extension of the
elbow. It is used in hand balancing and in any
pushing movement involving the upper extremity. The long head is an important extensor of the
shoulder joint.

Two muscles extend the elbow—the triceps
brachii and the anconeus. Push-ups demand strenuous contraction of these muscles. Dips on the
parallel bars are more difficult to perform. Bench-
pressing a barbell or a dumbbell is an excellent exercise. Overhead presses and triceps curls (elbow
extensions from an overhead position) emphasize
the triceps.

The triceps brachii should be stretched with
both the shoulder and the elbow in maximal
flexion.

FIG. 6.16 ● Triceps brachii muscle, posterior view. *O*, Origin; *I*, insertion.

Anconeus muscle   FIG. 6.17

(an-ko´ne-us)

Origin

Posterior surface of the lateral condyle of the
humerus

Insertion

Posterior surface of the olecranon process of the
ulna

Action

Extension of the elbow

Palpation

Posterolateral aspect of the proximal ulna to the olecranon process during resisted extension

Innervation

Radial nerve (C7, C8)

Application, strengthening, and flexibility

The chief function of the anconeus muscle is to
pull the synovial membrane of the elbow joint out
of the way of the advancing olecranon process
during extension of the elbow. It contracts along
with the triceps brachii. It is strengthened with
any elbow extension exercise against resistance.

Maximal elbow flexion stretches the anconeus.

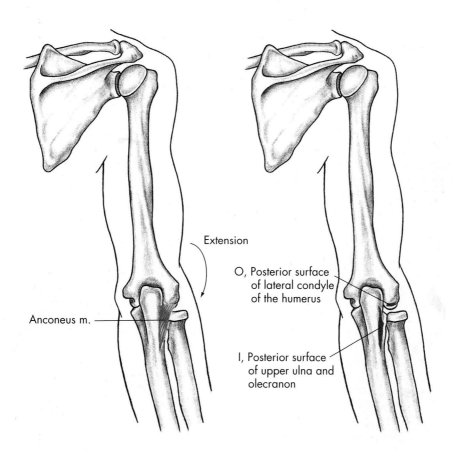

Extension

Anconeus m.

O, Posterior surface
of lateral condyle
of the humerus

I, Posterior surface
of upper ulna and
olecranon

FIG. 6.17 ● Anconeus muscle, posterior view. *O*, Origin; *I*, insertion.

Pronator teres muscle   FIG. 6.18

(pro-na´tor te´rez)

Origin

Distal part of the medial condyloid ridge of the humerus and medial side of the proximal ulna

Insertion

Middle third of the lateral surface of the radius

Action

Pronation of the forearm
Weak flexion of the elbow

Palpation

Anteromedial surface of the proximal forearm during resisted pronation

Innervation

Median nerve (C6, C7)

Application, strengthening, and flexibility

Typical movement of the pronator teres muscle is with the forearm pronating as the elbow flexes. Movement is weaker in flexion with supination. The use of the pronator teres alone in movement tends to bring the back of the hand to the face as it contracts. Pronation of the forearm with a dumbbell in the hand localizes action and develops the pronator teres muscle. The hammer exercise used for the supinator muscle may be modified to develop the pronator teres. In the beginning, the forearm is supported and the hand is free off the table edge. The hammer is again held suspended out of the ulnar side of the hand hanging toward the floor. The forearm is then pronated to the palm-down position to strengthen this muscle.

The elbow must be fully extended while taking the forearm into full supination to stretch the pronator teres.

Chapter 6

Pronator teres m.

O, Distal part of medial condyloid ridge of humerus, medial side of the proximal ulna

I, Middle third of lateral surface of radius

Pronation

FIG. 6.18 ● Pronator teres muscle, anterior view. *O*, Origin; *I*, insertion.

Pronator quadratus muscle   FIG. 6.19

(pro-na´tor kwad-ra´tus)

Origin
Distal fourth of the anterior side of the ulna

Insertion
Distal fourth of the anterior side of the radius

Action
Pronation of the forearm

Palpation
Cannot be palpated

Innervation
Median nerve (palmar interosseous branch) (C6, C7)

Application, strengthening, and flexibility

The pronator quadratus muscle works in pronating the forearm in combination with the triceps in extending the elbow. It is commonly used in turning a screwdriver, as in taking out a screw, when extension and pronation are needed. It is used also in throwing a screwball, when extension and pronation are needed. It may be developed with similar pronation exercises against resistance, as described for the pronator teres. The pronator quadratus is best stretched by using a partner to grasp the wrist and passively take the forearm into extreme supination.

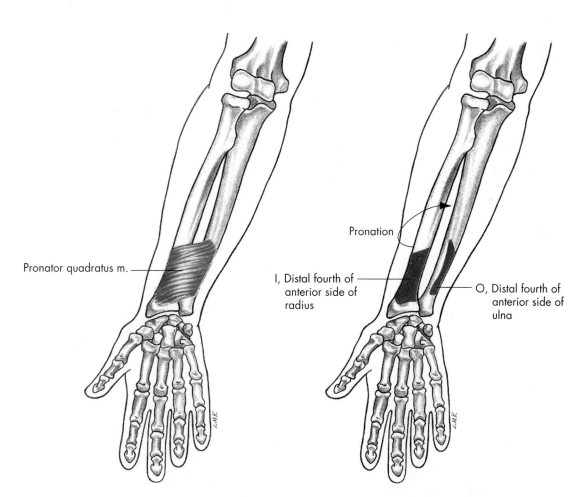

FIG. 6.19 ● Pronator quadratus muscle, anterior view. *O*, Origin; *I*, insertion.

Supinator muscle FIG. 6.20

(su′pi-na′tor)

Origin

Lateral epicondyle of the humerus and neighboring posterior part of the ulna

Insertion

Lateral surface of the proximal radius just below the head

Action

Supination of the forearm

Palpation

Cannot be palpated

Innervation

Radial nerve (C6)

Application, strengthening, and flexibility

The supinator muscle is called into play when movements of extension and supination are required, as when turning a screwdriver. The curve in throwing a baseball calls this muscle into play as the elbow is extended just before ball release. It is most isolated in activities that require supination with elbow extension, because the biceps brachii assist with supination most when the elbow is flexed.

The hands should be grasped and the forearms extended, in an attempt to supinate the forearms against the grip of the hands. This localizes, to a degree, the action of the supinator.

Strengthening this muscle begins with holding a hammer in the hand with the hammer head suspended from the ulnar side of the hand while the forearm is supported on a desk or table. The hammer should be hanging toward the floor, with the forearm supinated to the palm-up position.

The supinator is stretched when the forearm is maximally pronated.

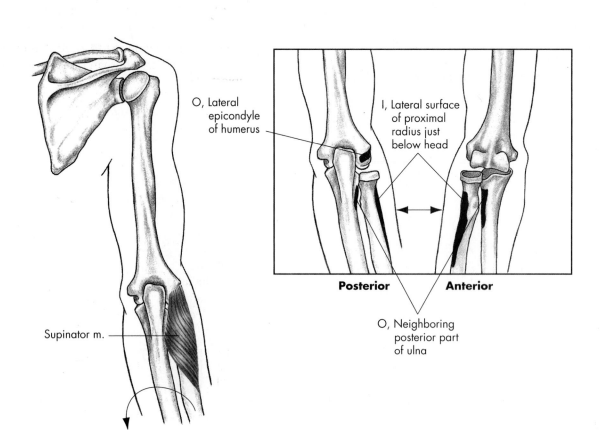

FIG. 6.20 ● Supinator muscle, posterior view. *O*, Origin; *I*, insertion.

Web sites

Anatomy & Physiology Tutorials:

www.gwc.maricopa.edu/class/bio201/index.htm

Radiologic Anatomy Browser:

radlinux1.usuf1.usuhs.mil/rad/iong/index.html

This site has numerous radiological views of the musculoskeletal system.

University of Arkansas Medical School Gross Anatomy for Medical Students:

anatomy.uams.edu/htmlpages/anatomyhtml/ gross.html

Dissections, anatomy tables, atlas images, links, etc.

Loyola University Medical Center: Structure of the Human Body:

www.meddean.luc.edu/lumen/MedEd/ GrossAnatomy/GA.html

An excellent site with many slides, dissections, tutorials, etc., for the study of human anatomy.

Wheeless' Textbook of Orthopaedics:

www.ortho-u.net/

This site has an extensive index of links to the fractures, joints, muscles, nerves, trauma, medications, medical topics, and lab tests, as well as links to orthopedic journals and other orthopedic and medical news.

Arthroscopy.Com:

www.arthroscopy.com/sports.htm

Patient information on various musculoskeletal problems of the upper and lower extremity

Premiere Medical Search Engine:

www.medsite.com

This site allows the reader to enter any medical condition and it will search the net to find relevant articles.

Virtual Hospital:

www.vh.org

Numerous slides, patient information, etc.

Worksheet exercises

As an aid to learning, for in-class and out-of-class assignments, or for testing, tear-out worksheets are found at the end of the text (pp. 328 and 329).

Skeletal worksheet (no. 1)

Draw and label on the worksheet the following muscles:
a. Biceps brachii
b. Brachioradialis
c. Brachialis
d. Pronator teres
e. Pronator quadratus
f. Supinator
g. Triceps brachii
h. Anconeus

Human figure worksheet (no. 2)

Label and indicate with arrows the following movements of the elbow and radioulnar joints:
1. Elbow joint
   a. Flexion
   b. Extension
2. Radioulnar joint
   a. Pronation
   b. Supination

Laboratory and review exercises

1. Locate the following parts of the humerus, radius, and ulna on a human skeleton and on a subject.
   a. Skeleton
      1. Medial epicondyle
      2. Lateral epicondyle
      3. Trochlea
      4. Capitulum
      5. Olecranon fossa
      6. Olecranon process
      7. Coronoid process
      8. Coronoid fossa
      9. Tuberosity of the radius
   b. Subject
      1. Medial epicondyle
      2. Lateral epicondyle
      3. Olecranon process
      4. Olecranon fossa
2. How and where can the following muscles be palpated on a human subject?
   a. Biceps brachii
   b. Brachioradialis
   c. Brachialis
   d. Pronator teres
   e. Supinator
   f. Triceps brachii
   g. Anconeus

3. Palpate and list the muscles primarily responsible for the following movements as you demonstrate each:
   a. Flexion
   b. Extension
   c. Pronation
   d. Supination
4. List the planes in which each of the following elbow and radioulnar joint movements occurs. List the respective axis of rotation for each movement in each plane.
   a. Flexion
   b. Extension
   c. Pronation
   d. Supination
5. Discuss the difference between chinning with the palms toward the face and chinning with the palms away from the face. Consider this muscularly and anatomically.
6. Analyze and list the differences in elbow and radioulnar joint muscle activity between turning a door knob clockwise and pushing the door open, versus turning the knob counterclockwise, pulling the door open.
7. Fill in the antagonistic muscle action chart below by listing the muscle(s) or parts of muscles that are antagonist in their actions to the muscles in the left column.
8. Fill in the muscle analysis chart below by listing the muscles primarily involved in each movement.

Antagonistic muscle action chart • Elbow and radioulnar joints

Agonist	Antagonist
Biceps brachii	
Brachioradialis	
Brachialis	
Pronator teres	
Supinator	
Triceps brachii	
Anconeus	

Muscle analysis chart • Elbow and radioulnar joints

Elbow and radioulnar joints	
Flexion	Extension
Pronation	Supination

References

Andrews JR, Wilk KE: *The athlete's shoulder,* New York, 1994, Churchill Livingstone.

Andrews JR, Zarins B, Wilk KE: *Injuries in baseball,* Philadelphia, 1998, Lippincott-Raven.

Back BR Jr, et al: Triceps rupture: a case report and literature review, *American Journal of Sports Medicine* 15:285, May–June 1987.

Gabbard CP, et al: Effects of grip and forearm position on flex arm hang performance, *Research Quarterly for Exercise and Sport,* July 1983.

Guarantors of Brain: *Aids to the examination of the peripheral nervous system,* ed 4, London, 2000, Saunders.

Herrick RT, Herrick S: Ruptured triceps in powerlifter presenting as cubital tunnel syndrome—a case report, *American Journal of Sports Medicine* 15:514, September–October 1987.

Hislop HJ, Montgomery J: *Daniels and Worthingham's muscle testing: techniques of manual examination,* ed 6, Philadelphia, 1995, Saunders.

Magee DJ: *Orthopedic physical assessment,* ed 4, Philadelphia, 2002, Saunders.

Rasch PJ: *Kinesiology and applied anatomy,* ed 7, Philadelphia, 1989, Lea & Febiger.

Sieg KW, Adams SP: *Illustrated essentials of musculoskeletal anatomy,* ed 2, Gainesville, FL, 1985, Megabooks.

Sisto DJ, et al: An electromyographic analysis of the elbow in pitching, *American Journal of Sports Medicine* 15:260, May–June 1987.

Smith LK, Weiss EL, Lehmkuhl LD: *Brunnstrom's clinical kinesiology,* ed 5, Philadelphia, 1996, Davis.

Springer SI: Racquetball and elbow injuries, *National Racquetball* 16:7, March 1987.

Van De Graaff KM: *Human anatomy,* ed 6, Dubuque, IA. 2002, McGraw-Hill.

Chapter

6

Chapter 7

The Wrist and Hand Joints

Objectives

- To identify on a human skeleton selected bony features of the wrist, hand, and fingers

- To label selected bony features on a skeletal chart

- To draw and label the muscles on a skeletal chart

- To palpate the muscles on a human subject while demonstrating their actions

- To list the planes of motion and their respective axes of rotation

- To organize and list the muscles that produce the primary movements of the wrist, hand, and fingers

---

Online Learning Center Resources

Visit *Manual of Structural Kinesiology's* Online Learning Center at **www.mhhe.com/floyd15e** for additional information and study material for this chapter, including:

- *Self-grading quizzes*
- *Anatomy flashcards*
- *Animations*

The joints of the wrist, hand, and fingers are often overlooked in their importance to us in comparison with the larger joints needed for ambulation. Even though the fine motor skills characteristic of this area are not essential in some sports, many sports with skilled activities require precise functioning of the wrist and hand. Several sports, such as archery, bowling, golf, baseball, and tennis, require the combined use of all of these joints.

Because of numerous muscles, bones, and ligaments, combined with relatively small joint size, the functional anatomy of the wrist and hand is complex and overwhelming to some. This complexity may be simplified by relating the functional anatomy to the major actions of the joints: flexion, extension, abduction, and adduction of the wrist and hand.

A large number of muscles are used in these movements. Anatomically and structurally, the human wrist and hand have highly developed, complex mechanisms capable of a variety of movements, which is a result of the arrangement of the 29 bones, more than 25 joints, and more than 30 muscles, of which 18 are intrinsic (both origin and insertion found in the hand) muscles.

For most students who use this text, an extensive knowledge of these intrinsic muscles is not necessary. However, athletic trainers, physical therapists, occupational therapists, chiropractors, anatomists, physicians, and nurses require a more extensive knowledge. The intrinsic muscles are listed, illustrated, and discussed to a limited degree at the end of this chapter. References at the end of this chapter provide additional sources from which to gain further information.

Our discussion is limited to a review of the muscles, joints, and movements involved in gross motor activities. The muscles included are those of the forearm and the extrinsic muscles of the wrist, hand, and fingers. The larger, more important extrinsic muscles of each joint are included, providing a limited knowledge of this area. The prescription of exercises for strengthening these muscles will be somewhat redundant, since there are primarily only four movements accomplished by their combined actions. An exercise that will strengthen most of these muscles is fingertip push-ups.

Bones

The wrist and hand contain 29 bones, including the radius and ulna (Fig. 7.1). Eight carpal bones in two rows of four bones form the wrist. The proximal row consists, from the radial (thumb) side to the ulnar (little finger) side, of the scaphoid (boat-shaped) or navicular as it is commonly known, the lunate (moon-shaped), the triquetrum (three-cornered), and the pisiform (pea-shaped) bones. The distal row, from the radial to ulnar side, consists of the trapezium (greater multangular), trapezoid (lesser multangular), capitate (head-shaped), and hamate (hooked) bones. These bones form a three-sided arch that is concave on the palmar side. This bony arch is spanned by the transverse carpal and volar carpal ligaments creating the carpal tunnel, which is frequently a source

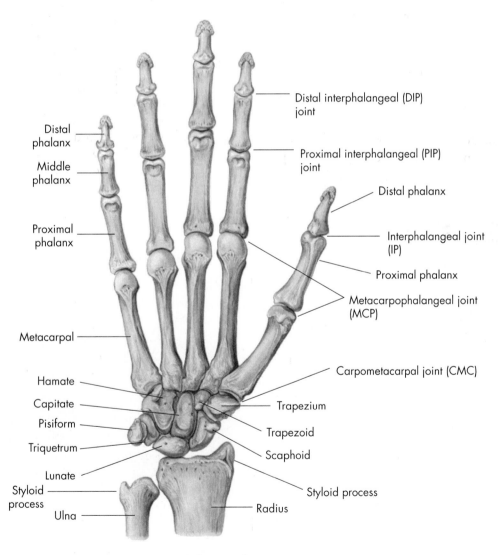

FIG. 7.1 ● Right wrist and hand, palmar surface.

From Anthony CP, Kolthoff NJ: *Textbook of anatomy and physiology,* ed 9, St. Louis, 1975, Mosby.

of problems known as carpal tunnel syndrome (see Fig. 7.8). Five metacarpal bones, numbered one to five from the thumb to the little finger, join the wrist bones. There are 14 phalanges (digits), three for each phalange except the thumb, which has only two. They are indicated as proximal, middle, and distal from the metacarpals. Additionally, the thumb has a sesamoid bone within its flexor tendon, and other sesamoids may occur in the fingers.

The medial epicondyle, medial condyloid ridge, and coranoid process serve as a point of origin for many of the wrist and finger flexors, whereas the lateral epicondyle and lateral supracondylar ridge serve as the point of origin for many extensors of the wrist and fingers (Figs. 6.1 and 6.2). Distally, the key bony landmarks for the muscles involved in wrist motion are the base of the second, third, and fifth metacarpals and the pisiform and hamate. The muscles of the fingers, which are also involved in wrist motion, insert on the base of the proximal, middle, and distal phalanxes (Figs. 7.1 and 7.2). The base of the first metacarpal, proximal and distal phalanxes of the thumb serve as key insertion points for the muscles involved in thumb motion (Fig. 7.1).

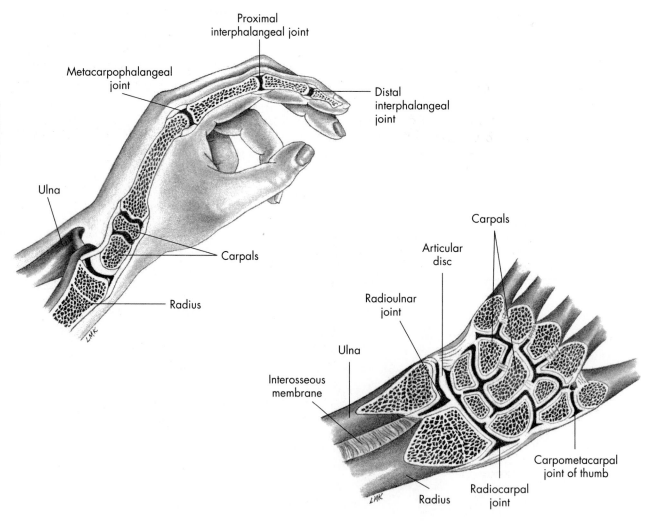

FIG. 7.2 ● Wrist and hand joint structures.

Joints

The wrist joint is classified as a condyloid-type joint, allowing flexion, extension, abduction (radial deviation), and adduction (ulnar deviation) (Fig. 7.2). Wrist motion occurs primarily between the distal radius and the proximal carpal row, consisting of the scaphoid, lunate, and triquetrum. The joint allows 70 to 90 degrees of flexion and 65 to 85 degrees of extension. The wrist can abduct 15 to 25 degrees and adduct 25 to 40 degrees (Fig. 7.3).

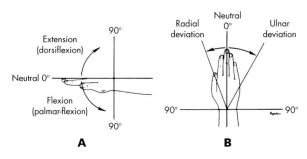

FIG. 7.3 ● ROM of the wrist. **A,** Flexion and extension. *Flexion* (palmar flexion): zero to ±80°. *Extension* (dorsiflexion): zero to ±70°; **B,** Radial and ulnar deviation. *Radial deviation* zero to 20°. *Ulnar deviation:* zero to 30°.

Each finger has three joints. The metacarpophalangeal (MCP) joints are classified as condyloid. In these joints, 0 to 40 degrees of extension and 85 to 100 degrees of flexion are possible. The proximal interphalangeal (PIP) joints, classified as ginglymus, can move from full extension to approximately 90 to 120 degrees of flexion.

The distal interphalangeal (DIP) joints, also classified as ginglymus, can flex 80 to 90 degrees from full extension (Fig. 7.5).

The thumb has only two joints, both of which are classified as ginglymus. The metacarpophalangeal (MCP) joint moves from full extension into 40 to 90 degrees of flexion. The interphalangeal (IP) joint can flex 80 to 90 degrees. The carpometacarpal (CMC) joint of the thumb is a unique saddle-type joint having 50 to 70 degrees of abduction. It can flex approximately 15 to 45 degrees and extend 0 to 20 degrees (Fig. 7.6).

Ligaments, too numerous to mention in this discussion, support and provide static stability to the many joints of the wrist and hand. Some of the finger ligaments are detailed in Fig. 7.4.

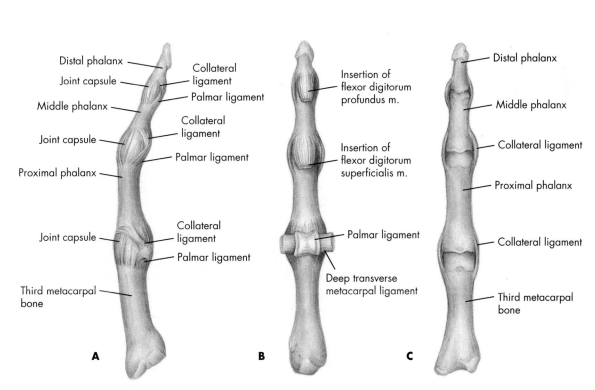

FIG. 7.4 ● Metacarpophalangeal and interphalangeal joints of ring finger. **A,** A lateral view; **B,** an anterior (palmar) view; and **C,** a posterior view.

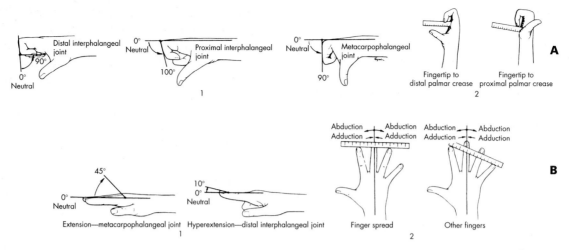

FIG. 7.5 ● ROM of the fingers. **A,** Flexion. *1,* Motion can be estimated or measured in degrees. *2,* Motion can be estimated by a ruler as the distance from the tip of the finger to the distal palmar crease (*left*) (measures flexion of the middle and distal joints) and the proximal palmar crease (*right*) (measures the distal, middle, and proximal joints of the fingers); **B,** Extension, abduction, and adduction. *1,* Extension and hyperextension. *2,* Abduction and adduction. These motions take place in the plane of the palm away from and to the long, or middle, finger of the hand. The spread of fingers can be measured from the tip of the index finger to the tip of the little finger (*right*). Individual fingers spread from tip to tip of indicated fingers (*left*).

Chapter 7

FIG. 7.6 ● ROM of the thumb. **A,** Abduction. *1,* zero starting position: the extended thumb alongside the index finger, which is in line with the radius. *Abduction* is the angle created between the metacarpal bones of the thumb and index finger. This motion may take place in two planes. *2,* Radial abduction or *extension* takes place parallel to the plane of the palm; **B,** Flexion. *1,* Zero starting position: the extended thumb. *2,* Flexion of the interphalangeal joint: zero to ±80°. *3,* Flexion of the metacarpophalangeal joint: zero to ±50°. *4,* Fexion of the carpometacarpal joint: zero to ±15°; **C,** Opposition. Zero starting position (*far left*): the thumb in line with the index fingers. *Opposition* is a composite motion consisting of three elements: (1) abduction, (2) rotation, and (3) flexion. Motion is usually considered complete when the tip of the thumb touches the tip of the fifth finger. Some consider the arc of opposition complete when the tip of the thumb touches the base of the fifth finger. Both methods are illustrated.

Movements

The common actions of the wrist are flexion, extension, abduction, and adduction (Fig. 7.7, *A–D*). The fingers can only flex and extend (Fig. 7.7, *E–F*), except at the metacarpophalangeal joints, where abduction and adduction (Fig. 7.7, *G–H*) are controlled by the intrinsic hand muscles. In the hand, the middle phalange is regarded as the reference point by which to differentiate abduction and adduction. Abduction of the index and middle fingers occurs when they move laterally toward the radial side of the forearm. Abduction of the ring and little fingers occurs when they move medially toward the ulnar side of the hand. Movement medially of the index and middle fingers toward the ulnar side of the forearm is adduction. Ring and little finger adduction occurs when these fingers move laterally toward the radial side of the hand. The thumb is abducted when it moves away from the palm and is adducted when it moves toward the palmar aspect of the second metacarpal. These movements, together with pronation and supination of the forearm, make possible the many fine, coordinated movements of the forearm, wrist, and hand.

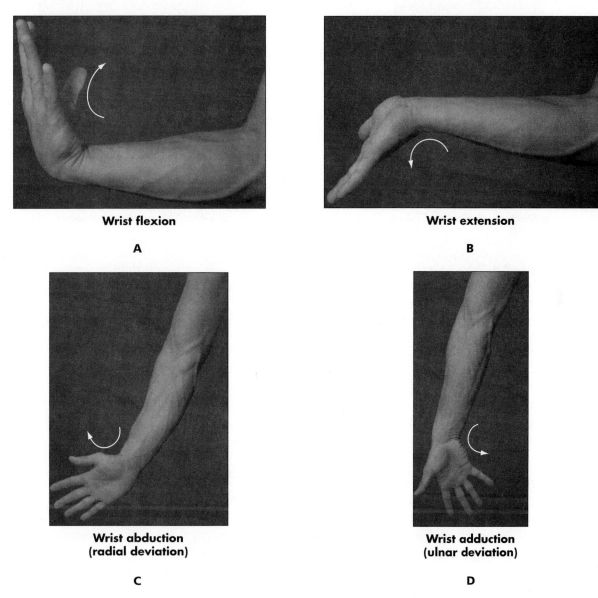

Wrist flexion

A

Wrist extension

B

Wrist abduction (radial deviation)

C

Wrist adduction (ulnar deviation)

D

FIG. 7.7 ● Wrist and hand movements. **A,** Wrist flexion; **B,** wrist extension; **C,** wrist abduction; **D,** wrist adduction.

Chapter **7**

Flexion of fingers and thumb, opposition

E

Extension of fingers and thumb, reposition

F

**Adduction of
metacarpophalangeal joints**

G

**Abduction of
metacarpophalangeal joints**

H

FIG. 7.7 continued ● Wrist and hand movements. **E,** flexion of the fingers and thumb, opposition; **F,** extension of the fingers and thumb, reposition; **G,** adduction of metacarpophalangeal joints; **H,** abduction of metacarpophalangeal joints.

Flexion (palmar flexion)

Movement of the palm of the hand and/or the phalanges toward the anterior or volar aspect of the forearm

Extension (dorsiflexion)

Movement of the back of the hand and/or the phalanges toward the posterior or dorsal aspect of the forearm; sometimes referred to as hyperextension

Abduction (radial deviation, radial flexion)

Movement of the thumb side of the hand toward the lateral aspect or radial side of the forearm; also, movement of the fingers away from the middle finger

Adduction (ulnar deviation, ulnar flexion)

Movement of the little finger side of the hand toward the medial aspect or ulnar side of the forearm; also, movement of the fingers back together toward the middle finger

Opposition

Movement of the thumb across the palmar aspect to oppose any or all of the phalanges

Reposition

Movement of the thumb as it returns to the anatomical position from opposition with the hand and/or fingers

Muscles   TABLE 7.1

The extrinsic muscles of the wrist and hand can be grouped according to function and location (Table 7.1). There are six muscles that move the wrist but do not cross the hand to move the fingers and thumb. The three wrist flexors in this group are the flexor carpi radialis, flexor carpi ulnaris, and palmaris longus—all of which have their origin on the medial epicondyle of the humerus. The extensors of the wrist have their origins on the lateral epicondyle and include the extensor carpi radialis longus, extensor carpi radialis brevis, and extensor carpi ulnaris (Figs. 6.7 and 6.9).

Another nine muscles function primarily to move the phalanges but are also involved in wrist joint actions because they originate on the forearm and cross the wrist. These muscles generally are weaker in their actions on the wrist. The flexor digitorum superficialis and the flexor digitorum profundus are finger flexors; however, they also assist in wrist flexion along with the flexor pollicis longus, which is a thumb flexor. The extensor digitorum, the extensor indicis, and the extensor digiti minimi are finger extensors but also assist in wrist extension, along with the extensor pollicis longus and the extensor pollicis brevis, which extend the thumb. The abductor pollicis longus abducts the thumb and assists in wrist abduction.

All of the wrist flexors generally have their origins on the anteromedial aspect of the proximal forearm and medial epicondyle of the humerus, whereas their insertions are on the anterior aspect of the wrist and hand. All of the flexor tendons except for the flexor carpi ulnaris and palmaris longus pass through the carpal tunnel, along with the median nerve. Conditions leading to swelling and inflammation in this area can result in increased pressure in the carpal tunnel, which interferes with normal function of the median nerve, leading to reduced motor and sensation function of its distribution (Fig. 7.8).

The wrist extensors generally have their origins on the posterolateral aspect of the proximal forearm and lateral humeral epicondyle, whereas their insertions are located on the posterior aspect of the wrist and hand. The flexor and extensor tendons at the distal forearm immediately proximal to the wrist are held in place on the palmar and dorsal aspects by transverse bands of tissue. These bands, respectively known as the flexor and extensor retinaculum, prevent these tendons from bowstringing during flexion and extension.

The wrist abductors are the flexor carpi radialis, extensor carpi radialis longus, extensor carpi radialis brevis, abductor pollicis longus, extensor pollicis longus, and extensor pollicis brevis. These muscles generally cross the wrist joint anterolaterally and posterolaterally to insert on the radial side of the hand. The flexor carpi ulnaris and extensor carpi ulnaris adduct the wrist and cross the wrist joint anteromedially and posteromedially to insert on the ulnar side of the hand.

Chapter

7

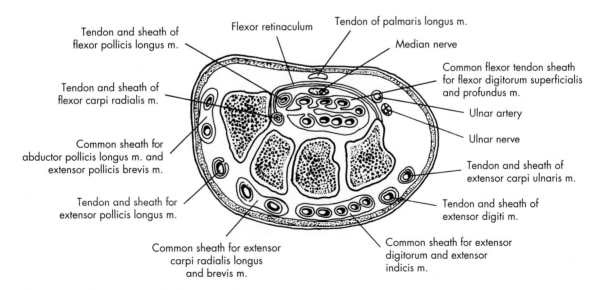

Tendon and sheath of flexor pollicis longus m.

Tendon and sheath of flexor carpi radialis m.

Common sheath for abductor pollicis longus m. and extensor pollicis brevis m.

Tendon and sheath for extensor pollicis longus m.

Common sheath for extensor carpi radialis longus and brevis m.

Flexor retinaculum

Tendon of palmaris longus m.

Median nerve

Common flexor tendon sheath for flexor digitorum superficialis and profundus m.

Ulnar artery

Ulnar nerve

Tendon and sheath of extensor carpi ulnaris m.

Tendon and sheath of extensor digiti m.

Common sheath for extensor digitorum and extensor indicis m.

FIG. 7.8 ● Cross-section of the right wrist. Note the carpal canal and the arrangement of the tendon sheaths.

TABLE 7.1 • Agonist muscles of the wrist and hand joints

	Muscle	Origin	Insertion	Action	Plane of motion	Palpation	Innervation
Anterior muscles (wrist flexors)	Flexor carpi radialis	Medial epicondyle of humerus	Base of 2nd and 3rd metacarpals on palmar surface	Flexion of the wrist	Sagittal	Anterior wrist surface, slightly lateral, in line with the 2nd and 3rd metacarpals	Median nerve (C6, C7)
				Abduction of the wrist	Frontal		
				Weak flexion of the elbow	Sagittal		
	Palmaris longus	Medial epicondyle of the humerus	Palmar aponeurosis of the 2nd, 3rd, 4th, and 5th metacarpals	Flexion of the wrist	Sagittal	Anteromedial and central aspect of the anterior forearm just proximal to the wrist, particularly with slight wrist flexion and opposition of thumb to the 5th finger	Median nerve (C6, C7)
				Weak flexion of the elbow			
	Flexor carpi ulnaris	Medial epicondyle of humerus and posterior aspect of proximal ulna	Base of 5th metacarpal (palmar surface), pisiform, and hamate	Flexion of the wrist	Sagittal	Anteromedial surface of the forearm, a few inches below the medial epicondyle of the humerus to just proximal to the wrist, with resisted flexion/adduction	Ulnar nerve (C8, T1)
				Adduction of the wrist	Frontal		
				Weak flexion of the elbow	Sagittal		
Anterior muscles (wrist and phalangeal flexors)	Flexor digitorum superficialis	Medial epicondyle of humerus Ulnar head: medial coronoid process Radial head: upper 2/3 of anterior border of the radius	Each tendon splits and attaches to the sides of middle phalanx of four fingers on palmar surface	Flexion of the fingers at the metacarpophalangeal and proximal interphalangeal joints	Sagittal	In depressed area between palmaris longus and flexor carpi ulnaris tendons, particularly with flexion of 3rd and 4th phalanges	Median nerve (C7, C8, T1)
				Flexion of the wrist			
				Weak flexion of the elbow			
	Flexor digitorum profundus	Proximal 3/4ths of anterior and medial ulna	Base of distal phalanges of four fingers	Flexion of the four fingers at the metacarpophalangeal, proximal interphalangeal, and distal interphalangeal joints	Sagittal	Over the palmar surface of the 2nd, 3rd, 4th, and 5th metacarpophalangeal joint during finger flexion against resistance	Median nerve (C8, T1) to 2nd and 3rd fingers; ulnar nerve (C8, T1) to 4th and 5th fingers
				Flexion of the wrist			
	Flexor pollicis longus	Middle anterior surface of the radius and the anterior medial border of the ulna just distal to the coronoid process.	Base of distal phalanx of thumb on palmar surface	Flexion of the thumb carpometacarpal, metacarpophalangeal, and interphalangeal joints	Sagittal	Anterior surface of the thumb, particularly on the proximal phalanx during thumb flexion	Median nerve palmar interosseous branch (C8, T1)
				Flexion of the wrist			

TABLE 7.1 (continued) • **Agonist muscles of the wrist and hand joints**

	Muscle	Origin	Insertion	Action	Plane of motion	Palpation	Innervation
Posterior muscles (wrist extensors)	Extensor carpi ulnaris	Lateral epicondyle of humerus and middle 1/2 of the posterior border of the ulna	Base of 5th metacarpal on dorsal surface	Extension of the wrist	Sagittal	Just lateral to the ulnar styloid process and crossing the posteromedial wrist, particularly with wrist extension/adduction	Radial nerve (C6, C7, C8)
				Adduction of the wrist	Frontal		
				Weak extension of the elbow	Sagittal		
	Extensor carpi radialis brevis	Lateral epicondyle of humerus	Base of 3rd metacarpal on dorsal surface	Extension of the wrist	Sagittal	Just proximal to the dorsal aspect of the wrist and approximately 1 cm medial to the radial styloid process, the tendon may be felt during extension and traced to base of 3rd metacarpal. Proximally, just medial to the bulk of the brachioradialis	Radial nerve (C6, C7)
				Abduction of the wrist	Frontal		
				Weak extension of the elbow	Sagittal		
	Extensor carpi radialis longus	Lower third of lateral supracondylar ridge of humerus and lateral epicondyle of the humerus	Base of 2nd metacarpal on dorsal surface	Extension of the wrist	Sagittal	Just proximal to the dorsal aspect of the wrist and approximately 1 cm medial to the radial styloid process, the tendon may be felt during extension and traced to base of 2nd metacarpal. Proximally, just medial to the bulk of the brachioradialis	Radial nerve (C6, C7)
				Abduction of the wrist	Frontal		
				Weak extension of the elbow	Sagittal		

Chapter

7

(continued)

TABLE 7.1 (continued) • **Agonist muscles of the wrist and hand joints**

	Muscle	Origin	Insertion	Action	Plane of motion	Palpation	Innervation
Posterior muscles (wrist and phalangeal extensors)	Extensor digitorum	Lateral epicondyle of humerus	Four tendons to bases of 2nd and 3rd phalanges of four fingers on dorsal surface	Extension of the 2nd, 3rd, 4th, and 5th phalanges at the metacarpophalangeal joints	Sagittal	With all four fingers extended, on the anterior surface of the distal forearm immediately medial to extensor pollicis longus tendon, then dividing into four separate tendons that are over the dorsal aspect of the hand and metacarpophalangeal joints	Radial nerve (C6, C7, C8)
				Extension of the wrist			
				Weak extension of the elbow			
	Extensor indicis	Middle to distal 1/3 of posterior ulna	Base of the middle and distal phalanxes of the 2nd phalange, dorsal surface	Extension of the index finger at the metacarpophalangeal joint	Sagittal	Posterior aspect of the distal forearm and dorsal surface of the hand just medial to the extensor digitorum tendon of the index finger	Radial nerve (C6, C7, C8)
				Weak wrist extension			
	Extensor digiti minimi	Lateral epicondyle of humerus	Base of the middle and distal phalanxes of the 5th phalange (dorsal surface)	Extension of the little finger at the metacarpophalangeal joint	Sagittal	Passing over the dorsal aspect of the distal radioulnar joint, particularly with relaxed flexion of other fingers and alternating 5th finger extension and relaxation	Radial nerve (C6, C7, C8)
				Weak wrist extension			
	Extensor pollicis longus	Posterior lateral surface of the lower middle ulna	Base of distal phalanx of thumb on dorsal surface	Extension of the thumb	Sagittal	Dorsal aspect of the hand to its insertion on the base of the distal phalanx	Radial nerve (C6, C7, C8)
				Extension of the wrist			
	Extensor pollicis brevis	Posterior surface of lower middle radius	Base of proximal phalanx of thumb on dorsal surface	Extension of the thumb at the metacarpophalangeal joint	Sagittal	Just lateral to the extensor pollicis longus tendon on the dorsal side of the hand to its insertion on the proximal phalanx	Radial nerve (C6, C7)
				Weak wrist extension			
Posterior muscles	Abductor pollicis longus	Posterior aspect of radius and midshaft of the ulna	Base of 1st metacarpal on dorsal surface	Abduction of the thumb at the carpometacarpal joint	Frontal	Lateral aspect of the wrist joint just proximal to the 1st metacarpal	Radial nerve (C6, C7)
				Abduction of the wrist			

The intrinsic muscles of the hand (see Table 7.2 and Fig. 7.26) have their origins and insertions on the bones of the hand. Grouping of the intrinsic muscles into three groups according to location is helpful in understanding and learning these muscles. On the radial side there are four muscles of the thumb—the opponens pollicis, the abductor pollicis brevis, the flexor pollicis brevis, and the adductor pollicis. On the ulnar side, there are three muscles of the little finger—the opponens digiti minimi, the abductor digiti minimi, and the flexor digiti minimi brevis. In the remainder of the hand, there are 11 muscles, which can be further grouped as the four lumbricals, the three palmar interossei, and the four dorsal interossei.

Wrist and hand muscles—location
Anteromedial at the elbow and forearm and anterior at the hand (7.9 A–C)
Primarily wrist flexion
    Flexor carpi radialis
    Flexor carpi ulnaris
    Palmaris longus
Primarily wrist and phalangeal flexion
    Flexor digitorum superficialis
    Flexor digitorum profundus
    Flexor pollicis longus

Posterolateral at the elbow and forearm and posterior at the hand (7.9 D)
Primarily wrist extension
    Extensor carpi radialis longus
    Extensor carpi radialis brevis
    Extensor carpi ulnaris
Primarily wrist and phalangeal extension
    Extensor digitorum
    Extensor indicis
    Extensor digiti minimi
    Extensor pollicis longus
    Extensor pollicis brevis
    Abductor pollicis longus

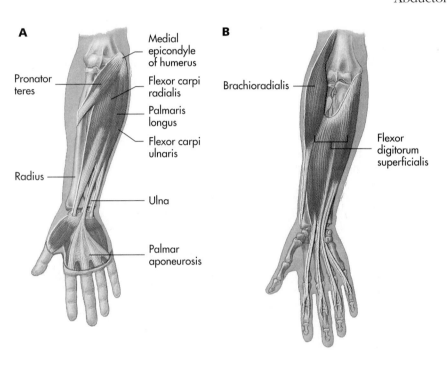

A

Pronator teres

Radius

Medial epicondyle of humerus

Flexor carpi radialis

Palmaris longus

Flexor carpi ulnaris

Ulna

Palmar aponeurosis

B

Brachioradialis

Flexor digitorum superficialis

FIG. 7.9 ● Muscles of the forearm. **A,** Anterior view of the right forearm (superficial). Brachioradialis muscle is removed; **B,** Anterior view of the right forearm (deeper than **A**). Pronator teres, flexor carpi radialis and ulnaris, and palmaris longus muscles are removed; **C,** Anterior view of the right forearm (deeper than **A** or **B**). Brachioradialis, pronator teres, flexor carpi radialis and ulnaris, palmaris longus, and flexor digitorum superficialis muscles are removed; **D,** Deep muscles of the right posterior forearm, Extensor digitorum, extensor digiti minimi, and extensor carpi ulnaris muscles are cut to reveal deeper muscles.

Chapter
7

C

Lateral epicondyle of humerus

Radius

Supinator

Flexor pollicis longus

Pronator quadratus

Medial epicondyle of humerus

Ulna

Flexor digitorum profundus

Lumbricales

D

Medial epicondyle of humerus

Anconeus

Extensor digiti minimi (cut)

Extensor carpi ulnaris (cut)

Extensor indicis

Cut tendons of extensor digitorum

Extensor digitorum (cut and reflected)

Supinator (deep)

Extensor carpi radialis longus

Extensor carpi radialis brevis

Abductor pollicis longus

Extensor pollicis longus

Extensor pollicis brevis

Nerves

The muscles of the wrist and hand are all innervated from the radial, median, and ulnar nerves of the brachial plexus as illustrated in Figs. 6.11, 6.12, and 7.10. The radial nerve, originating from C6, C7, and C8, provides innervation for the extensor carpi radialis brevis and extensor carpi radialis longus. It then branches to become the posterior interosseous nerve which supplies the extensor carpi ulnaris, extensor digitorum, extensor digiti minimi, abductor pollicis longus, extensor pollicis longus, extensor pollicis brevis, and extensor indicis. The median nerve, arising from C6, C7, C8, and T1, innervates the flexor carpi radialis, palmaris longus, flexor digitorum superficialis. It then branches to become the anterior interosseous nerve, which innervates the flexor digitorum profundus for the index and long finger as well as the flexor pollicis longus. Regarding the intrinsic muscles of the hand, the median nerve innervates the abductor pollicis brevis, flexor pollicis brevis (superficial head), opponens pollicis, and the first and second lumbrical. The ulnar nerve, branching from C8 and T1, supplies the flexor digitorum profundus for the fourth and fifth fingers and the flexor carpi ulnaris. Additionally, it innervates the remaining intrinsic muscles of the hand (the deep head of the flexor pollicis brevis, adductor pollicis, palmar interossei, dorsal interossei, third and fourth lumbrical, opponens digiti minimi, abductor digiti minimi, and flexor digiti minimi brevis). Sensation to the ulnar side of the hand, ulnar one-half of the ring finger and the entire little finger are provided by the ulnar nerve.

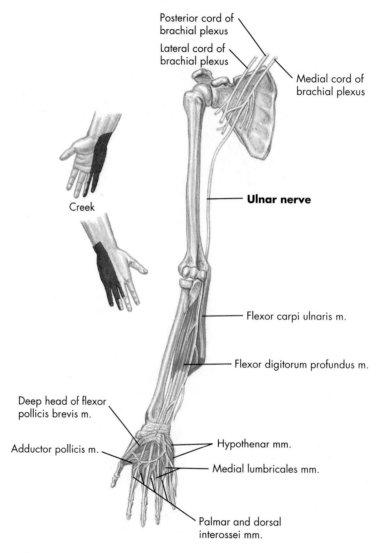

Posterior cord of brachial plexus

Lateral cord of brachial plexus

Medial cord of brachial plexus

Ulnar nerve

Creek

Flexor carpi ulnaris m.

Flexor digitorum profundus m.

Deep head of flexor pollicis brevis m.

Adductor pollicis m.

Hypothenar mm.

Medial lumbricales mm.

Palmar and dorsal interossei mm.

FIG. 7.10 ● Muscular and cutaneous distribution of the ulnar nerve.

Flexor carpi radialis muscle   FIG. 7.11

(fleks´or kar´pi ra´di-a´lis)

Origin

Medial epicondyle of the humerus

Insertion

Base of the second and third metacarpals, anterior (palmar surface)

Action

Flexion of the wrist
Abduction of the wrist
Weak flexion of the elbow

Palpation

Anterior surface of the wrist, slightly lateral, in line with the second and third metacarpals

Innervation

Median nerve (C6, C7)

Application, strengthening, and flexibility

The flexor carpi radialis, flexor carpi ulnaris, and palmaris longus are the most powerful of the wrist flexors. They are brought into play during any activity that requires wrist curling or stabilization of the wrist against resistance, particularly if the forearm is supinated.

The flexor carpi radialis may be developed by performing wrist curls against a handheld resistance. This may be accomplished when the supinated forearm is supported by a table, with the hand and wrist hanging over the edge to allow full range of motion. The extended wrist is then flexed or curled up to strengthen this muscle.

To stretch the flexor carpi radialis, the elbow must be fully extended with the forearm supinated while a partner passively extends and adducts the wrist.

Flexor carpi radialis m.

Flexion

Abduction

O, Medial epicondyle of the humerus

I, Base of second and third metacarpal, anterior (palmar surface)

FIG. 7.11 ● Flexor carpi radialis muscle, anterior view. *O*, Origin; *I*, insertion.

Palmaris longus muscle   FIG. 7.12

(pal-ma´ris long´gus)

Origin

Medial epicondyle of the humerus

Insertion

Palmar aponeurosis of the second, third, fourth, and fifth metacarpals

Action

Flexion of the wrist
Weak flexion of the elbow

Palpation

Anteromedial and central aspect of the anterior forearm just proximal to the wrist, particularly with slight wrist flexion and opposition of thumb to the 5th finger

Innervation

Median nerve (C6, C7)

Application, strengthening, and flexibility

Unlike the flexor carpi radialis and flexor carpi ulnaris, which are not only wrist flexors but also abductors and adductors, respectively, the palmaris longus is involved only in wrist flexion because of its central location on the anterior forearm and wrist. It may also be strengthened with any type of wrist-curling activity, such as the ones described for the flexor carpi radialis muscle.

Maximal elbow and wrist extension stretches the palmaris longus.

FIG. 7.12 ● Palmaris longus muscle, anterior view. *O*, Origin; *I*, insertion.

Flexor carpi ulnaris muscle   FIG. 7.13

(fleks´or kar´pi ul-na´ris)

Origin

Medial epicondyle of the humerus
Posterior aspect of the proximal ulna

Insertion

Pisiform, hamate, and base of the fifth metacarpal
  (palmar surface)

Action

Flexion of the wrist
Adduction of the wrist, together with the extensor
  carpi ulnaris muscle
Weak flexion of the elbow

Palpation

Anteromedial surface of the forearm, a few inches
  below the medial epicondyle of the humerus to
  just proximal to the wrist, with resisted flexion/
  adduction

Innervation

Ulnar nerve (C8, T1)

Application, strengthening, and flexibility

The flexor carpi ulnaris is very important in wrist
flexion or curling activities. In addition, it is one
of only two muscles involved in wrist adduction
or ulnar flexion. It may be strengthened with any
type of wrist-curling activity against resistance,
such as those described for the flexor carpi radialis muscle.

To stretch the flexor carpi ulnaris, the elbow
must be fully extended with the forearm supinated
while a partner passively extends and abducts the
wrist.

FIG. 7.13 ● Flexor carpi ulnaris muscle, anterior view. *O*, Origin; *I*, insertion.

Extensor carpi ulnaris muscle   FIG. 7.14

(eks-ten´sor kar´pi ul-na´ris)

Origin

Lateral epicondyle of the humerus
Middle two-fourths of the posterior border of
the ulna

Insertion

Base of the fifth metacarpal (dorsal surface)

Action

Extension of the wrist
Adduction of the wrist together with the flexor
carpi ulnaris muscle
Weak extension of the elbow

Palpation

Just lateral to the ulnar styloid process and crossing
the posteromedial wrist, particularly with wrist
extension/adduction

Innervation

Radial nerve (C6–C8)

Application, strengthening, and flexibility

Besides being a powerful wrist extensor, the extensor carpi ulnaris muscle is the only muscle other than the flexor carpi ulnaris involved in wrist adduction or ulnar deviation. The extensor carpi ulnaris, the extensor carpi radialis brevis, and the extensor carpi radialis longus are the most powerful of the wrist extensors. Any activity requiring wrist extension or stabilization of the wrist against resistance, particularly if the forearm is pronated, depends greatly on the strength of these muscles. They are often brought into play with the backhand in racquet sports.

The extensor carpi ulnaris may be developed by performing wrist extension against a handheld resistance. This may be accomplished with the pronated forearm being supported by a table with the hand hanging over the edge to allow full range of motion. The wrist is then moved from the fully flexed position to the fully extended position against the resistance.

Stretching the extensor carpi ulnaris requires the elbow to be extended with the forearm pronated while the wrist is passively flexed and slightly abducted.

FIG. 7.14 ● Extensor carpi ulnaris muscle, posterior view. *O*, Origin; *I*, insertion.

O, Lateral epicondyle
of humerus

Extensor
carpi
ulnaris m.

O, Middle two-fourths
of the posterior
border of the ulna

Extension

Adduction

I, Base of fifth
metacarpal
(dorsal surface)

Extensor carpi radialis brevis muscle   FIG. 7.15

(eks-ten´sor kar´pi ra´di-a´lis bre´vis)

Origin

Lateral epicondyle of the humerus

Insertion

Base of the third metacarpal (dorsal surface)

Action

Extension of the wrist
Abduction of the wrist
Weak extension of the elbow

Palpation

Dorsal side of the forearm, which is difficult to
  palpate

Just proximal to the dorsal aspect of the wrist and
  approximately 1 cm medial to the radial styloid
  process, the tendon may be felt during extension
  and traced to base of 3rd metacarpal. Proximally,
  just medial to the bulk of the brachioradialis

Innervation

Radial nerve (C6, C7)

Application, strengthening, and flexibility

The extensor carpi radialis brevis is important in
any sports activity that requires powerful wrist extension, such as golf or tennis. Wrist extension
exercises, such as those described for the extensor carpi ulnaris, are appropriate for development
of the muscle.

Stretching the extensor carpi radialis brevis and
longus requires the elbow to be extended with
the forearm pronated while the wrist is passively
flexed and slightly adducted.

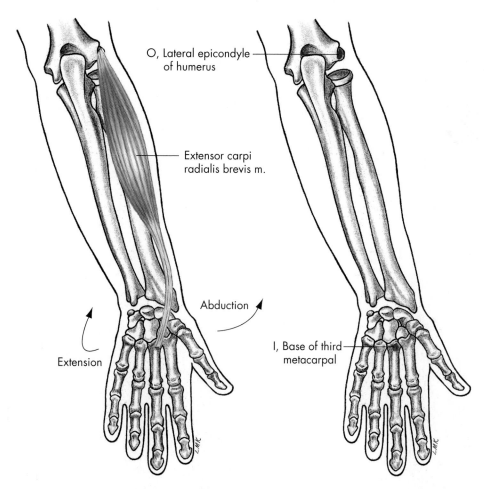

FIG. 7.15 ● Extensor carpi radialis brevis muscle, posterior view. *O,* Origin; *I,* insertion.

Extensor carpi radialis longus muscle   FIG. 7.16

(eks-ten´sor kar´pi ra´di-a´lis long´gus)

Origin

Lower third of lateral supracondylar ridge of
humerus and lateral epicondyle of the humerus

Insertion

Base of the second metacarpal (dorsal surface)

Action

Extension of the wrist
Abduction of the wrist
Weak extension of the elbow

Palpation

Just proximal to the dorsal aspect of the wrist and
approximately 1 cm medial to the radial styloid
process, the tendon may be felt during extension
and traced to base of 2nd metacarpal. Proximally,
just medial to the bulk of the brachioradialis

Innervation

Radial nerve (C6, C7)

Application, strengthening, and flexibility

The extensor carpi radialis longus, like the extensor carpi radialis brevis, is also important in any
sports activity that requires powerful wrist extension. In addition, both muscles are involved in
abduction of the wrist. The extensor carpi radialis
longus may be developed with the same wrist extension exercises as described for the extensor
carpi ulnaris muscle.

The extensor carpi radialis longus is stretched
in the same manner as the extensor carpi radialis
brevis.

Chapter 7

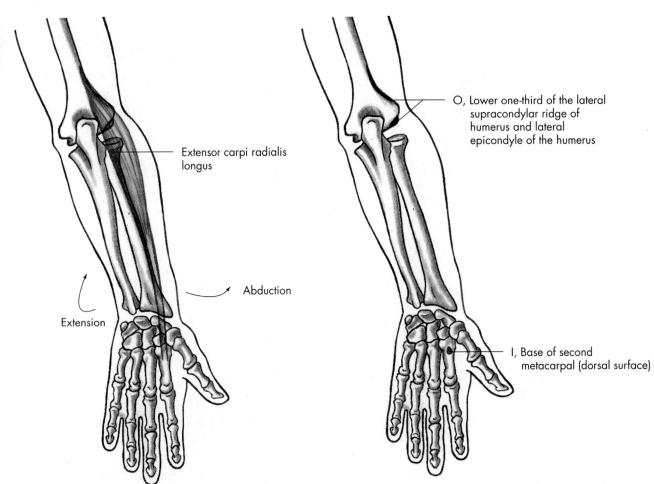

Extensor carpi radialis longus

Abduction

Extension

O, Lower one-third of the lateral
supracondylar ridge of
humerus and lateral
epicondyle of the humerus

I, Base of second
metacarpal (dorsal surface)

FIG. 7.16 ● Extensor carpi radialis longus muscle, posterior view. *O*, Origin; *I*, insertion.

Flexor digitorum superficialis muscle FIG. 7.17

(fleks´or dij-i-to´rum su´per-fish-e-al´is)

Origin

Medial epicondyle of the humerus
Ulnar head: medial coronoid process
Radial head: upper two-thirds of anterior border
  of radius

Insertion

Each tendon splits and attaches to the sides of the
  middle phalanx of four fingers (palmar surface)

Action

Flexion of the fingers at the metacarpophalangeal
  and proximal interphalangeal joints
Flexion of the wrist
Weak flexion of the elbow

FIG. 7.17 ● Flexor digitorum superficialis
muscle, anterior view. *O,* Origin; *I,* insertion.

Palpation

In depressed area between palmaris longus and
  flexor carpi ulnaris tendons, particularly with
  flexion of 3rd and 4th phalanges

Innervation

Median nerve (C7, C8, and T1)

Application, strengthening, and flexibility

The flexor digitorum superficialis muscle, also
known as the flexor digitorum sublimis, divides
into four tendons on the palmar aspect of the wrist
and hand to insert on each of the four fingers. The
flexor digitorum superficialis and the flexor digitorum profundus are the only muscles involved in
flexion of all four fingers. Both of these muscles
are vital in any type of gripping activity.

Squeezing a sponge rubber ball in the palm of
the hand, along with other gripping and squeezing
activities, can be used to develop these muscles.

The flexor digitorum superficialis is stretched by
passively extending the elbow, wrist, metacarpophalangeal, and proximal interphalangeal joints
while maintaining the forearm in full supination.

Flexor digitorum
superficialis

Flexion of wrist

Flexion of fingers

O, Medial epicondyle
of the humerus.
Ulnar head:
medial coronoid
process. Radial
head: upper
two-thirds of
anterior
border of
radius

I, Split tendons attach to sides
  of middle phalanx of four
  fingers (palmar surface)

Flexor digitorum profundus muscle   FIG. 7.18

(fleks´or dij-i-to´rum pro-fun´dus)

Origin

Proximal three-fourths of the anterior and medial ulna

Insertion

Base of the distal phalanxes of the four fingers

Action

Flexion of the four fingers at the metacarpophalangeal, proximal interphalangeal, and distal interphalangeal joints
Flexion of the wrist

Palpation

Over the palmar surface of the 2nd, 3rd, 4th, and 5th metacarpophalangeal joint during finger flexion against resistance

Innervation

Median nerve (C8, T1) to the second and third fingers
Ulnar nerve (C8, T1) to the fourth and fifth fingers

Application, strengthening, and flexibility

Both the flexor digitorum profundus muscle and the flexor digitorum superficialis muscle assist in wrist flexion because of their palmar relationship to the wrist. The flexor digitorum profundus is used in any type of gripping, squeezing, or hand-clenching activity, such as gripping a racket or climbing a rope.

The flexor digitorum profundus muscle may be developed through these activities, in addition to the strengthening exercises described for the flexor digitorum superficialis muscle.

The flexor digitorum profundus is stretched similarly to the flexor digitorum superficialis, except that the distal interphalangeal joints must be passively extended in addition to the elbow, wrist, metacarpophalangeal, and proximal interphalangeal joints while maintaining the forearm in full supination.

FIG. 7.18 ● Flexor digitorum profundus muscle, anterior view. *O,* Origin; *I,* insertion.

Flexor pollicis longus muscle   FIG. 7.19

(fleks´or pol´i-sis long´gus)

Origin

Middle anterior surface of the radius and the anterior medial border of the ulna just distal to the coronoid process

Insertion

Base of the distal phalanx of the thumb (palmar surface)

Action

Flexion of the thumb carpometacarpal, metacarpophalangeal, and interphalangeal joints
Flexion of the wrist

Palpation

Anterior surface of the thumb, particularly on the proximal phalanx during thumb flexion

Innervation

Median nerve, palmar interosseous branch (C8, T1)

Application, strengthening, and flexibility

The primary function of the flexor pollicis longus muscle is flexion of the thumb, which is vital in gripping and grasping activities of the hand. Because of its palmar relationship to the wrist, it provides some assistance in wrist flexion.

It may be strengthened by pressing a sponge rubber ball into the hand with the thumb and by many other gripping or squeezing activities.

The flexor pollicis longus is stretched by passively extending the entire thumb while simultaneously maintaining maximal wrist extension.

Chapter

7

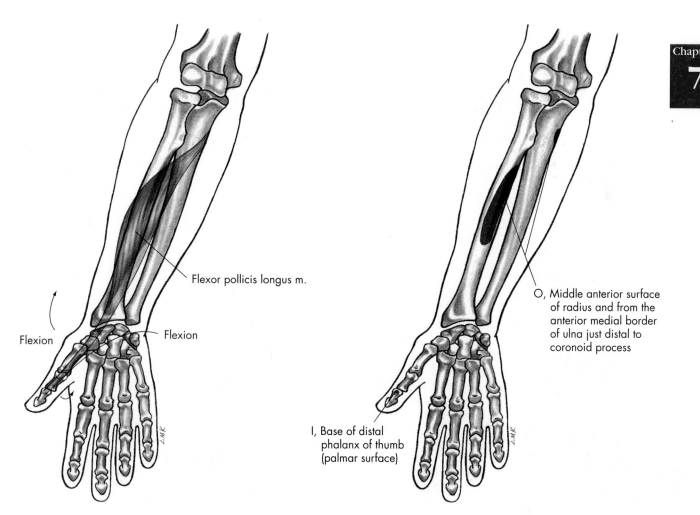

Flexor pollicis longus m.

Flexion

Flexion

O, Middle anterior surface of radius and from the anterior medial border of ulna just distal to coronoid process

I, Base of distal phalanx of thumb (palmar surface)

FIG. 7.19 ● Flexor pollicis longus muscle, anterior view. *O*, Origin; *I*, insertion.

Extensor digitorum muscle · FIG. 7.20

(eks-ten´sor dij-i-to´rum)

Origin

Lateral epicondyle of the humerus

Insertion

Four tendons to bases of middle and distal
  phalanges of four fingers (dorsal surface)

Action

Extension of the second, third, fourth, and fifth
  phalanges at the metacarpophalangeal joints
Extension of the wrist
Weak extension of the elbow

Palpation

With all four fingers extended, on the anterior
  surface of the distal forearm immediately medial to
  extensor pollicis longus tendon, then dividing into
  four separate tendons that are over the dorsal
  aspect of the hand and metacarpophalangeal joints

Innervation

Radial nerve (C6–C8)

Application, strengthening, and flexibility

The extensor digitorum, also known as the extensor digitorum communis, is the only muscle involved in extension of all four fingers. This muscle divides into four tendons on the dorsum of the wrist to insert on each of the fingers. It also assists with wrist extension movements. It may be developed by applying manual resistance to the dorsal aspect of the flexed fingers and then extending the fingers fully. When performed with the wrist in flexion, this exercise increases the workload on the extensor digitorum.

To stretch the extensor digitorum, the fingers must be maximally flexed at the metacarpophalangeal, proximal interphalangeal, and distal interphalangeal joints while the wrist is fully flexed.

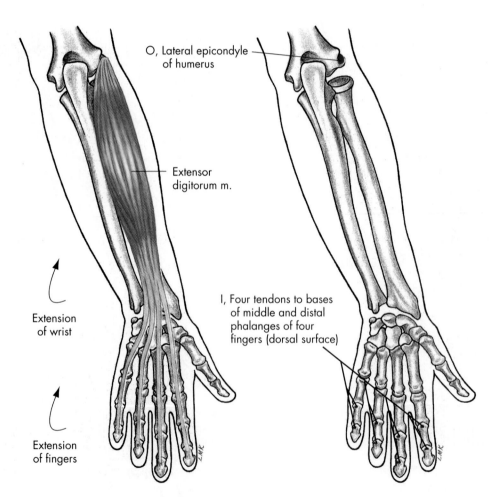

FIG. 7.20 ● Extensor digitorum muscle, posterior view. *O,* Origin; *I,* insertion.

Extensor indicis muscle   FIG. 7.21
(eks-ten´sor in´di-sis)

Origin
Middle to distal one-third of the posterior ulna

Insertion
Base of the middle and distal phalanxes of second phalange (dorsal surface)

Action
Extension of the index finger at the metacarpophalangeal joint

Weak wrist extension

Palpation
Posterior aspect of the distal forearm and dorsal surface of the hand just medial to the extensor digitorum tendon of the index finger

Innervation
Radial nerve (C6–C8)

Application, strengthening, and flexibility

The extensor indicis muscle is the pointing muscle. That is, it is responsible for extending the index finger, particularly when the other fingers are flexed. It also provides weak assistance to wrist extension and may be developed through exercises similar to those described for the extensor digitorum.

The extensor indicis is stretched by passively taking the index finger into maximal flexion at its metacarpophalangeal, proximal interphalangeal, and distal interphalangeal joints while fully flexing the wrist.

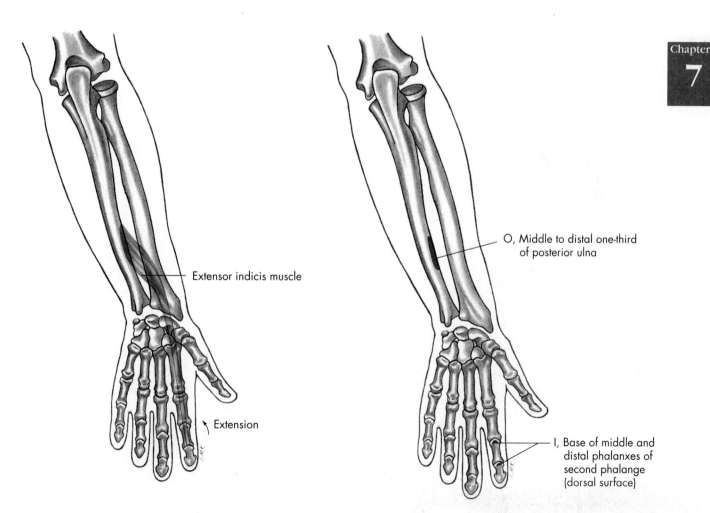

Extensor indicis muscle

Extension

O, Middle to distal one-third of posterior ulna

I, Base of middle and distal phalanxes of second phalange (dorsal surface)

FIG. 7.21 ● Extensor indicis muscle, posterior view. *O*, Origin; *I*, insertion.

Extensor digiti minimi muscle   FIG. 7.22
(eks-ten´sor dij´i-ti min´im-i)

Origin
Lateral epicondyle of the humerus

Insertion
Base of the middle and distal phalanxes of the fifth phalange (dorsal surface)

Action
Extension of the little finger at the metacarpophalangeal joint

Weak wrist extension

Palpation
Passing over the dorsal aspect of the distal radio-ulnar joint, particularly with relaxed flexion

of other fingers and alternating 5th finger extension and relaxation

Innervation
Radial nerve (C6–C8)

Application, strengthening, and flexibility

The primary function of the extensor digiti minimi muscle is to assist the extensor digitorum in extending the little finger. Because of its dorsal relationship to the wrist, it also provides weak assistance in wrist extension. It is strengthened with the same exercises described for the extensor digitorum.

The extensor digiti minimi is stretched by passively taking the little finger into maximal flexion at its metacarpophalangeal, proximal interphalangeal, and distal interphalangeal joints while fully flexing the wrist.

Extensor digiti minimi m.

Extension

O, Lateral epicondyle of humerus

I, Base of middle and distal phalanxes of fifth phalange (dorsal surface)

FIG. 7.22 ● Extensor digiti minimi muscle, posterior view. *O*, Origin; *I*, insertion.

Extensor pollicis longus muscle   FIG. 7.23

(eks-ten´sor pol´i-sis long´gus)

Origin

Posterior lateral surface of the lower middle ulna

Insertion

Base of the distal phalanx of the thumb (dorsal surface)

Action

Extension of the wrist
Extension of the thumb

Palpation

Dorsal aspect of the hand to its insertion on the base of the distal phalanx

Innervation

Radial nerve (C6–C8)

Application, strengthening, and flexibility

The primary function of the extensor pollicis longus muscle is extension of the thumb, although it does provide weak assistance in wrist extension.

It may be strengthened by extending the flexed thumb against manual resistance. It is stretched by passively taking the entire thumb into maximal flexion at its carpometacarpal, metacarpophalangeal, and interphalangeal joints while fully flexing the wrist.

The tendons of the extensor pollicis longus and extensor pollicis brevis, along with the tendon of the abductor pollicis brevis, forms the anatomical snuffbox, which is the small depression that develops between these two tendons when they contract. The name "anatomical snuffbox" originates from tobacco users placing their snuff in this depression.

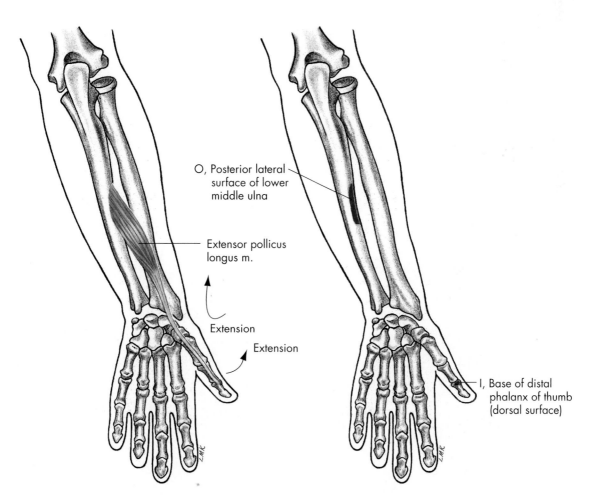

O, Posterior lateral surface of lower middle ulna

Extensor pollicus longus m.

Extension

Extension

I, Base of distal phalanx of thumb (dorsal surface)

FIG. 7.23 ● Extensor pollicis longus muscle, posterior view. *O*, Origin; *I*, insertion.

Extensor pollicis brevis muscle   FIG. 7.24

(eks-ten´sor pol´i-sis bre´vis)

Origin

Posterior surface of the lower middle radius

Insertion

Base of the proximal phalanx of the thumb (dorsal surface)

Action

Extension of the thumb at the metacarpophalangeal joint

Weak wrist extension

Palpation

Extensor pollicis brevis

Just lateral to the extensor pollicis longus tendon on the dorsal side of the hand to its insertion on the proximal phalanx

Innervation

Radial nerve (C6, C7)

Application, strengthening, and flexibility

The extensor pollicis brevis assists the extensor pollicis longus in extending the thumb. Because of its dorsal relationship to the wrist, it, too, provides weak assistance in wrist extension.

It may be strengthened through the same exercises described for the extensor pollicis longus muscle. It is stretched by passively taking the first carpometacarpal joint and the metacarpophalangeal joint of the thumb into maximal flexion while fully flexing the wrist.

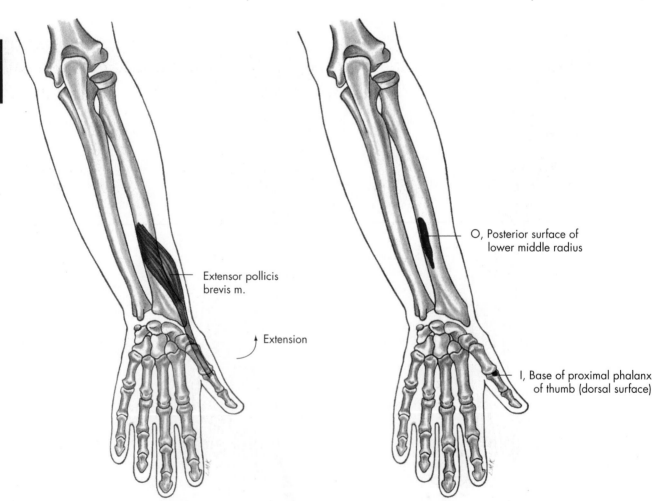

Extensor pollicis brevis m.

↑ Extension

O, Posterior surface of lower middle radius

I, Base of proximal phalanx of thumb (dorsal surface)

FIG. 7.24 ● Extensor pollicis brevis muscle, posterior view. *O,* Origin; *I,* insertion.

Abductor pollicis longus muscle   FIG. 7.25

(ab-duk´tor pol´i-sis lon´gus)

Origin

Posterior aspect of the radius and midshaft of the ulna

Insertion

Base of the first metacarpal (dorsal surface)

Action

Abduction of the thumb at the carpometacarpal joint

Abduction of the wrist

Palpation

Lateral aspect of the wrist joint just proximal to the first metacarpal

Innervation

Radial nerve (C6, C7)

Application, strengthening, and flexibility

The primary function of the abductor pollicis longus muscle is abduction of the thumb, although it does provide some assistance in abduction of the wrist. It may be developed by abducting the thumb from the adducted position against a manually applied resistance. Stretching of the abductor pollicis longus is accomplished by fully flexing and adducting the entire thumb across the palm with the wrist fully adducted.

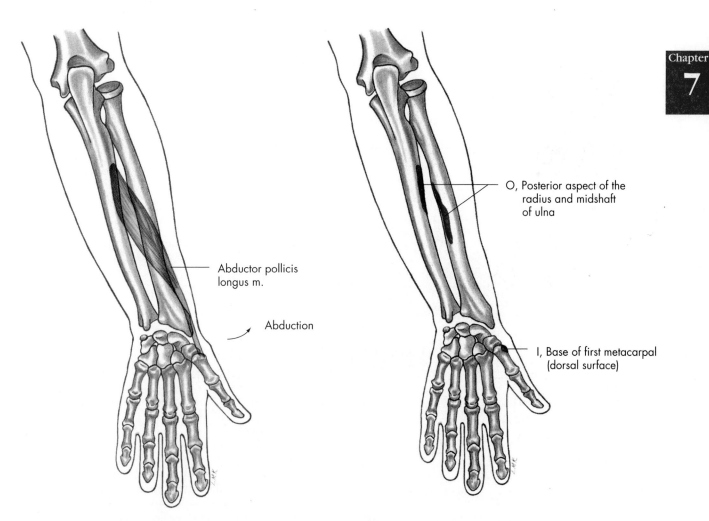

Abductor pollicis longus m.

Abduction

O, Posterior aspect of the radius and midshaft of ulna

I, Base of first metacarpal (dorsal surface)

FIG. 7.25 ● Abductor pollicis longus muscle, posterior view. *O*, Origin; *I*, insertion.

Intrinsic muscles of the hand

The intrinsic hand muscles may be grouped according to location as well as according to the parts of the hand they control (Fig. 7.26). The abductor pollicis brevis, opponens pollicis, flexor pollicis brevis, and adductor pollicis make up the thenar eminence—the muscular pad on the palmar surface of the first metacarpal. The hypothenar eminence is the muscular pad that forms the ulnar border on the palmar surface of the hand and is made up of the abductor digiti minimi, flexor digiti minimi brevis, and opponens digiti minimi. The intermediate muscles of the hand consist of three palmar interossei, four dorsal interossei, and four lumbrical muscles.

Four intrinsic muscles act on the carpometacarpal joint of the thumb. The opponens pollicis is the muscle that causes opposition in the thumb metacarpal. The abductor pollicis brevis abducts the thumb metacarpal and is assisted in this action by the flexor pollicis brevis, which also flexes the thumb metacarpal. The metacarpal of the thumb is adducted by the adductor pollicis. Both the flexor pollicis brevis and the adductor pollicis flex the proximal phalanx of the thumb.

The three palmar interossei are adductors of the second, fourth, and fifth phalanges. The four dorsal interossei both flex and abduct the index, middle, and ring proximal phalanxes, in addition to assisting with extension of the middle and distal phalanxes of these fingers. The third dorsal interossei also adducts the middle finger. The four lumbricals flex the index, middle, ring, and little proximal phalanxes and extend the middle and distal phalanxes of these fingers.

Three muscles act on the little finger. The opponens digiti minimi causes opposition of the little finger metacarpal. The abductor digiti minimi abducts the little finger metacarpal, and the flexor digiti minimi brevis flexes this metacarpal.

Refer to Table 7.2 for further details regarding the intrinsic muscles of the hand.

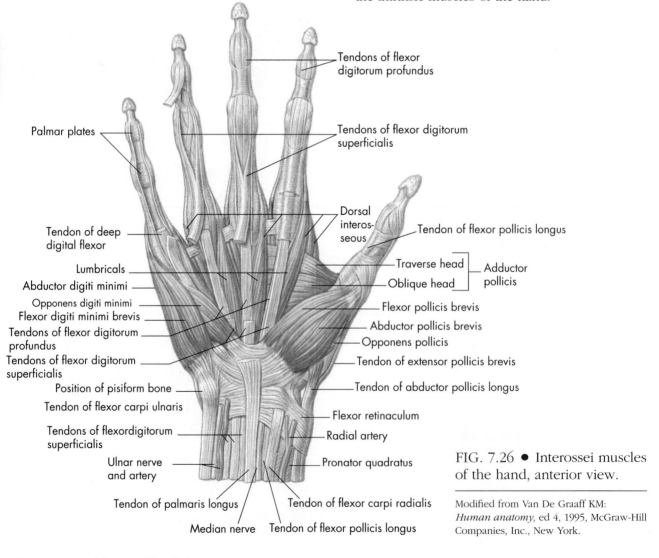

FIG. 7.26 ● Interossei muscles of the hand, anterior view.

Modified from Van De Graaff KM: *Human anatomy,* ed 4, 1995, McGraw-Hill Companies, Inc., New York.

TABLE 7.2 • Intrinsic muscles of the hand

	Muscle	Origin	Insertion	Action	Palpation	Innervation
Thenar muscles	Opponens pollicis	Anterior surface of transverse carpal ligament, trapezium	Lateral border of 1st metacarpal	CMC opposition of thumb	Palmar aspect of 1st metacarpal with opposition of fingertips to thumb	Median nerve (C6, C7)
	Abductor pollicis brevis	Anterior surface of transverse carpal ligament, trapezium, scaphoid	Base of 1st proximal phalanx	CMC abduction of thumb	Radial aspect of palmar surface of 1st metacarpal with 1st CMC abduction	Median nerve (C6, C7)
	Flexor pollicis brevis	Superficial head: trapezium and transverse carpal ligament Deep head: ulnar aspect of 1st metacarpal	Base of proximal phalanx of 1st metacarpal	CMC flexion and abduction; MCP flexion of thumb	Medial aspect of thenar eminence just proximal to 1st MCP joint with 1st MCP flexion against resistance	Superficial head: median nerve (C6, C7) Deep head: ulnar nerve (C8, T1)
Intermediate muscles	Adductor pollicis	Transverse head: anterior shaft of 3rd metacarpal Oblique head: base of 2nd and 3rd metacarpals, capitate, trapezoid	Ulnar aspect of base of proximal phalanx of 1st metacarpal	CMC adduction; MCP flexion of thumb	Palmar surface between 1st and 2nd metacarpal with 1st CMC adduction	Ulnar nerve (C8, T1)
	Palmar interossei	Shaft of 2nd, 4th, and 5th metacarpals and extensor expansions	Bases of 2nd, 4th, and 5th proximal phalanxes and extensor expansions	MCP adduction of 2nd, 4th, and 5th phalanges	Cannot be palpated	Ulnar nerve (C8, T1)
	Dorsal interossei	Two heads on shafts on adjacent metacarpals	Bases of 2nd, 3rd, and 4th proximal phalanxes and extensor expansions	MCP flexion and abduction; PIP/DIP extension of 2nd, 3rd, and 4th phalanges; MCP adduction of 3rd phalange	Dorsal surface between 1st and 2nd metacarpals, between shafts of 2nd through 5th metacarpals with active abduction/adduction of 2nd, 3rd, and 4th MCP joints	Ulnar nerve, palmar branch (C8, T1)
	Lumbricales	Flexor digitorum profundus tendon in center of palm	Extensor expansions on radial side of 2nd, 3rd, 4th, and 5th proximal phalanxes	MCP flexion and PIP/DIP extension of 2nd, 3rd, 4th, and 5th phalanges	Cannot be palpated	1st and 2nd: median nerve (C6, C7) 3rd and 4th: ulnar nerve (C8, T1)
Hypothenar muscles	Opponens digiti minimi	Hook of hamate and adjacent transverse carpal ligament	Medial border of 5th metacarpal	MCP opposition of 5th phalange	On radial aspect of hypothenar eminence with opposition of 5th phalange to thumb	Ulnar nerve (C8, T1)
	Abductor digiti minimi	Pisiform and flexor carpi ulnaris tendon	Ulnar aspect of base of 5th proximal phalanx	MCP abduction of 5th phalange	Ulnar aspect of hypothenar eminence with 5th MCP abduction	Ulnar nerve (C8, T1)
	Flexor digiti minimi brevis	Hook of hamate and adjacent transverse carpal ligament	Ulnar aspect of base of 5th proximal phalanx	MCP flexion of 5th phalange	Palmar surface of 5th metacarpal, lateral to opponens digiti minimi with 5th MCP flexion against resistance	Ulnar nerve (C8, T1)

Chapter

7

Web sites

Anatomy & Physiology Tutorials:

www.gwc.maricopa.edu/class/bio201/index.htm

Radiologic Anatomy Browser:

http://radlinux1.usuf1.usuhs.mil/rad/iong/index.html

This site has numerous radiological views of the musculoskeletal system.

University of Arkansas Medical School Gross Anatomy for Medical Students:

anatomy.uams.edu/htmlpages/anatomyhtml/gross.html

Dissections, anatomy tables, atlas images, links, etc.

Loyola University Medical Center: Structure of the Human Body:

www.meddean.luc.edu/lumen/MedEd/GrossAnatomy/GA.html

An excellent site with many slides, dissections, tutorials, etc., for the study of human anatomy.

Wheeless's Textbook of Orthopaedics:

www.ortho-u.net/

This site has an extensive index of links to the fractures, joints, muscles, nerves, trauma, medications, medical topics, and lab tests, as well as links to orthopedic journals and other orthopedic and medical news.

Arthroscopy.Com:

www.arthroscopy.com/sports.htm

Patient information on various musculoskeletal problems of the upper and lower extremity

Electronic Textbook of Hand Surgery:

www.e-hand.com/default.htm

Slides and illustrations of upper extremity musculoskeletal anatomy

Premiere Medical Search Engine:

www.medsite.com

This site allows the reader to enter any medical condition and it will search the net to find relevant articles.

Virtual Hospital:

www.vh.org

Numerous slides, patient information, etc.

Dynamic Human version 2.0 CD-ROM: The Visual Guide to Anatomy & Physiology:

www.mhhe.com/biosci/ap/dynamichuman2/

Web site that accompanies this CD-ROM

Worksheet exercises

As an aid to learning, for in-class or out-of-class assignments, or for testing, tear-out worksheets are found at the end of the text (pp. 330 and 331).

Skeletal worksheet (no. 1)

Draw and label on the worksheet the following muscles:
a. Flexor pollicis longus
b. Flexor carpi radialis
c. Flexor carpi ulnaris
d. Extensor digitorum
e. Extensor pollicis longus
f. Extensor carpi ulnaris

Human figure worksheet (no. 2)

Label and indicate with arrows the following movements of the wrist and hand:
a. Flexion
b. Extension
c. Abduction (ulnar flexion)
d. Adduction (radial flexion)

Laboratory and review exercises

1. Locate the following parts of the humerus, radius, ulna, carpals, and metacarpals on a human skeleton and on a subject:
   a. Skeleton
      1. Medial epicondyle
      2. Lateral epicondyle
      3. Trochlea
      4. Capitulum
      5. Coronoid process
      6. Tuberosity of the radius
      7. Styloid process—radius
      8. Styloid process—ulna
      9. First and third metacarpals
      10. Wrist bones
      11. First phalanx of third metacarpal
   b. Subject
      1. Medial epicondyle
      2. Lateral epicondyle
      3. Pisiform
      4. Scaphoid (navicular)
2. How and where can the following muscles be palpated on a human subject?
   a. Flexor pollicis longus
   b. Flexor carpi radialis
   c. Flexor carpi ulnaris
   d. Extensor digitorum communis
   e. Extensor pollicis longus
   f. Extensor carpi ulnaris

3. Demonstrate the action and list the muscles primarily responsible for these movements at the wrist joint:
   a. Flexion
   b. Extension
   c. Abduction
   d. Adduction
4. List the planes in which each of the following wrist, hand, and finger joint movements occur. List the respective axis of rotation for each movement in each plane.
   a. Abduction
   b. Adduction
   c. Flexion
   d. Extension
5. Discuss why the thumb is the most important part of the hand.
6. How should boys and girls be taught to do push-ups? Justify your answer.
   a. Hands flat on the floor
   b. Fingertips
7. With a laboratory partner, determine how and why maintaining full flexion of all the fingers is impossible when passively moving the wrist into maximal flexion. Is it also difficult to maintain maximal extension of all the finger joints while passively taking the wrist into full extension?
8. Fill in the muscle analysis chart below by listing the muscles primarily involved in each movement.

Muscle analysis chart • Wrist, hand, and fingers

Wrist and hand	
Flexion	Extension
Adduction	Abduction
Fingers—metacarpophalangeal joints	
Flexion	Extension
Fingers—proximal interphalangeal joints	
Flexion	Extension
Fingers—distal interphalangeal joints	
Flexion	Extension
Thumb	
Flexion	Extension

References

Gabbard CP, et al: Effects of grip and forearm position on flex arm hang performance, *Research Quarterly for Exercise and Sport,* July 1983.

Gench BE, Hinson MM, Harvey PT: *Anatomical kinesiology,* Dubuque, IA, 1995, Eddie Bowers.

Guarantors of Brain: *Aids to the examination of the peripheral nervous system,* ed 4, London, 2000, Saunders.

Herrick RT, Herrick S: Ruptured triceps in powerlifter presenting as cubital tunnel syndrome—a case report, *American Journal of Sports Medicine* 15:514, September–October 1987.

Hislop HJ, Montgomery J: *Daniels and Worthingham's muscle testing: techniques of manual examination,* ed 6, Philadelphia, 1995, Saunders.

Lindsay DT: *Functional human anatomy,* St. Louis, 1996, Mosby.

Luttgens K, Hamilton N: *Kinesiology: scientific basis of human motion,* ed 10, New York, 2002, McGraw-Hill.

Magee DJ: *Orthopedic physical assessment,* ed 4, Philadelphia, 2002, Saunders.

Norkin CC, Levangie PK: *Joint structure and function—a comprehensive analysis,* Philadelphia, 1983, Davis.

Norkin CC, White DJ: *Measurement of joint motion: a guide to goniometry,* Philadelphia, 1985, Davis.

Rasch PJ: *Kinesiology and applied anatomy,* ed 7, Philadelphia, 1989, Lea & Febiger.

Seeley RR, Stephens TD, Tate P: *Anatomy & physiology,* ed 6, Dubuque, IA, 2003, McGraw-Hill.

Sieg KW, Adams SP: *Illustrated essentials of musculoskeletal anatomy,* ed 2, Gainesville, FL, 1985, Megabooks.

Sisto DJ, et al: An electromyographic analysis of the elbow in pitching, *American Journal of Sports Medicine* 15:260, May–June 1987.

Smith LK, Weiss EL, Lehmkuhl LD: *Brunnstrom's clinical kinesiology,* ed 5, Philadelphia, 1996, Davis.

Springer SI: Racquetball and elbow injuries, *National Racquetball* 16:7, March 1987.

Stone RJ, Stone JA: *Atlas of the skeletal muscles,* 1990, McGraw-Hill Companies, Inc., New York.

Van De Graaff KM: *Human anatomy,* ed 6, Dubuque, IA, 2002, McGraw-Hill.

Muscular Analysis of Upper Extremity Exercises

Objectives

● To analyze the joint movements and muscles used in simple exercises

● To learn and understand the concept of open versus closed kinetic chain

● To learn to group individual muscles into units that produce certain joint movements

● To begin to think of exercises that increase the strength and endurance of individual muscle groups

---

Online Learning Center Resources

Visit *Manual of Structural Kinesiology's* Online Learning Center at **www.mhhe.com/floyd15e** for additional information and study material for this chapter, including:

- *Self-grading quizzes*
- *Anatomy flashcards*
- *Animations*

The upper extremity is often one of the body's weakest areas when considering the number of muscles involved. American boys and girls are extremely weak in the upper shoulder area. A majority are unable to do one traditional chin-up (pull-up), whereby the subject, grasping a horizontal bar with the palms toward the face and feet off the floor, pulls the body up until the chin is over the bar. As a result of this widespread weakness, the exercise had to be modified to secure more meaningful results. The modification involved the feet being on the floor and the body being pulled up to touch the bar.*

Strength and endurance in this part of the human body are essential for improved appearance and posture, as well as for more efficient skill performance. Specific exercises and activities to condition this area should be intelligently selected by becoming thoroughly familiar with the muscles involved.

At this stage, simple exercises are used to begin teaching individuals how to group muscles to produce joint movement. Some of these simple introductory exercises are included in this chapter.

The early analysis of exercise makes the study of structural kinesiology more meaningful as students come to better understand the importance of individual muscles and groups of muscles in bringing about joint movements in various exercises. Chapter 13 contains analysis of exercises for the entire body, with emphasis on the trunk and lower extremities. Contrary to what most beginning

---

*Pate R, et al: The national children and youth fitness study, II. The modified pull-up test, *Journal of Physical Education, Recreation and Dance* 58:71, 1987.

students in structural kinesiology believe, muscular analysis of activities is not difficult once the basic concepts are understood.

Concepts for analysis

In analyzing activities, it is important to understand that muscles are usually grouped according to their concentric function and work in paired opposition to an antagonistic group. An example of this *aggregate* muscle grouping to perform a given joint action is seen with the quadriceps all working to cause knee extension in opposition to the hamstrings, which all work together to cause knee flexion. An often confusing aspect is that, depending on the activity, these muscle groups can function to control the exact opposite actions by contracting eccentrically. That is, through eccentric contractions, the quadriceps may control knee flexion, and the hamstrings may control knee extension. Students should be able to view an activity and to not only determine which muscles are performing the movement, but also know what type of contraction is occurring and what kind of exercises are appropriate for developing the muscles. Chapter 2 provides a review of how muscles contract to work in groups to function in joint movement.

Analysis of movement

When analyzing various exercises and sport skills, it is essential to break down all of the movements into phases. The number of phases, usually three to five, will vary, depending on the skill. Practically all sport skills will have at least a preparatory phase, a movement phase, and a follow-through phase. Many will also begin with a stance phase and end with a recovery phase. The names of the phases will vary from skill to skill to fit in with the terminology used in various sports, and may also vary depending upon the body part involved. In some cases, these major phases may also be divided even further, as with baseball, where the preparatory phase for the pitching arm is broken into early cocking and late cocking.

The *stance phase* allows the athlete to assume a comfortable and balanced body position from which to initiate the sport skill. The emphasis is on setting the various joint angles in the correct positions with respect to one another and to the sport surface. Generally, with respect to the subsequent phases, the stance phase is a relatively static phase with fairly short ranges of motion involved.

The *preparatory phase,* often referred to as the cocking or wind-up phase, is used to lengthen the appropriate muscles so that they will be in position to generate more force and momentum as they concentrically contract in the next phase. It is the most critical phase in leading toward the desired result of the activity and becomes more dynamic as the need for explosiveness increases.

The *movement phase,* sometimes known as the acceleration, action, motion, or contact phase, is the action part of the skill. It is the phase in which the summation of force is generated directly to the ball, sport object, or opponent, and is usually characterized by near-maximal concentric activity in the involved muscles.

The *follow-through phase* begins immediately after the climax of the movement phase, in order to bring about negative acceleration of the involved limb or body segment. In this phase, often referred to as the deceleration phase, the velocity of the body segment progressively decreases, usually over a wide range of motion. This velocity decrease is usually attributable to high eccentric activity in the muscles that were antagonist to the muscles used in the movement phase. Generally, the greater the acceleration in the movement phase, the greater the length and the importance of the follow-though phase. Occasionally, some athletes may begin the follow-through too soon, thereby cutting short the movement phase and having a less-than-desirable result in the activity.

The *recovery phase* is used after follow-through to regain balance and positioning to be ready for the next sport demand. To a degree, the muscles used eccentrically in the follow-through phase to decelerate the body or body segment will be used concentrically in recovery to bring about the initial return to a functional position.

Skill analysis can be seen with the example of a baseball pitch in Fig. 8.1. The stance phase begins when the player assumes a position with the ball in the glove before receiving the signal from the catcher. The pitcher begins the preparatory phase by extending the throwing arm posteriorly and rotating the trunk to the right in conjunction with left hip flexion. The right shoulder girdle is fully retracted in combination with abduction and maximum external rotation of the glenohumeral joint to complete this phase. Immediately following, the movement phase begins with forward movement of the arm and continues until ball release. At ball release, the follow-through phase begins as the arm continues moving in the same direction established by the movement phase until

Stance

Preparatory

Movement

Follow-through

FIG. 8.1 ● Skill analysis phases—baseball pitch.

the velocity decreases to the point that the arm can safely change movement direction. This deceleration of the body, and especially the arm, is accomplished by high amounts of eccentric activity. At this point, the recovery phase begins, enabling the player to reposition to field the batted ball. In this example, reference has been made briefly only to the throwing arm, but there are many similarities in other overhand sports skills, such as the tennis serve, javelin throw, and volleyball serve. In actual practice, the movements of each joint in the body should be analyzed into the various phases.

Upper extremity activities

Children seem to have an innate desire to climb, swing, and hang. Such movements use the muscles of the hands, wrists, elbows, and shoulder joints. But the opportunity to perform these types of activities is limited in our modern culture. Unless emphasis is placed on the development of this area of our bodies by physical education

teachers in elementary schools, for both boys and girls, it will continue to be muscularly the weakest area of our bodies. Weakness in the upper extremities can impair skill development and performance in many common enjoyable recreational activities, such as golf, tennis, softball, and racquetball. Athletes enjoy what they can do well, and they can be taught to enjoy activities that will increase the strength of this part of the body. These and other such activities are ones that can be enjoyed throughout the entire adult life; therefore, adequate skill development built on an appropriate base of muscular strength and endurance is essential for enjoyment and prevention of injury.

Often, we perform typical strengthening exercises in the weight room, such as the bench press, overhead press, and biceps curl. While being good exercises, these all concentrate primarily on the muscles of the anterior upper extremity. This can lead to an overdevelopment of these muscles with respect to the posterior muscles. As a result, individuals may become strong and tight anteriorly and weak and flexible posteriorly. It is for these reasons that one must be able to analyze specific strengthening exercises and determine the muscles involved so that overall muscular balance is addressed through appropriate exercise prescription.

Chapter
8

The kinetic chain concept

As you have learned, our extremities consist of several bony segments linked by a series of joints. These bony segments and their linkage system of joints may be likened to a chain. Just as with a chain, any one link in the extremity may be moved individually without significantly affecting the other links if the chain is open or not attached at one end. However, if the chain is securely attached or closed, substantial movement of any one link cannot occur without substantial and subsequent movement of the other links.

In the body, an extremity may be seen as representing an *open kinetic chain* if the distal end of the extremity is not fixed to any surface. This arrangement allows any one joint in the extremity to move or function separately without necessitating movement of other joints in the extremity. Examples in the upper extremity would be a shoulder shrug, deltoid raise (shoulder abduction), or biceps curl. Lower extremity examples include seated hip flexion, knee extension, and ankle dorsiflexion exercises. In all of these examples, the core of the body and the proximal segment is stabilized while the distal segment is free to move in space through a single plane. These types of exercises are beneficial in isolating a particular joint to concentrate on specific muscle groups; however, they are not very functional in that most physical activity, particularly for the lower extremity, requires multiple-joint activity involving numerous muscle groups simultaneously.

If the distal end of the extremity is fixed, as in a push-up, dip, squat, or dead lift, the extremity represents a *closed kinetic chain*. In this closed system, movement of one joint cannot occur without causing predictable movements of the other joints in the extremity. Closed-chain activities are very functional and involve the body moving in relation to the relatively fixed distal segment. The advantage of these types of exercise are that multiple joints are involved and numerous muscle groups must participate in causing and controlling the multiple-plane movements, which strongly correlate to most physical activities.

Consideration of the open versus closed kinetic chain through analysis of skilled movements is helpful in determining appropriate conditioning exercises to improve performance. Generally, closed kinetic chain exercises are more functional and applicable to the demands of sports and physical activity. Most sports involve closed-chain activities in the lower extremities and open-chain activities in the upper extremities. However, there are many exceptions, and closed-chain conditioning exercises may be beneficial for extremities primarily involved in open-chain sporting activities. Open-chain exercises are useful in concentrating on the development of a specific muscle group at a single joint.

Analysis of upper body exercises

Presented over the next several pages are brief analyses of several common upper body exercises. Students are encouraged to follow and perhaps expand on the approach used to analyze other upper body activities. All muscles listed in the analysis are contracting concentrically unless specifically noted to be contracting eccentrically or isometrically.

Valsalva maneuver

Many people bear down by holding the breath without thinking when attempting to lift something heavy. This bearing down, known as the Valsalva maneuver, is accomplished by trying to exhale against a closed epiglottis (the flap of cartilage behind the tongue that shuts the air passage when swallowing) and is thought by many to enhance one's lifting ability. It is mentioned here to caution against its use due to the dramatic increase in blood pressure followed by an equally dramatic drop in blood pressure it causes. Using the Valsalva manever can cause lightheadedness and fainting and lead to complications in people with heart disease. Instead of using the Valsalva maneuver, one should always be sure to use rhythmic and consistent breathing. It is usually advisable to exhale during the lifting or contracting phase and inhale during the lowering or recovery phase.

Shoulder pull

Description

In a standing or sitting position, the subject interlocks the fingers in front of the chest and then attempts to pull them apart (Fig. 8.2). This contraction is maintained for 5 to 20 seconds.

FIG. 8.2 ● Shoulder pull.

Analysis

In this type of exercise, there is little or no movement of the contracting muscles. In certain isometric exercises, contraction of the antagonistic muscles is as strong as contraction of the muscles attempting to produce the force for movement. The muscle groups contracting to produce a movement are designated the *agonists*. In the exercise just described, the agonists in the right upper extremity are antagonistic to the agonists in the left upper extremity, and vice versa (Table 8.1). This exercise results in isometric contractions of the wrist and hand, elbow, shoulder joint, and shoulder girdle muscles. The strength of the contraction depends on the angle of pull and the leverage of the joint involved. Thus, it is not the same at each point.

Isometric exercises vary in the number of muscles contracting, depending on the type of exercise and the joints at which movement is attempted. The shoulder pull exercise produces some contraction of antagonistic muscles at four sets of joints.

TABLE 8.1 • Shoulder pull

Joint	This entire exercise is isometric in design, so that all contractions presented are isometric			
	Action	Agonists	Action	Agonists
Wrist and hand	Extension	Resisted by flexors of wrists and hand Agonists—wrist and hand extensors Antagonists—wrist and hand extensors	Flexion	Resisted by extensors of wrist and hand Agonists—wrist and hand flexors Antagonists—wrist and hand extensors
Elbow joint	Extension	Resisted by flexors of wrist, elbow, and hand Agonists—triceps brachii, anconeus Antagonists—biceps, brachii, brachialis, brachioradialis	Flexion	Resisted by extensors of wrist, elbow, and hand Agonists—biceps brachii, brachialis, brachioradialis Antagonists—triceps brachii, anconeus
Shoulder joint	Abduction	Resisted by adductors of shoulder joint Agonists—deltoid and supraspinatus Antagonists—teres major, latissimus dorsi, pectoralis major	Adduction	Resisted by abductors of shoulder joint Agonists—teres major, latissimus dorsi, pectoralis major Antagonists—deltoid and supraspinatus
Shoulder girdle	Adduction and depression	Resisted by abductors of shoulder girdle Agonists—rhomboid and trapezius Antagonists—serratus anterior, pectoralis major, trapezius (upper)	Abduction and elevation	Resisted by adductors of shoulder girdle Agonists—serratus anterior, pectoralis minor, trapezius (upper) Antagonists—rhomboid and trapezius

Arm curl

Description

With the subject in a standing position, the dumb-bell is held in the hands with the palms to the front. The dumbbell is lifted until the elbow is completely flexed (Fig. 8.3). Then it is returned to the starting position.

Analysis

This exercise is divided into two phases for analysis: (1) lifting phase to flexed position and (2) lowering phase to extended position (Table 8.2). NOTE: An assumption is made that no movement occurs in the shoulder joint and shoulder girdle.

A   **B**

FIG. 8.3 ● Arm curl. **A,** Beginning position in extension; **B,** flexed position.

TABLE 8.2 • **Arm curl**

Joint	Lifting phase to flexed position		Lowering phase to extended position	
	Action	Agonists	Action	Agonists
Wrist and hand	Flexion*	Wrist and hand flexors (isometric contraction) Flexor carpi radialis Flexor carpi ulnaris Palmaris longus Flexor digitorum profundus Flexor digitorum superficialis Flexor pollicis longus	Flexion*	Wrist and hand flexors (isometric contraction) Flexor carpi radialis Flexor carpi ulnaris Palmaris longus Flexor digitorum profundus Flexor digitorum superficialis Flexor pollicis longus
Elbow	Flexion	Elbow flexors Biceps brachii Brachialis Brachioradialis	Extension	Elbow flexors (eccentric contraction) Biceps brachii Brachialis Brachioradialis

***Note:** The wrist is in a position of slight extension to facilitate greater active finger flexion in gripping the dumbbell. (The flexors remain isometrically contracted throughout the entire exercise, to hold the dumbbell.)

Triceps extension

Description

The subject uses the opposite hand to assist in maintaining the arm in a shoulder-flexed position. The subject then, grasping the dumbbell and beginning in full elbow flexion, extends the elbow until the arm and forearm are straight. The shoulder joint and shoulder girdle are stabilized by the opposite hand. Consequently, no movement is assumed to occur in these areas (Fig. 8.4).

Analysis

This exercise is divided into two phases for analysis: (1) lifting phase to extended position and (2) lowering phase to flexed position (Table 8.3). NOTE: An assumption is made that no movement occurs in the shoulder joint and shoulder girdle.

A　　　　　　　　**B**

FIG. 8.4 ● Triceps extension. **A,** Beginning position in flexion; **B,** extended position.

TABLE 8.3 • Triceps extension

Joint	Lifting phase to extended position			Lowering phase to flexed position		
	Action		Agonists	Action		Agonists
Wrist and hand	Flexion*		Wrist and hand flexors (isometric contraction) Flexor carpi radialis Flexor carpi ulnaris Palmaris longus Flexor digitorum profundus Flexor digitorum superficialis Flexor pollicis longus	Flexion*		Wrist and hand flexors (isometric contraction) Flexor carpi radialis Flexor carpi ulnaris Palmaris longus Flexor digitorum profundus Flexor digitorum superficialis Flexor pollicis longus
Elbow	Extension		Elbow extensors Triceps brachii Anconeus	Flexion		Elbow extensors (eccentric contraction) Triceps brachii Anconeus

***Note:** The wrist is in a position of slight extension to facilitate greater active finger flexion in gripping the dumbbell. (The flexors remain isometrically contracted throughout the entire exercise, to hold the dumbbell.)

Barbell press

Description

This exercise is sometimes referred to as the *overhead* or *military press*. The barbell is held in a position high in front of the chest, with palms facing forward, feet comfortably spread, and back and legs straight (Fig. 8.5, *A*). From this position, the barbell is pushed upward until fully overhead, and then it is returned to the starting position (Fig. 8.5, *B*).

Analysis

This exercise is separated into two phases for analysis: (1) lifting phase to full overhead position and (2) lowering phase to starting position (Table 8.4).

A

B

FIG. 8.5 ● Barbell press. **A,** Starting position; **B,** full overhead position.

TABLE 8.4 • **Barbell press**

| Joint | Lifting phase to full overhead position | | Lowering phase to starting position | |
	Action	Agonists	Action	Agonists
Wrist and hand	Flexion*	Wrist and hand flexors (isometric contraction) 　Flexor carpi radialis 　Flexor carpi ulnaris 　Palmaris longus 　Flexor digitorum profundus 　Flexor digitorum superficialis 　Flexor pollicis longus	Flexion*	Wrist and hand flexors (isometric contraction) 　Flexor carpi radialis 　Flexor carpi ulnaris 　Palmaris longus 　Flexor digitorum profundus 　Flexor digitorum superficialis 　Flexor pollicis longus
Elbow	Extension	Elbow extensors 　Triceps brachii 　Anconeus	Flexion	Elbow extensors (eccentric contraction) 　Triceps brachii 　Anconeus
Shoulder	Flexion	Shoulder joint flexors 　Pectoralis major (clavicular head or upper fibers) 　Anterior deltoid 　Coracobrachialis 　Biceps brachii	Extension	Shoulder joint flexors (eccentric contraction) 　Pectoralis major (clavicular head or upper fibers) 　Anterior deltoid 　Coracobrachialis 　Biceps brachii
Shoulder girdle	Upward rotation and elevation	Shoulder girdle upward rotators and elevators 　Trapezius 　Levator scapulae 　Serratus anterior	Downward rotation and depression	Shoulder girdle upward rotators and elevators (eccentric contraction) 　Trapezius 　Levator scapulae 　Serratus anterior

***Note:** The wrist is in a position of slight extension to facilitate greater active finger flexion in gripping the bar.

Chapter 8

Chest press (bench press)

Description

The subject lies on the exercise bench in the supine position, grasps the barbell, and presses the weight upward through the full range of arm and shoulder movement (Fig. 8.6). Then the weight is lowered to the starting position.

Analysis

This exercise can be divided into two phases for analysis: (1) lifting phase to upward position and (2) lowering phase to starting position (Table 8.5).

A   **B**

FIG. 8.6 ● Chest press (bench press). **A,** Starting position; **B,** up position.

TABLE 8.5 • Chest press (bench press)

Joint	Lifting phase to upward position		Lowering phase to starting position	
	Action	Agonists	Action	Agonists
Wrist and hand	Flexion*	Wrist and hand flexors (isometric contraction) Flexor carpi radialis Flexor carpi ulnaris Palmaris longus Flexor digitorum profundus Flexor digitorum superficialis Flexor pollicis longus	Flexion*	Wrist and hand flexors (isometric contraction) Flexor carpi radialis Flexor carpi ulnaris Palmaris longus Flexor digitorum profundus Flexor digitorum superficialis Flexor pollicis longus
Elbow	Extension	Elbow extensors Triceps brachii Anconeus	Flexion	Elbow extensors (eccentric contraction) Triceps brachii Anconeus
Shoulder	Flexion and horizontal adduction	Shoulder flexors and horizontal adductors Pectoralis major Anterior deltoid Coracobrachialis Biceps brachii	Extension and horizontal abduction	Shoulder joint flexors and horizontal adductors (eccentric contraction) Pectoralis major Anterior deltoid Coracobrachialis Biceps brachii
Shoulder girdle	Abduction	Shoulder girdle abductors Serratus anterior Pectoralis minor	Adduction	Shoulder girdle abductors (eccentric contraction) Serratus anterior Pectoralis minor

*Note: The wrist is in a position of slight extension to facilitate greater active finger flexion in gripping the bar.

Chin-up (pull-up)

Description

The subject grasps a horizontal bar or ladder with the palms toward the face (Fig. 8.7, *A*). From a hanging position on the bar, the subject pulls up until the chin is over the bar (Fig. 8.7, *B*) and returns to the starting position (Fig. 8.7, *C*).

Analysis

This exercise is separated into two phases for analysis: (1) pulling up phase to chinning position and (2) lowering phase to starting position (Table 8.6).

A   **B**   **C**

FIG. 8.7 ● Pull-up. **A,** Straight-arm hang; **B,** chin over bar; **C,** bent-arm hang on way up or down.

TABLE 8.6 • **Chin-up (pull-up)**

Joint	Pulling up phase to chinning position		Lowering phase to starting position	
	Action	Agonists	Action	Agonists
Wrist and hand	Flexion	Wrist and hand flexors (isometric contraction) 　Flexor carpi radialis 　Flexor carpi ulnaris 　Palmaris longus 　Flexor digitorum profundus 　Flexor digitorum superficialis 　Flexor pollicis longus	Flexion	Wrist and hand flexors (isometric contraction) 　Flexor carpi radialis 　Flexor carpi ulnaris 　Palmaris longus 　Flexor digitorum profundus 　Flexor digitorum superficialis 　Flexor pollicis longus
Elbow	Flexion	Elbow flexors 　Biceps brachii 　Brachialis 　Brachioradialis	Extension	Elbow flexors (eccentric contraction) 　Biceps brachii 　Brachialis 　Brachioradialis
Shoulder	Extension	Shoulder joint extensors 　Latissimus dorsi 　Teres major 　Posterior deltoid 　Pectoralis major 　Triceps brachii (long head)	Flexion	Shoulder joint extensors (eccentric contraction) 　Latissimus dorsi 　Teres major 　Posterior deltoid 　Pectoralis major 　Triceps brachii (long head)
Shoulder girdle	Adduction, depression, and downward rotation	Shoulder girdle adductors, depressors, and downward rotators 　Trapezius (lower and middle) 　Pectoralis minor 　Rhomboids	Elevation, abduction, and upward rotation	Shoulder girdle adductors, depressors, and downward rotators (eccentric contraction) 　Trapezius (lower and middle) 　Pectoralis minor 　Rhomboids

Chapter

8

Latissimus pull (lat pull)

Description

From a sitting position, the subject reaches up and grasps a horizontal bar (Fig. 8.8, *A*). The bar is pulled down to a position behind the neck and shoulders (Fig. 8.8, *B*). Then it is returned slowly to the starting position.

Analysis

This exercise is separated into two phases for analysis: (1) pull-down phase to behind-the-shoulders position, and (2) return phase to starting position (Table 8.7).

A

B

FIG. 8.8 ● Latissimus pull (lat pull). **A,** Starting position; **B,** downward position.

TABLE 8.7 • Latissimus pull (lat pull)

| Joint | Pull-down phase to behind-the-shoulders position | | Return phase to starting position | |
	Action	Agonists	Action	Agonists

Wrist and hand	Flexion	Wrist and hand flexors (isometric contraction)
		   Flexor carpi radialis
		   Flexor carpi ulnaris
		   Palmaris longus
		   Flexor digitorum profundus
		   Flexor digitorum superficialis
		   Flexor pollicis longus
			Flexion	Wrist and hand flexors (isometric contraction)
				   Flexor carpi radialis
				   Flexor carpi ulnaris
				   Palmaris longus
				   Flexor digitorum profundus
				   Flexor digitorum superficialis
				   Flexor pollicis longus

Elbow	Flexion	Elbow flexors
		   Biceps brachii
		   Brachialis
		   Brachioradialis
			Extension	Elbow flexors (eccentric contraction)
				   Biceps brachii
				   Brachialis
				   Brachioradialis

Shoulder	Adduction	Shoulder joint adductors
		   Pectoralis major
		   Posterior deltoid
		   Latissimus dorsi
		   Teres major
		   Subscapularis
			Abduction	Shoulder joint adductors (eccentric contraction)
				   Pectoralis major
				   Posterior deltoid
				   Latissimus dorsi
				   Teres major
				   Subscapularis

Shoulder girdle	Adduction, depression, and downward rotation	Shoulder girdle adductors, depressors, and downward rotators
		   Trapezius (lower and middle)
		   Pectoralis minor
		   Rhomboids
			Abduction, elevation, and upward rotation	Shoulder girdle adductors, depressors, and downward rotators (eccentric contraction)
				   Trapezius (lower and middle)
				   Pectoralis minor
				   Rhomboids

Chapter

8

Push-up (fingertip)

Description

The subject lies on the floor in a prone position with the legs together, the fingertips touching the floor, and the hands pointed forward and approximately under the shoulders (Fig. 8.9, *A*). Keeping the back and legs straight, the subject pushes up to the up position and returns to the starting position (Fig. 8.9, *B*).

Analysis

This exercise is separated into two phases for analysis: (1) pushing phase to up position and (2) lowering phase to starting position (Table 8.8).

Chin-ups and push-ups are excellent exercises for the shoulder area, shoulder girdle, shoulder joint, elbow joint, and wrist and hand (see Figs. 8.7 and 8.9). The use of free weights, machines, and other conditioning exercises helps develop strength and endurance for this part of the body.

A

B

FIG. 8.9 • Push-up. **A,** Starting position; **B,** up position.

TABLE 8.8 • **Push-up (fingertip)**

Joint	Pushing phase to up position		Lowering phase to starting position	
	Action	Agonists	Action	Agonists
Wrist and hand	Flexion	Wrist and hand flexors (isometric contraction) Flexor carpi radialis Flexor carpi ulnaris Palmaris longus Flexor digitorum profundus Flexor digitorum superficialis Flexor pollicis longus	Flexion	Wrist and hand flexors (isometric contraction) Flexor carpi radialis Flexor carpi ulnaris Palmaris longus Flexor digitorum profundus Flexor digitorum superficialis Flexor pollicis longus
Elbow	Extension	Elbow extensors Triceps brachii Anconeus	Flexion	Elbow extensors (eccentric contraction) Triceps brachii Anconeus
Shoulder	Horizontal Adduction	Shoulder joint horizontal adductors Pectoralis major Anterior deltoid Biceps brachii Coracobrachialis	Horizontal abduction	Shoulder joint horizontal adductors (eccentric contraction) Pectoralis major Anterior deltoid Biceps brachii Coracobrachialis
Shoulder girdle	Abduction	Shoulder girdle abductors Serratus anterior Pectoralis minor	Adduction	Shoulder girdle abductors (eccentric contraction) Serratus anterior Pectoralis minor

Prone row

Description

This exercise is sometimes referred to as a bent-over row. The subject is lying prone on a table or kneeling on a bench so that the involved arm is free from contact with the floor (Fig. 8.10, *A*). When kneeling, the subject uses the contralateral arm to support the body. The dumbbell is held in the hand with arm and the shoulder hanging straight to the floor. From this position, the subject adducts the shoulder girdle and horizontally abducts the shoulder joint (Fig. 8.10, *B*). Then the dumbbell is lowered slowly to the starting position.

Analysis

This exercise is separated into two phases for analysis: (1) pull-up phase to horizontal abducted position, and (2) lowering phase to starting position (Table 8.9).

FIG. 8.10 ● Prone row.

TABLE 8.9 • **Prone row**

| Joint | Pull-up phase to horizontal abducted position | | Lowering phase to starting position | |
	Action	Agonists	Action	Agonists
Wrist and hand	Flexion	Wrist and hand flexors (isometric contraction) Flexor carpi radialis Flexor carpi ulnaris Palmaris longus Flexor digitorum profundus Flexor digitorum superficialis Flexor pollicis longus	Flexion	Wrist and hand flexors (isometric contraction) Flexor carpi radialis Flexor carpi ulnaris Palmaris longus Flexor digitorum profundus Flexor digitorum superficialis Flexor pollicis longus
Elbow	Flexion	Passive flexion occurs as the arm becomes parallel to the floor due to gravity	Extension	Passive extension occurs as the arm becomes perpendicular to the floor due to gravity
Shoulder	Horizontal abduction	Shoulder joint horizontal abductors Posterior deltoid Infraspinatus Teres minor Latissimus dorsi	Horizontal Adduction	Shoulder joint horizontal abductors (eccentric contraction) Posterior deltoid Infraspinatus Teres minor Latissimus dorsi
Shoulder girdle	Adduction	Shoulder girdle adductors Trapezius (lower and middle) Rhomboids	Abduction	Shoulder girdle adductors (eccentric contraction) Trapezius (lower and middle) Rhomboids

Web sites

American College of Sports Medicine:

www.acsm.org

Scientific research, education, and practical applications of sports medicine and exercise science to maintain and enhance physical performance, fitness, health, and quality of life

Concept II:

www.concept2.com

Information on the technique of rowing and the muscles used

Fitness World:

www.fitnessworld.com

The information at this site is about fitness in general and includes access to *Fitness Management* magazine.

National Council of Strength & Fitness:

www.ncsf.org

Personal Training Certification & Continuing Education for the Fitness Professional

National Strength and Conditioning Association:

www.nsca-lift.org

Information on the profession of strength and conditioning specialists and personal trainers

NSCA Certification Commission:

www.nsca-cc.org

The certifying body for the National Strength and Conditioning Association

Presidents Council on Physical Fitness and Sports:

www.fitness.gov

Information and links from the U.S. government on fitness

Worksheet exercises

As an aid to learning, for in-class and out-of-class assignments, or for testing, a tear-out worksheet is found at the end of the text (p. 332).

Upright row exercise worksheet (no. 1)

List the movements that occur in each joint as the subject lifts the weight in performing upright rows. For each joint movement, list the muscles primarily responsible and denote whether they are contracting concentrically or eccentrically.

Dips exercise worksheet (no. 2)

List the movements that occur in each joint as the subject moves the body in performing dips. For each joint movement, list the muscles primarily responsible and denote whether they are contracting concentrically or eccentrically.

Laboratory and review exercises

1. Analyze other conditioning exercises that involve the shoulder areas, such as dips, upright rows, shrugs, and inclined presses.
2. Observe and analyze shoulder muscular activities of children on playground equipment.
3. Discuss how you would teach boys and girls who cannot perform one chin-up to learn to do chin-ups. Additionally, discuss how you would teach subjects who cannot perform one push-up to do push-ups.
4. Should boys and girls attempt to do chin-ups and push-ups to see whether they have adequate strength in the shoulder area?
5. Test yourself doing chin-ups and push-ups to determine your strength and muscular endurance in the shoulder area.
6. What, if any, benefit would result from doing fingertip push-ups as opposed to push-ups with the hands flat on the floor?
7. Stand slightly farther than arm's length from a wall with your hands facing forward at shoulder-level height. Push your hand straight in front of your shoulder until the elbow is extended fully and the glenohumeral joint is flexed 90 degrees by performing each of the following movements before proceeding to the next:
   • Glenohumeral flexion to 90 degrees
   • Full elbow extension
   • Wrist extension to 70 degrees
   Analyze the movements and the muscles responsible for each movement at the shoulder girdle, glenohumeral joint, elbow, and wrist.
8. Now face a wall and stand about 6 inches from it. Place both hands on the wall at shoulder level and put your nose and chest against the wall. Keeping your palms in place on the wall, slowly push your body from the wall as in a push-up until your chest is as far away from the wall as possible without removing your palms from the wall surface. Analyze the movements and the muscles responsible for each movement at the shoulder girdle, glenohumeral joint, elbow, and wrist.

9. What is the difference between the two exercises in questions #7 and #8? Can you perform #8 one step at a time, as you did in #7?
10. Analyze each exercise in the exercise analysis chart below. Use one row for each joint involved that actively moves during the exercise. Do not include joints where there is no active movement or where the joint is maintained in one position isometrically.

Exercise analysis chart

Exercise	Phase	Joint, movement occurring	Force causing movement (muscle or gravity)	Force resisting movement (muscle or gravity)	Functional muscle group, type of contraction
Barbell press (overhead or military press)	Lifting phase				
	Lowering phase				
Chest press (bench press)	Lifting phase				
	Lowering phase				
Chin-up (pull-up)	Pulling up phase				
	Lowering phase				
Latissimus pull (lat pull)	Pull-down phase				
	Return phase				
Push-up	Pushing phase				
	Lowering phase				
Prone row (bent-over row)	Pull-up phase				
	Lowering phase				

Chapter 8

References

Adrian M: Isokinetic exercise, *Training and Conditioning* 1:1, June 1991.

Andrews JR, Wilk KE: *The athlete's shoulder,* New York, 1994, Churchill Livingstone.

Andrews JR, Zarins B, Wilk KE: *Injuries in baseball,* Philadelphia, 1998, Lippincott-Raven.

Booher JM Thibodeau GA: *Athletic injury assessment,* ed 4, Dubuque, IA, 2000, McGraw-Hill.

Bouche J: Three essential lifts for high school players, *Scholastic Coach* 56:42, April 1987.

Brzycki M: Rx for a safe productive strength program, *Scholastic Coach* 57:70, September 1987.

Ellenbecker TS, Davies GJ: *Closed kinetic chain exercise: a comprehensive guide to multiple-joint exercise,* Champaign, IL, 2001, Human Kinetics.

Epley B: Getting elementary muscles, *Coach and Athlete* 44:60, November–December 1981.

Geisler P: Kinesiology of the full golf swing—implications for intervention and rehabilitation, *Sports Medicine Update* 11:9, #2, 1996.

Hamilton N, Luttgens K: *Kinesiology: scientific basis of human motion,* ed 10, Boston, 2002, McGraw-Hill.

Matheson O, et al: Stress fractures in athletes, *American Journal of Sports Medicine* 15:46, January–February 1987.

National Strength and Conditioning Association; Baechle TR, Earle RW: *Essentials of strength training and conditioning,* ed 2, Champaign, IL, 2000, Human Kinetics.

Northrip JW, Logan GA, McKinney WC: *Analysis of sport motion: anatomic and biomechanic perpectives,* ed 3, 1983, McGraw-Hill Companies, Inc., New York.

Schlitz J: The athlete's daily dozen stretches, *Athletic Journal* 66:20, November 1985.

Smith LK, Weiss EL, Lehmkuhl LD: *Brunnstrom's clinical kinesiology,* ed 5, Philadelphia, 1996, Davis.

Steindler A: *Kinesiology of the human body,* Springfield, IL, 1970, Charles C Thomas.

The Hip Joint and Pelvic Girdle

Objectives

- To identify on a human skeleton or subject selected bony features of the hip joint and pelvic girdle

- To label on a skeletal chart selected bony features of the hip joint and pelvic girdle

- To draw on a skeletal chart the individual muscles of the hip joint

- To demonstrate, using a human subject, all of the movements of the hip joint and pelvic girdle and list their respective planes of movement and axes of motion

- To palpate on a human subject the muscles of the hip joint and pelvic girdle

- To list and organize the primary muscles that produce movement of the hip joint and pelvic girdle and list their antagonists

---

Online Learning Center Resources

Visit *Manual of Structural Kinesiology's* Online Learning Center at **www.mhhe.com/floyd15e** for additional information and study material for this chapter, including:

- *Self-grading quizzes*
- *Anatomy flashcards*
- *Animations*

The hip, or acetabular femoral joint, is a relatively stable joint due to its bony architecture, strong ligaments, and large, supportive muscles. It functions in weight bearing and locomotion, which is enhanced significantly by its wide range of motion, which provides the ability to run, cross-over cut, side-step cut, jump, and make many other directional changes.

Bones   FIGS. 9.1 to 9.3

The hip joint is the ball-and-socket joint that consists of the head of the femur connecting with the acetabulum of the pelvic girdle. The pelvic girdle consists of a right and left pelvic bone joined together posteriorly by the sacrum. The femur is the longest bone in the body. The sacrum can be considered an extension of the spinal column with five fused vertebrae. Extending inferior to the sacrum is the coccyx. The pelvic bones are made up of three bones: the ilium, the ischium, and the pubis. At birth and during growth and development, they are three distinct bones. At maturity, they are fused to form one pelvic bone.

The pelvic bone can be divided roughly into three areas, starting from the acetabulum:

Upper two-fifths = ilium
Posterior and lower two-fifths = ischium
Anterior and lower one-fifth = pubis

In studying the muscles of the hip and thigh, it is helpful to focus on the important bony landmarks, keeping in mind their purpose as key attachment points for the muscles. The anterior pelvis serves to provide points of origin for muscles generally involved in flexing the hip. Specifically, the tensor fasciae latae arises from the anterior iliac crest, the

Iliac crest

Base of sacrum

Sacroiliac joints

Sacrum

Ilium

Iliac fossa

Anterior superior
iliac spine

Pectineal line

Anterior inferior
iliac spine

Femoral head

Acetabulum

Greater trochanter

Femoral neck

Coccyx

Obturator foramen

Intertrochanteric
line

Lesser trochanter

Pubis

Ischial tuberosity

Inferior pubic ramus

Femur

Ischium

Symphysis pubis

Pubic crest

Superior pubic ramus

Adductor tubercle

Lateral epicondyle

Medial epicondyle

Lateral femoral condyle

Patella

Medial femoral condyle

Lateral tibial condyle

Medial tibial condyle

Gerdy's tubercle

Fibular head

Fibula

Tibial tuberosity

Tibia

FIG. 9.1 ● Right pelvis and femur, anterior view.

sartorius originates on the anterior superior iliac spine, and the rectus femoris originates on the anterior inferior iliac spine. Laterally, the gluteus medius and minimus, which abduct the hip, originate just below the iliac crest. Posteriorly, the gluteus maximus originates on the posterior iliac crest as well as the posterior sacrum and coccyx. Posteroinferiorly, the ischial tuberosity serves as the

point of origin for the hamstrings, which extend the hip. Medially, the pubis and its inferior ramus serve as the point of origin for the hip adductors, which include the adductor magnus, adductor longus, adductor brevis, pectineus, and gracilis.

The proximal thigh generally serves as a point of insertion for some of the short muscles of the hip and as the origin for three of the knee extensors.

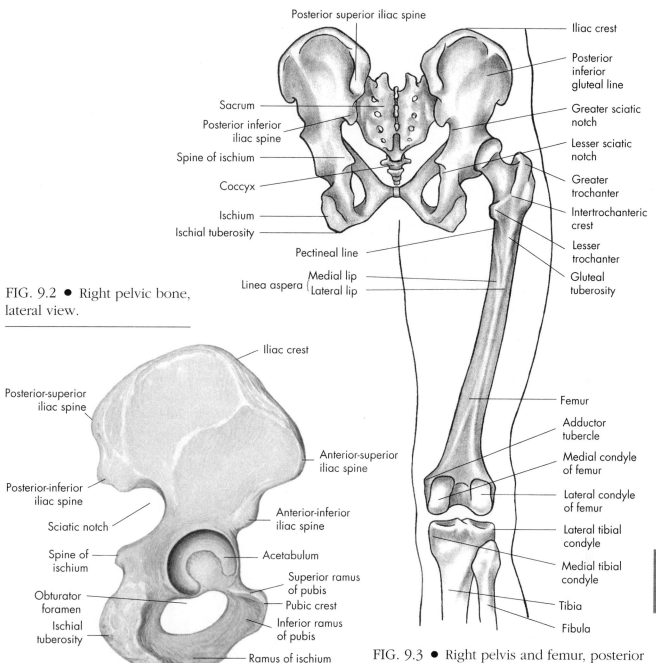

Posterior superior iliac spine

Iliac crest

Posterior inferior gluteal line

Greater sciatic notch

Sacrum

Posterior inferior iliac spine

Lesser sciatic notch

Spine of ischium

Greater trochanter

Coccyx

Intertrochanteric crest

Ischium

Lesser trochanter

Ischial tuberosity

Gluteal tuberosity

Pectineal line

Medial lip
Linea aspera { Lateral lip

FIG. 9.2 ● Right pelvic bone, lateral view.

Iliac crest

Posterior-superior iliac spine

Anterior-superior iliac spine

Posterior-inferior iliac spine

Sciatic notch

Anterior-inferior iliac spine

Spine of ischium

Acetabulum

Obturator foramen

Superior ramus of pubis

Pubic crest

Ischial tuberosity

Inferior ramus of pubis

Ramus of ischium

Femur

Adductor tubercle

Medial condyle of femur

Lateral condyle of femur

Lateral tibial condyle

Medial tibial condyle

Tibia

Fibula

FIG. 9.3 ● Right pelvis and femur, posterior view.

Most notably, the greater trochanter is the point of insertion for all of the gluteal muscles and most of the six deep external rotators. Although not palpable, the lesser trochanter serves as the bony landmark upon which the iliopsoas inserts. Anteriorly, the three vasti muscles of the quadriceps originate proximally. Posteriorly, the linea aspera serves as the insertion for the hip adductors.

Distally, the patella serves as a major bony landmark to which all four quadriceps muscles insert. The remainder of the hip muscles insert on the proximal tibia or fibula. The sartorius, gracilis, and semitendinosus insert on the upper anteromedial surface of the tibia just below the medial condyle, after crossing the knee posteromedially. The semimembranosus inserts posteromedially on the medial tibial condyle. Laterally, the biceps femoris inserts primarily on the head on the fibula, with some fibers attaching on the lateral tibial condyle. Anterolaterally, Gerdy's tubercle provides the insertion point for the iliotibial tract of the tensor fasciae latae.

Chapter
9

Joints   FIGS. 9.1 to 9.5

In the anterior area, the pelvic bones are joined to form the symphysis pubis, an amphiarthrodial joint. In the posterior area, the sacrum is located between the two pelvic bones and forms the sacroiliac joints. Strong ligaments unite these bones to form rigid, slightly movable joints. The bones are large and heavy and for the most part are covered by thick, heavy muscles. Very minimal oscillating-type movements can occur in these joints, as in walking or in hip flexion when lying on one's back. However, movements usually involve the entire pelvic girdle and hip joints. In walking, there is hip flexion and extension with rotation of the pelvic girdle, forward in hip flexion and backward in hip extension. Jogging and running result in faster movements and in a greater range of movement.

Sport skills such as kicking a football or soccer ball are other good examples of hip and pelvic movements. Pelvic rotation helps increase the length of the stride in running; in kicking, it can result in a greater range of motion, which translates to a greater distance or more speed to the kick.

Except for the glenohumeral joint, the hip is one of the most mobile joints of the body, largely because of its multiaxial arrangement. Unlike the glenohumeral, the hip joint's bony architecture provides a great deal of stability, resulting in relatively few hip joint subluxations and dislocations.

The hip joint is classified as an enarthrodial-type joint and is formed by the femoral head inserting into the socket provided by the acetabulum of the pelvis. An extremely strong and dense ligamentous capsule, illustrated in Figs. 9.4 and 9.5, reinforces the joint, especially anteriorly. Anteriorly, the iliofemoral, or Y, ligament prevents hip hyperextension. The teres ligament attaches from deep in the acetabulum to a depression in the head of the femur and slightly limits adduction. The pubofemoral ligament is located anteromedially and inferiorly and limits excessive extension and abduction. Posteriorly, the triangular ischiofemoral ligament extends from the ischium below to the trochanteric fossa of the femur and limits internal rotation.

Because of individual differences, there is some disagreement about the exact possible range of each movement in the hip joint, but the ranges are generally 0 to 130 degrees of flexion, 0 to 30 degrees of extension, 0 to 35 degrees of abduction, 0 to 30 degrees of adduction, 0 to 45 degrees

FIG. 9.4 ● Right hip joint, anterior ligaments.

FIG. 9.5 ● Right hip joint, posterior ligaments.

of internal rotation, and 0 to 50 degrees of external rotation (Fig. 9.6).

The pelvic girdle moves back and forth within three planes for a total of six different movements. To avoid confusion, it is important to analyze the pelvic girdle activity to determine the exact location of the movement. All pelvic girdle rotation actually results from motion at one or more of the following locations: the right hip, the left hip, the lumbar spine. Although it is not essential for movement to occur in all three of these areas, it must occur in at least one for the pelvis to rotate in any direction. Table 9.1 lists the motions at the hips and lumbar spine that can often accompany rotation of the pelvic girdle.

FIG. 9.6 ● Active motion of the hip. **A,** Flexion is measured in degrees from a supine position. The knee can be extended or flexed; **B,** Extension or hyperextension is normally measured with the knee extended; **C,** Abduction can be measured in a supine or sidelying position; adduction is best measured with the athlete lying supine; **D,** Internal and external rotation can be evaluated in a supine or prone position.

TABLE 9.1 • Motions accompanying pelvic rotation

Pelvic rotation	Lumbar spine motion	Right hip motion	Left hip motion
Anterior rotation	Extension	Flexion	Flexion
Posterior rotation	Flexion	Extension	Extension
Right lateral rotation	Left lateral flexion	Abduction	Adduction
Left lateral rotation	Right lateral flexion	Adduction	Abduction
Right transverse rotation	Left lateral rotation	Internal rotation	External rotation
Left transverse rotation	Right lateral rotation	External rotation	Internal rotation

Movements   FIGS. 9.7 and 9.8

Anterior and posterior pelvic rotation occur in the sagittal or anteroposterior plane, whereas right and left lateral rotation occur in the lateral or frontal plane. Right transverse (clockwise) rotation and left transverse (counterclockwise) rotation occur in the horizontal or transverse plane of motion.

Hip flexion: movement of the femur straight anteriorly toward the pelvis

Hip extension: movement of the femur straight posteriorly away from the pelvis; sometimes referred to as hyperextension

Hip abduction: movement of the femur laterally to the side away from the midline

Hip adduction: movement of the femur medially toward the midline

Hip external rotation: rotary movement of the femur laterally around its longitudinal axis away from the midline; lateral rotation

Hip internal rotation: rotary movement of the femur medially around its longitudinal axis toward the midline; medial rotation

Hip diagonal abduction: movement of the femur in a diagonal plane away from the midline of the body

Hip diagonal adduction: movement of the femur in a diagonal plane toward the midline of the body

Anterior pelvic rotation: anterior movement of the upper pelvis; the iliac crest tilts forward in a sagittal plane; anterior tilt

Posterior pelvic rotation: posterior movement of the upper pelvis; the iliac crest tilts backward in a sagittal plane; posterior tilt

Left lateral pelvic rotation: in the frontal plane, the left pelvis moves inferiorly in relation to the right pelvis; either the left pelvis rotates downward or the right pelvis rotates upward; left lateral tilt

Right lateral pelvic rotation: in the frontal plane, the right pelvis moves inferiorly in relation to the

Flexion

A

Extension

B

Abduction

C

Adduction

D

FIG. 9.7 ● Movements of the hip.

External rotation
E

Internal rotation
F

Diagonal abduction
G

Diagonal adduction
H

FIG. 9.7 (continued) ● Movements of the hip.

Anterior pelvic rotation
A

Posterior pelvic rotation
B

Right lateral pelvic rotation
C

Right transverse pelvic rotation
D

FIG. 9.8 ● Pelvic girdle motions.

left pelvis; either the right pelvis rotates downward or the left pelvis rotates upward; right lateral tilt

Left transverse pelvic rotation: in a horizontal plane of motion, rotation of the pelvis to the body's left; the right iliac crest moves anteriorly in relation to the left iliac crest, which moves posteriorly

Right transverse pelvic rotation: in a horizontal plane of motion, rotation of the pelvis to the body's right; the left iliac crest moves anteriorly in relation to the right iliac crest, which moves posteriorly

Muscles FIGS. 9.9 to 9.11

At the hip joint, there are seven two-joint muscles that have one action at the hip and another at the knee. The muscles actually involved in hip and pelvic girdle motions depend largely on the direction of the movement and the position of the body

Chapter 9

FIG. 9.9 ● **A,** Superficial muscles of the right upper leg, anterior surface; **B,** superficial muscles of the right upper leg, posterior surface.

Modified from Anthony CP, Kolthoff NJ: *Textbook of anatomy and physiology,* ed 9, St. Louis, 1975, Mosby.

Anterior

Rectus femoris   Vastus medialis

Vastus lateralis

Vastus intermedius

Femur

Lateral

Sartorius

Intermuscular septum

Adductor longus

Adductor brevis   **Medial**

Gracilis

Adductor magnus

Biceps femoris short head

Biceps femoris long head

Semimembranosus

Semitendinosus

Posterior

FIG. 9.10 ● Cross-section of the left thigh at the midsection.

in relation to the earth and its gravitational forces. In addition, it should be noted that the body part that moves the most will be the part least stabilized. For example, when standing on both feet and contracting the hip flexors, the trunk and pelvis will rotate anteriorly, but, when lying supine and contracting the hip flexors, the thighs will move forward into flexion on the stable pelvis.

In another example, the hip flexor muscles are used in moving the thighs toward the trunk, but the extensor muscles are used eccentrically when the pelvis and the trunk move downward slowly on the femur and concentrically when the trunk is

raised on the femur—this, of course, in rising to the standing position.

In the downward phase of the knee-bend exercise, the movement at the hips and knees is flexion. The muscles primarily involved are the hip and knee extensors in eccentric contraction.

Hip joint and pelvic girdle muscles—location

Muscle location largely determines the muscle action. Seventeen or more muscles are found in the area (the six external rotators are counted as one muscle). Most hip joint and pelvic girdle muscles are large and strong.

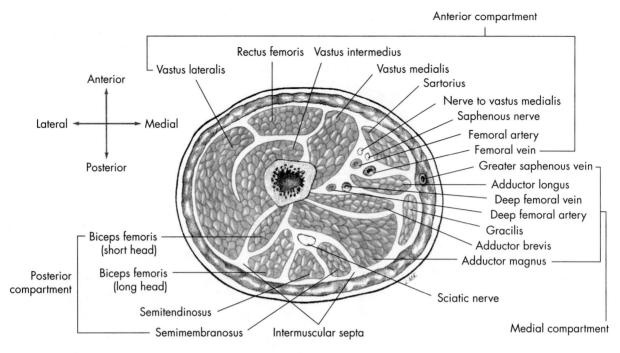

FIG. 9.11 ● Transverse section of the left midthigh, detailing the anterior, posterior, and medial compartments.

Anterior
    Primarily hip flexion
        Iliopsoas (iliacus and psoas)
        Pectineus
        Rectus femoris*†
        Sartorius†
Lateral
    Primarily hip abduction
        Gluteus medius
        Gluteus minimus
        External rotators
        Tensor fasciae latae†
Posterior
    Primarily hip extension
        Gluteus maximus
        Biceps femoris*†
        Semitendinosus*†
        Semimembranosus*†
        External rotators (six deep)
Medial
    Primarily hip adduction
        Adductor brevis
        Adductor longus
        Adductor magnus
        Gracilis†

*Two-joint muscles, knee actions are discussed in Chapter 8.
†Two-joint muscles.

Muscle identification

In developing a thorough and practical knowledge of the muscular system, it is essential that individual muscles be understood. Figs. 9.9, 9.10, 9.12, 9.13, 9.14, and 9.15 illustrate groups of muscles that work together to produce joint movement. While viewing the muscles in these figures, correlate them with Table 9.2.

The muscles of the pelvis that act on the hip joint may be divided into two regions—the iliac and gluteal regions. The iliac region contains the iliopsoas muscle, which flexes the hip. The iliopsoas actually is three different muscles—the iliacus, the psoas major, and the psoas minor. The 10 muscles of the gluteal region function primarily to extend and rotate the hip. Located in the gluteal region are the gluteus maximus, gluteus medius, gluteus minimi, and tensor fasciae latae, and the six deep external rotators—piriformis, obturator externus, obturator internus, gemellus superior, gemellus inferior, and quadratus femoris.

The thigh is divided into three compartments by the intermuscular septa (Fig. 9.11). The anterior compartment contains the rectus femoris, vastus medialis, vastus intermedius, vastus lateralis, and sartorius. The hamstring muscle group, consisting of the biceps femoris, semitendinosus, and semimembranosus, is located in the posterior compartment. The medial compartment contains the thigh muscles primarily responsible for adduction of the hip, which are the adductor brevis, adductor longus, adductor magnus, pectineus, and gracilis.

FIG. 9.12 ● Muscles of the right anterior pelvic and thigh regions.

FIG. 9.13 ● Muscles of the right medial thigh.

TABLE 9.2 • Agonist muscles of the hip joint

	Muscle	Origin	Insertion	Action	Plane of motion	Palpation	Innervation
Anterior	Iliacus	Inner surface of the ilium	Lesser trochanter of the femur and shaft just below	Flexion of the hip	Sagittal	Difficult to palpate; anterior aspect of hip approximately 1.5 inches below center of inguinal ligament with active hip flexion/extension of supine subject, immediately lateral to pectineus	Lumbar nerve and femoral nerve (L2–L4)
				External rotation of the femur	Transverse		
	Psoas major and minor	Lower borders of the transverse processes (L1–L5), sides of the bodies of the last thoracic vertebrae (T12), the lumbar vertebrae (L1–L5), intervertebral fibrocartilages, and base of the sacrum	Lesser trochanter of the femur and shaft just below Psoas minor: Pectineal line and iliopectineal eminence	Flexion of the hip	Sagittal		
				External rotation of the femur	Transverse		
	Rectus femoris	Anterior inferior iliac spine of the ilium and groove (posterior) above the acetabulum	Superior aspect of the patella tendon to the tibial tuberosity	Flexion of the hip	Sagittal	Straight down anterior thigh from anterior inferior iliac spine to patella, particularly during resisted hip flexion/knee extension	Femoral nerve (L2–L4)
				Extension of the knee			
	Sartorius	Anterior superior iliac spine and notch just below the spine	Anterior medial surface of the tibia just below the condyle	Flexion of the hip	Sagittal	From the anterior superior iliac spine to the medial tibial condyle during combined resistance of hip flexion/external rotation/abduction and knee flexion in a supine position	Femoral nerve (L2, L3)
				Flexion of the knee			
				External rotation of the thigh as it flexes the hip and knee	Transverse		
	Pectineus	Space 1 inch wide on the front of the pubis just above the crest	Rough line leading from the lesser trochanter down to the linea aspera	Flexion of the hip	Sagittal	Difficult to palpate; anterior aspect of hip approximately 1.5 inches below center of inguinal ligament with active hip flexion/extension of supine subject, immediately medial to iliopsoas	Femoral nerve (L2–L4)
				Adduction of the hip	Frontal		
				Internal rotation of the hip	Transverse		

Chapter 9

TABLE 9.2 (continued) • **Agonist muscles of the hip joint**

	Muscle	Origin	Insertion	Action	Plane of motion	Palpation	Innervation
Medial	Adductor brevis	Front of the inferior pubic ramus just below the origin of the adductor longus	Lower two-thirds of the pectineal line of the femur and the upper half of the medial lip of the linea aspera	Adduction of the hip	Frontal	Very difficult to palpate and differentiate from adductor longus which is immediately inferior	Obturator nerve (L3, L4)
				External rotation as it adducts the hip	Transverse		
	Adductor longus	Anterior pubis just below its crest	Middle third of the linea aspera	Adduction of the hip	Frontal	Just inferior to the pubic bone on upper medial side of thigh with resisted adduction	Obturator nerve (L3, L4)
				Assists in flexion of the hip	Sagittal		
	Adductor magnus	Edge of the entire pubic ramus and the ischium and ischial tuberosity	Whole length of the linea aspera, inner condyloid ridge, and adductor tubercle	Adduction of the hip	Frontal	Medial aspect of thigh from ischial tuberosity to adductor tubercle with resisted adduction from abducted position	Anterior: obturator nerve (L2–L4) Posterior: sciatic nerve (L4, L5, S1–S3)
				External rotation as the hip adducts	Transverse		
	Gracilis	Anteromedial edge of the descending ramus of the pubis	Anterior medial surface of the tibia below the condyle	Adduction of the hip	Frontal	A thin tendon on anteromedial thigh with knee flexion and resisted adduction	Obturator nerve (L2–L4)
				Flexion of the knee	Sagittal		
				Internal rotation of the hip	Transverse		

(*continued*)

TABLE 9.2 (continued) • Agonist muscles of the hip joint

	Muscle	Origin	Insertion	Action	Plane of motion	Palpation	Innervation
Posterior	Biceps femoris	Long head: ischial tuberosity. Short head: lower half of the linea aspera, and lateral condyloid ridge	Head of the fibula and lateral condyle of the tibia	Extension of the hip	Sagittal	Posterolateral aspect of distal thigh with combined knee flexion and external rotation against resistance	Long head: sciatic nerve—tibial division (S1–S3) Short head: sciatic nerve—peroneal division (L5, S1, S2)
				Flexion of the knee			
				External rotation of the hip	Transverse		
				External rotation of the knee			
	Semi-tendi-nosus	Ischial tuberosity	Upper anterior medial surface of the tibia just below the condyle	Extension of the hip	Sagittal	Posteromedial aspect of distal thigh with combined knee flexion and internal rotation against resistance	Sciatic nerve—tibial division (L5, S1, S2)
				Flexion of the knee			
				Internal rotation of the hip	Transverse		
				Internal rotation of the knee			
	Semimem-branosus	Ischial tuberosity	Posteromedial surface of the medial tibial condyle	Extension of the hip	Sagittal	Largely covered by other muscles, the tendon can be felt at the posteromedial aspect of the knee with combined knee flexion and internal rotation against resistance	Sciatic nerve—tibial division (L5, S1, S2)
				Flexion of the knee			
				Internal rotation of the hip	Transverse		
				Internal rotation of the knee			
	Gluteus maximus	Posterior 1/4 of the crest of the ilium, posterior surface of the sacrum and coccyx near the ilium, and fascia of the lumbar area	Oblique ridge on the lateral surface of the greater trochanter and the iliotibial band of the fasciae latae	Extension of the hip	Sagittal	Running downward and laterally between posterior iliac crest superiorly, anal cleft medially, and gluteal fold inferiorly, emphasized with hip extension and external rotation	Inferior gluteal nerve (L5, S1, S2)
				External rotation of the hip	Transverse		
				Lower fibers, which assist in adduction	Frontal		

Chapter 9

TABLE 9.2 (continued) • Agonist muscles of the hip joint

	Muscle	Origin	Insertion	Action	Plane of motion	Palpation	Innervation
Lateral	Gluteus medius	Lateral surface of the ilium just below the crest	Posterior and middle surfaces of the greater trochanter of the femur	Abduction of the hip	Frontal	Slightly in front of and a few inches above the greater trochanter with active elevation of opposite pelvis from a standing position	Superior gluteal nerve (L4, L5, S1)
				External rotation as the hip abducts (posterior fibers)			
				Internal rotation (anterior fibers)	Transverse		
	Gluteus minimus	Lateral surface of the ilium just below the origin of the gluteus medius	Anterior surface of the greater trochanter of the femur	Abduction of the hip	Frontal	Covered by tensor fasciae latae between anterior iliac crest and greater trochanter during internal rotation and abduction	Superior gluteal nerve (L4, L5, S1)
				Hip internal rotation as femur is abducted	Transverse		
	Tensor fasciae latae	Anterior iliac crest and surface of the ilium just below the crest	One fourth of the way down the thigh into the iliotibial tract, which in turn inserts onto Gerdy's tubercle of the anterolateral tibial condyle	Abduction of the hip	Frontal	Between anterior iliac crest and greater trochanter during internal rotation and abduction	Superior gluteal nerve (L4, L5, S1)
				Flexion of the hip	Sagittal		
				Internal rotation of the hip as it flexes	Transverse		

(continued)

FIG. 9.14 • Muscles of the right posterior thigh.

FIG. 9.15 • Muscles of the lateral right thigh.

TABLE 9.2 (continued) • Agonist muscles of the hip joint

	Muscle	Origin	Insertion	Action	Plane of motion	Palpation	Innervation
Deep posterior	Piriformis	Anterior sacrum, posterior portions of the ischium, and obturator foramen	Superior and posterior aspect of the greater trochanter	Hip external rotation	Transverse	With subject prone and gluteus maximus relaxed, palpate deeply between posterior superior greater trochanter and sacrum while passively internally/externally rotating femur	First and second sacral nerve (S1, S2)
	Gemellus superior	Ischial spine	Posterior aspect of the greater trochanter immediately below piriformis	Hip external rotation	Transverse	With subject prone and gluteus maximus relaxed, palpate deeply between posterior superior greater trochanter and ischial spine while passively internally/externally rotating femur	Sacral nerve (L5, S1, S2)
	Gemellus inferior	Ischial tuberosity	Posterior aspect of the greater trochanter with obturator internus	Hip external rotation	Transverse	With subject prone and gluteus maximus relaxed, palpate deeply between posterior greater trochanter and ischial tuberosity while passively internally/externally rotating femur	Branches from sacral plexus (L4, L5, S1, S2)
	Obturator internus	Margin of obturator foramen	Posterior aspect of the greater trochanter with gamellus superior	Hip external rotation	Transverse	With subject prone and gluteus maximus relaxed, palpate deeply between posterior superior greater trochanter and obturator foramen while passively internally/externally rotating femur	Branches from sacral plexus (L4, L5, S1, S2)
	Obturator externus	Inferior margin of obturator foramen	Posterior aspect of the greater trochanter immediately below obturator internus	Hip external rotation	Transverse	With subject prone and gluteus maximus relaxed, palpate deeply between inferior posterior greater trochanter and obturator foramen while passively internally/externally rotating femur	Obturator nerve (L3, L4)
	Quadratus femoris	Ischial tuberosity	Intertrochanteric ridge of femur	Hip external rotation	Transverse	With subject prone and gluteus maximus relaxed, palpate deeply between inferior posterior greater trochanter and ischial tuberosity while passively internally/externally rotating femur	Branches from sacral plexus (L4, L5, S1)

Chapter
9

Nerves

The muscles of the hip and pelvic girdle are all innervated from the lumbar and sacral plexus, known collectively as the lumbosacral plexus.

The lumbar plexus (Fig. 9.16) is formed by the anterior rami of spinal nerves L1 through L4 and some fibers from T12. The lower abdomen and the anterior and medial portions of the lower extremity are innervated by nerves arising from the

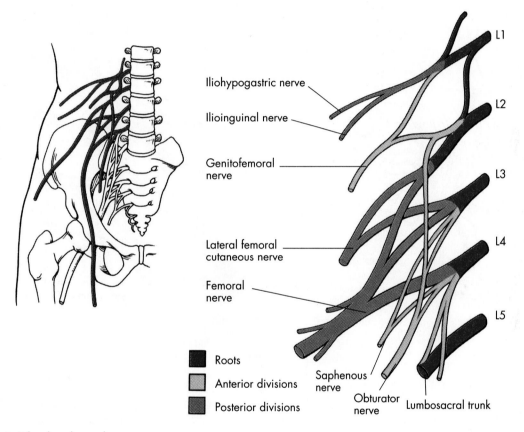

FIG. 9.16 ● The lumbar plexus.

lumbar plexus. The sacral plexus (Fig. 9.17) is formed by the anterior rami of L4, L5, and S1 through S4. The lower back, pelvis, perineum, posterior surface of the thigh and leg, and dorsal and plantar surfaces of the foot are innervated by nerves arising from the sacral plexus.

The major nerves of significance arising from the lumbar plexus to innervate the muscles of the

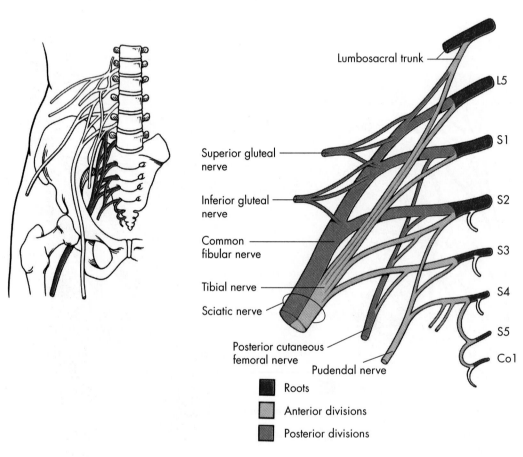

FIG. 9.17 ● The sacral plexus.

hip are the femoral and obturator nerves. The femoral nerve (Fig. 9.18) arises from the posterior division of the lumbar plexus and innervates the anterior muscles of the thigh, including the iliopsoas, rectus femoris, vastus medialis, vastus intermedius, vastus lateralis, pectineus, and sartorius. It also provides sensation to the anterior and lateral thigh and the medial leg and foot. The obturator nerve (Fig. 9.19) arises from the anterior division of the lumbar plexus and provides innervation to the hip adductors, such as the adductor brevis, adductor longus, adductor magnus, and gracilis, as well as the obturator externus. The obturator nerve provides sensation to the medial thigh.

The nerves arising from the sacral plexus that innervate the muscles of the hip are the superior gluteal, inferior gluteal, sciatic, and branches from the sacral plexus. The superior gluteal nerve arises from L4, L5, and S1 to innervate the gluteus medius, gluteus minimus, and tensor fasciae latae. The inferior gluteal nerve arises from L5, S1, and S2 to supply the gluteus maximus. Branches from

FIG. 9.18 ● Muscular and cutaneous distribution of the femoral nerve.

FIG. 9.19 ● Muscular and cutaneous distribution of the obturator nerve.

the sacral plexus innervate the piriformis (S1, S2), gemellus superior (L5, S1, S2), gemellus inferior and obturator internus (L4, L5, S1, S2), and quadratus femoris (L4, L5, S1).

The sciatic nerve is composed of the tibial and common peroneal (fibular) nerves, which are wrapped together in a connective tissue sheath until reaching approximately midways down the posterior thigh. The sciatic nerve tibial division (Fig. 9.20) innervates the semitendinosus, semimembranosus, biceps femoris (long head), and adductor magnus. The sciatic nerve supplies sensation to the anterolateral and posterolateral lower leg as well as most of the dorsal and plantar aspect of the foot. The tibial division provides sensation for the posterolateral lower leg and plantar aspect of the foot, while the peroneal division provides sensation to the anterolateral lower leg and dorsum of the foot. Both of these nerves continue down the lower extremity to provide motor and sensory function to the muscles of the lower leg; this will be addressed in Chapters 10 and 11.

FIG. 9.20 ● Muscular and cutaneous distribution of the tibial nerve.

Iliopsoas muscle   FIG. 9.21

(il´e-o-so´as)

Origin

Iliacus: inner surface of the ilium

Psoas major and minor: lower borders of the transverse processes (L1–L5), sides of the bodies of the last thoracic vertebrae (T12), the lumbar vertebrae (L1–L5), intervertebral fibrocartilages, and base of the sacrum

Insertion

Iliacus and psoas major: lesser trochanter of the femur and the shaft just below

Psoas minor: pectineal line and iliopectineal eminence

Action

Flexion of the hip

External rotation of the femur

Palpation

Difficult to palpate; anterior aspect of hip approximately 1.5 inches below center of inguinal ligament with active hip flexion/extension of supine subject, immediately lateral to pectineus

Innervation

Lumbar nerve and femoral nerve (L2–L4)

Application, strengthening, and flexibility

The iliopsoas is commonly referred to as if it were one muscle, but it is actually composed of the iliacus, the psoas major, and the psoas minor. Some anatomy texts make this distinction and list each muscle individually.

The iliopsoas muscle is powerful in actions such as raising the legs from the floor while in a supine position. The psoas major's origin in the lower back tends to move the lower back anteriorly or, in the supine position, pulls the lower back up as it raises the legs. For this reason, lower back problems are often aggravated by this activity, and bilateral 6-inch leg raises are usually not recommended. The abdominals are the muscles that can be used to prevent this lower back strain by pulling up on the front of the pelvis, thus flattening the back. Leg raising is primarily hip flexion and not abdominal action. Backs may be injured by strenuous and prolonged leg-raising exercises. The iliopsoas contracts strongly, both concentrically and eccentrically, in sit-ups, particularly if the hip is not flexed.

The iliopsoas may be exercised by supporting the arms on a dip bar or parallel bars and then flexing the hips to lift the legs. This may be done initially with the knees flexed in a tucked position to lessen the resistance. As the muscle becomes more developed, the knees can be straightened, which increases the resistance arm length to add more resistance. This concept of increasing or decreasing the resistance by modifying the resistance arm is explained further in Chapter 13.

To stretch the iliopsoas, the hip must be extended so that the femur is behind the plane of the body. In order to somewhat isolate the iliopsoas, full knee flexion should be avoided. Slight additional stretch may be applied by internally rotating the hip while it is extended.

Chapter 9

FIG. 9.21 • Iliopsoas muscle, anterior view. *O*, Origin; *I*, insertion.

Psoas muscle

Iliacus muscle

Flexion
External rotation

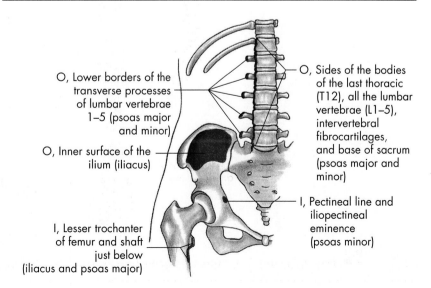

O, Lower borders of the transverse processes of lumbar vertebrae 1–5 (psoas major and minor)

O, Inner surface of the ilium (iliacus)

I, Lesser trochanter of femur and shaft just below (iliacus and psoas major)

O, Sides of the bodies of the last thoracic (T12), all the lumbar vertebrae (L1–5), intervertebral fibrocartilages, and base of sacrum (psoas major and minor)

I, Pectineal line and iliopectineal eminence (psoas minor)

Sartorius muscle   FIG. 9.22

(sar-to´ri-us)

Origin

Anterior superior iliac spine and notch just below
the spine

Insertion

Anterior medial surface of the tibia just below the
condyle

Action

Flexion of the hip
Flexion of the knee
External rotation of the thigh as it flexes the hip and
knee

Palpation

From the anterior superior iliac spine to the medial
tibial condyle during combined resistance of hip
flexion/external rotation/abduction and knee flexion in a supine position

Innervation

Femoral nerve (L2–L3)

Application, strengthening, and flexibility

Pulling from the anterior superior iliac spine and
the notch just below it, the tendency again is to
tilt the pelvis anteriorly (down in front) as this
muscle contracts. The abdominal muscles must
prevent this tendency by posteriorly rotating the
pelvis (pulling up in front), thus flattening the
lower back.

The sartorius, a two-joint muscle, is effective as
a hip flexor or as a knee flexor. It is weak when
both actions take place at the same time. Observe
that, in attempting to cross the knees when in a
sitting position, one customarily leans well back,
thus raising the origin to lengthen this muscle,
making it more effective in flexing and crossing
the knees. With the knees held extended, the sartorius becomes a more effective hip flexor. It is
the longest muscle in the body and is strengthened when hip flexion activities are performed as
described for developing the iliopsoas. Stretching
may be accomplished by a partner passively taking the hip into extreme extension, adduction,
and internal rotation with the knee extended.

Hip flexion

External
rotation

Sartorius m.

Knee flexion

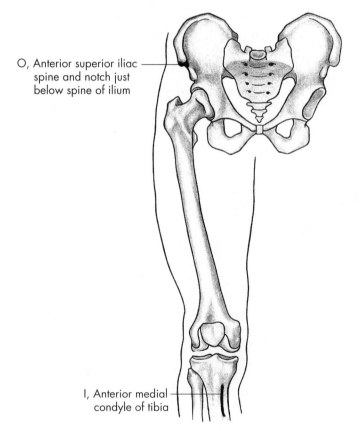

O, Anterior superior iliac
spine and notch just
below spine of ilium

I, Anterior medial
condyle of tibia

FIG. 9.22 ● Sartorius muscle, anterior view. *O*, Origin; *I*, insertion.

Rectus femoris muscle   FIG. 9.23

(rek´tus fem´or-is)

Origin

Anterior inferior iliac spine of the ilium and groove
 (posterior) above the acetabulum

Insertion

Superior aspect of the patella and patellar tendon to
 the tibial tuberosity

Action

Flexion of the hip
Extension of the knee

Palpation

Any place on the anterior surface of the femur

Innervation

Femoral nerve (L2–L4)

Application, strengthening, and flexibility

Pulling from the anterior inferior iliac spine of the
ilium, the rectus femoris muscle has the same tendency to anteriorly rotate the pelvis (down in front
and up in back). Only the abdominal muscles can
prevent this from occurring. In speaking of the hip
flexor group in general, it may be said that many
people permit the pelvis to be permanently tilted
forward as they get older. The relaxed abdominal
wall does not hold the pelvis up; therefore, an increased lumbar curve results.

Generally, a muscle's ability to exert force
decreases as it shortens. This explains why the
rectus femoris muscle is a powerful extensor of
the knee when the hip is extended but is weak
when the hip is flexed. This muscle is exercised,
along with the vastus group, in running, jumping,
hopping, and skipping. In these movements, the
hips are extended powerfully by the gluteus maximus and the hamstring muscles, which counteract the tendency of the rectus femoris muscle to
flex the hip while it extends the knee. It can be
remembered as one of the quadriceps muscle
group. The rectus femoris is developed by performing hip flexion exercises or knee extension
exercises against manual resistance.

The rectus femoris is best stretched in a side-
lying position by having a partner take the knee
into full flexion and simultaneously take the hip
into extension.

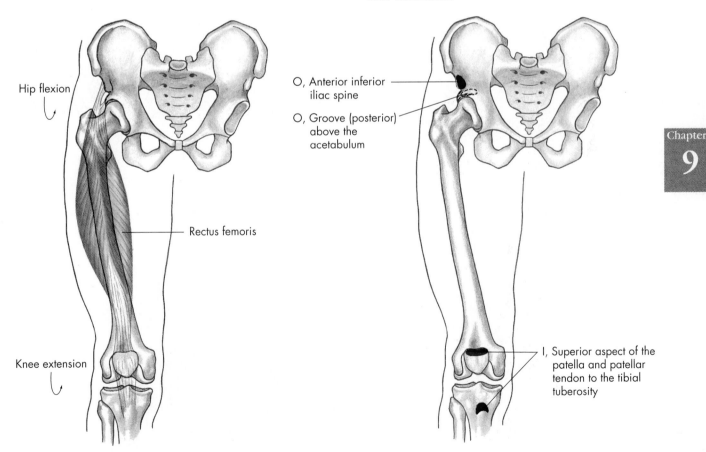

Hip flexion

Rectus femoris

Knee extension

O, Anterior inferior
iliac spine

O, Groove (posterior)
above the
acetabulum

I, Superior aspect of the
patella and patellar
tendon to the tibial
tuberosity

FIG. 9.23 ● Rectus femoris muscle, anterior view. *O,* Origin; *I,* insertion.

Tensor fasciae latae muscle   FIG. 9.24

(ten´sor fas´i-e la´te)

Origin

Anterior iliac crest and surface of the ilium just
  below the crest

Insertion

One-fourth of the way down the thigh into the
  iliotibial tract, which in turn inserts onto Gerdy's
  tubercle of the anterolateral tibial condyle

Action

Abduction of the hip
Flexion of the hip
Tendency to rotate the hip internally as it flexes

Palpation

Between anterior iliac crest and greater trochanter
  during internal rotation and abduction

Innervation

Superior gluteal nerve (L4–L5, S1)

Application, strengthening, and flexibility

The tensor fasciae latae muscle aids in preventing
external rotation of the hip as it is flexed by other
flexor muscles.

The tensor fasciae latae muscle is used when
flexion and internal rotation take place. This is a
weak movement but is important in helping direct
the leg forward so that the foot is placed straight
forward in walking and running. Thus, from the
supine position, raising the leg with definite internal rotation of the femur will call it into action.

The tensor fasciae latae may be developed by
performing hip abduction exercises against gravity and resistance while in a side-lying position.
This is done simply by abducting the hip that is
up and then slowly lowering it back to rest
against the other leg. Stretch may be applied by
remaining on the side and having a partner passively move the downside hip into full extension,
adduction, and external rotation.

Hip flexion

Tensor fasciae
latae m.

Hip abduction

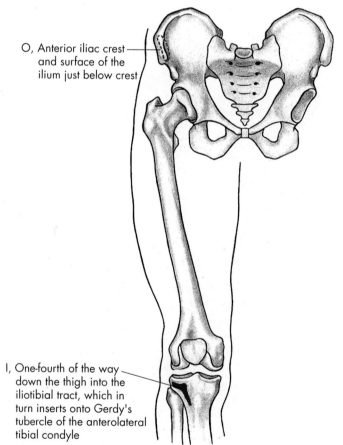

O, Anterior iliac crest
and surface of the
ilium just below crest

I, One-fourth of the way
down the thigh into the
iliotibial tract, which in
turn inserts onto Gerdy's
tubercle of the anterolateral
tibial condyle

FIG. 9.24 ● Tensor fasciae latae muscle, anterior view. *O*, Origin; *I*, insertion.

Gluteus maximus muscle   FIG. 9.25

(glu´te-us maks´i-mus)

Origin

Posterior one-fourth of the crest of the ilium, posterior surface of the sacrum and coccyx near the ilium, and fascia of the lumbar area

Insertion

Oblique ridge on the lateral surface of the greater trochanter and the iliotibial band of the fasciae latae

Action

Extension of the hip
External rotation of the hip
Lower fibers, which assist in adduction

Palpation

Running downward and laterally between posterior iliac crest superiorly, anal cleft medially, and gluteal fold inferiorly, emphasized with hip extension and external rotation

Innervation

Inferior gluteal nerve (L5, S1–S2)

Application, strengthening, and flexibility

The gluteus maximus muscle comes into action when movement between the pelvis and the femur approaches and goes beyond 15 degrees of extension. As a result, it is not used extensively in ordinary walking. It is important in extension of the thigh with external rotation.

Strong action of the gluteus maximus muscle is seen in running, hopping, skipping, and jumping. Powerful extension of the thigh is secured in the return to standing from a squatting position, especially if a barbell with weights is placed on the shoulders.

Hip extension exercises from a forward-leaning or prone position may be used to develop this muscle. This muscle is most emphasized when the hip starts from a flexed position and moves to full extension, with the knee flexed 30 degrees or more to reduce the hamstrings' involvement in the action.

The gluteus maximus is stretched in the supine position with full hip flexion to the ipsilateral axilla and then to the contralateral axilla with the knee in flexion. Simultaneous internal hip rotation accentuates this stretch.

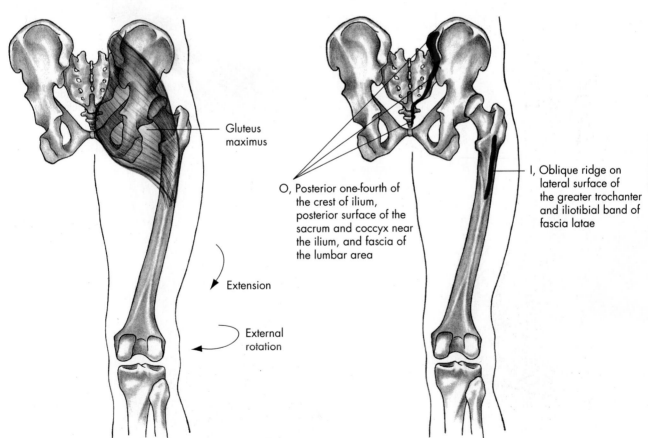

FIG. 9.25 ● Gluteus maximus muscle, posterior view. *O,* Origin; *I,* insertion.

Gluteus medius muscle   FIG. 9.26

(glu´te-us me´di-us)

Origin

Lateral surface of the ilium just below the crest

Insertion

Posterior and middle surfaces of the greater
   trochanter of the femur

Action

Abduction of the hip
External rotation as the hip abducts (posterior fibers)
Internal rotation (anterior fibers)

Palpation

Slightly in front of and a few inches above the
   greater trochanter with active elevation of opposite
   pelvis from a standing position

Innervation

Superior gluteal nerve (L4–L5, S1)

Application, strengthening, and flexibility

Typical action of the gluteus medius and gluteus
minimus muscles is seen in walking. As the weight
of the body is suspended on one leg, these muscles prevent the opposite pelvis from sagging.
Weakness in the gluteus medius and gluteus
minimus can result in the Trendelenburg gait.
With this weakness, the individual's opposite
pelvis will sag on weight bearing because the hip
abductors cannot maintain proper alignment.

Hip external rotation exercises performed
against resistance can provide some strengthening for the gluteus medius, but it is best strengthened by performing the side-lying leg raises or
hip abduction exercises as described for the tensor fasciae latae. The gluteus medius is best
stretched by moving the hip into extreme adduction in front of the opposite extremity and then
behind it.

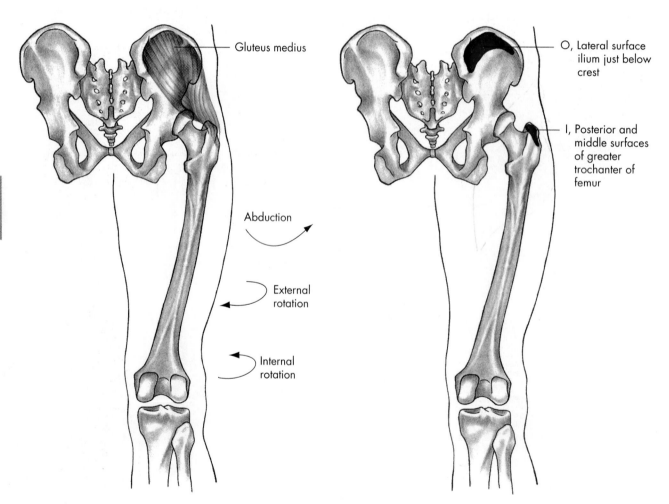

FIG. 9.26 ● Gluteus medius muscle, posterior view. *O*, Origin; *I*, insertion.

Gluteus minimus muscle   FIG. 9.27

(glu´te-us min´i-mus)

Origin

Lateral surface of the ilium just below the origin of the gluteus medius

Insertion

Anterior surface of the greater trochanter of the femur

Action

Abduction of the hip
Internal rotation as the femur abducts

Palpation

Covered by tensor fasciae latae between anterior iliac crest and greater trochanter during internal rotation and abduction

Innervation

Superior gluteal nerve (L4–L5, S1)

Application, strengthening, and flexibility

Both the gluteus minimus and the gluteus medius are used in powerfully maintaining proper hip abduction while running. As a result, both of these muscles are exercised effectively in running, hopping, and skipping, in which weight is transferred forcefully from one foot to the other. As the body ages, the gluteus medius and gluteus minimus muscles tend to lose their effectiveness. The spring of youth, as far as the hips are concerned, resides in these muscles. To have great drive in the legs, these muscles must be fully developed.

The gluteus minimus is best strengthened by performing hip abduction exercises similar to the ones described for the tensor fasciae latae and gluteus medius muscles. It may also be developed by performing hip internal rotation exercises against manual resistance. Stretching of this muscle is accomplished by extreme hip adduction with slight external rotation.

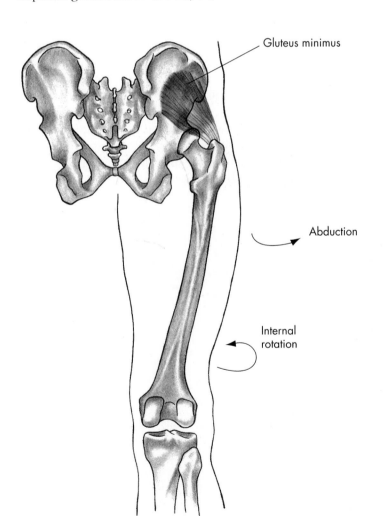

Gluteus minimus

Abduction

Internal rotation

O, Lateral surface of ilium below the origin of gluteus medius

I, Anterior surface of greater trochanter of femur

FIG. 9.27 ● Gluteus minimus muscle, posterior view. *O*, Origin; *I*, insertion.

The six deep lateral rotator muscles—

FIG. 9.28

piriformis (pi-ri-for´mis),
gemellus superior (je-mel´us su-pe´ri-or),
gemellus inferior (je-mel´us in-fe´ri-or),
obturator externus (ob-tu-ra´tor eks-ter´nus),
obturator internus (ob-tu-ra´tor in-ter´nus),
quadratus femoris (kwad-ra´tus fem´or-is)

Origin
Anterior sacrum, posterior portions of the ischium, and obturator foramen

Insertion
Superior and posterior aspect of the greater trochanter

Action
External rotation of the hip

Palpation
Although not directly palpable, deep palpation is possible with the subject prone during relaxation of the gluteus maximus while passively using the lower leg flexed at the knee to internally and externally rotate the femur

Innervation
Piriformis: first or second sacral nerve (S1–S2)
Gemellus superior: sacral nerve (L5, S1–S2)
Gemellus inferior: branches from sacral plexus (L4–L5, S1–S2)
Obturator externus: obturator nerve (L3–L4)
Obturator internus: branches from sacral plexus (L4–L5, S1–S2)
Quadratus femoris: branches from sacral plexus (L4–L5, S1)

Application, strengthening, and flexibility

The six lateral rotators are used powerfully in movements of external rotation of the femur, as in sports in which the individual takes off on one leg from a preliminary internal rotation. Throwing a baseball and swinging a baseball bat, in which there is rotation of the hip, are typical examples.

Standing on one leg and forcefully turning the body away from that leg is accomplished by contraction of these muscles, and it may be repeated for strengthening purposes. A partner may provide resistance as development progresses. The six deep lateral rotators may be stretched in the supine position with a partner passively internally rotating and slightly flexing the hip.

Of special note, the sciatic nerve usually passes just inferior to the piriformis muscle but may pass through it. As a result, tightness in the piriformis muscle may contribute to compression on the sciatic nerve. The piriformis may be stretched by having the subject lie on the uninvolved side with a partner passively taking the hip into full internal rotation combined with hip adduction and slight to moderate hip flexion.

FIG. 9.28 ● The six deep lateral rotator muscles, posterior view: piriformis, gemellus superior, gemellus inferior, obturator externus, obturator internus, and quadratus femoris.

Semitendinosus muscle   FIG. 9.29

(sem´i-ten-di-no´sus)

Origin

Ischial tuberosity

Insertion

Anterior medial surface of the tibia just below the condyle

Action

Extension of the hip
Flexion of the knee
Internal rotation of the hip
Internal rotation of the flexed knee

Palpation

Posteromedial aspect of distal thigh with combined knee flexion and internal rotation against resistance

Innervation

Sciatic nerve—tibial division (L5, S1–S2)

Application, strengthening, and flexibility

This two-joint muscle is most effective when contracting to either extend the hip or flex the knee. When there is extension of the hip and flexion of the knee at the same time, both movements are weak. When the trunk is bent forward with the knees straight, the hamstring muscles have a powerful pull on the rear pelvis and tilt it down in back by full contraction. If the knees are flexed when this movement takes place, one can observe that the work is done chiefly by the gluteus maximus muscle.

On the other hand, when the muscles are used in powerful flexion of the knees, as in hanging by the knees from a bar, the flexors of the hip come into play to raise the origin of these muscles and make them more effective as knee flexors. By full extension of the hips in this movement, the knee flexion movement is weakened. These muscles are used in ordinary walking as extensors of the hip and allow the gluteus maximus to relax in the movement.

The semitendinosus is best developed through knee flexion exercises against resistance. Commonly known as hamstring curls or leg curls, they may be performed in a prone position on a knee table or standing with ankle weights attached. This muscle is emphasized when performing hamstring curls while attempting to maintain the knee joint in internal rotation. This internally rotated position brings its insertion in alignment with its origin.

The semitendinosus is stretched by maximally extending the knee while flexing the internally rotated and slightly abducted hip.

FIG. 9.29 ● Semitendinosus muscle, posterior view. *O*, Origin; *I*, insertion.

Semimembranosus muscle   FIG. 9.30

(sem´i-mem´bra-no´sus)

Origin
Ischial tuberosity

Insertion
Posteromedial surface of the medial tibial condyle

Action
Extension of the hip
Flexion of the knee
Internal rotation of the hip
Internal rotation of the flexed knee

Palpation
Largely covered by other muscles, the tendon can be felt at the posteromedial aspect of the knee with combined knee flexion and internal rotation against resistance

Innervation
Sciatic nerve—tibial division (L5, S1–S2)

Application, strengthening, and flexibility

Both the semitendinosus and semimembranosus are responsible for internal rotation of the knee, along with the popliteus muscle, which is discussed in the next chapter. Because of the manner in which they cross the joint, the muscles are very important in providing dynamic medial stability to the knee joint.

The semimembranosus is best developed by performing leg curls. Internal rotation of the knee throughout the range accentuates the activity of this muscle. The semimembranosus is stretched in the same manner as the semitendinosus.

FIG. 9.30 ● Semimembranosus muscle, posterior view. *O*, Origin; *I*, insertion.

Biceps femoris muscle   FIG. 9.31

(bi´seps fem´or-is)

Origin

Long head: ischial tuberosity
Short head: lower half of the linea aspera, and
   lateral condyloid ridge

Insertion

Lateral condyle of the tibia and head of the fibula

Action

Extension of the hip
Flexion of the knee
External rotation of the hip
External rotation of the flexed knee

Palpation

Posterolateral aspect of distal thigh with combined
   knee flexion and external rotation against resistance

Innervation

Long head: sciatic nerve—tibial division (S1–S3)
Short head: sciatic nerve—peroneal division
   (L5, S1–S2)

Application, strengthening, and flexibility

The semitendinosus, semimembranosus, and biceps femoris muscles are known as the hamstrings. These muscles, together with the gluteus
maximus muscle, are used in extension of the hip
when the knees are straight or nearly so. Thus, in
running, jumping, skipping, and hopping, these
muscles are used together. The hamstrings are
used without the aid of the gluteus maximus,
however, when one is hanging from a bar by the
knees. Similarly, the gluteus maximus is used
without the aid of the hamstrings when the knees
are flexed while the hips are being extended. This
occurs when rising from a knee-bend position to
a standing position.

The biceps femoris is best developed through
hamstring curls as described for the semitendinosus, but it is emphasized more if the knee is
maintained in external rotation throughout the
range of motion, which brings the origin and insertion more in line with each other. The biceps
femoris is stretched by maximally extending the
knee while flexing the externally rotated and
slightly adducted hip.

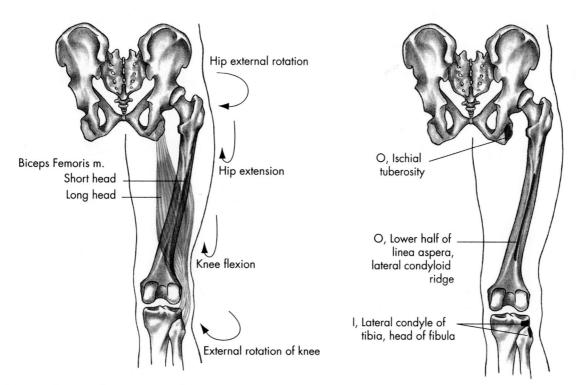

FIG. 9.31 ● Biceps femoris muscle, posterior view. *O*, Origin; *I*, insertion.

Adductor brevis muscle   FIG. 9.32

(ad-duk´tor bre´vis)

Origin

Front of the inferior pubic ramus just below the
origin of the longus

Insertion

Lower two-thirds of the pectineal line of the femur
and the upper half of the medial lip of the linea
aspera

Action

Adduction of the hip
External rotation as it adducts the hip

Palpation

Very difficult to palpate and differentiate from adductor longus, which is immediately inferior

Innervation

Obturator nerve (L3–L4)

Application, strengthening, and flexibility

The adductor brevis muscle, along with the other
adductor muscles, provides powerful movement
of the thighs toward each other. Squeezing the
legs together toward each other against resistance
is effective in strengthening the adductor brevis.
Abducting the extended and internally rotated hip
provides stretching of the adductor brevis.

Adductor brevis m.

Adduction

External rotation

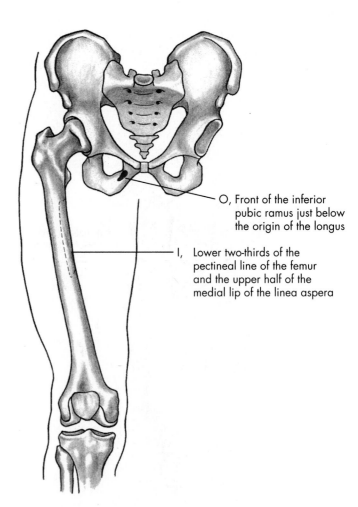

O, Front of the inferior
pubic ramus just below
the origin of the longus

I, Lower two-thirds of the
pectineal line of the femur
and the upper half of the
medial lip of the linea aspera

FIG. 9.32 ● Adductor brevis muscle, anterior view. *O*, Origin; *I*, insertion.

Chapter 9

Adductor longus muscle   FIG. 9.33
(ad-duk´tor long´gus)

Origin
Anterior pubis just below its crest

Insertion
Middle third of the linea aspera

Action
Adduction of the hip
Assists in flexion of the hip

Palpation
Just inferior to the pubic bone on upper medial side
    of thigh with resisted adduction

Innervation
Obturator nerve (L3–L4)

Application, strengthening, and flexibility
The muscle may be strengthened by using the scissors exercise, which requires the subject to sit on the floor with the legs spread wide while a partner puts his or her legs or arms inside each lower leg to provide resistance. As the subject attempts to adduct his or her legs together, the partner provides manual resistance throughout the range of motion. This exercise may be used for either one or both legs. The adductor longus is stretched in the same manner as the adductor brevis.

Adductor longus m.

Adduction

O, Anterior pubis
just below its crest

I, Middle third
of linea aspera

FIG. 9.33 ● Adductor longus muscle, anterior view. *O*, Origin; *I*, insertion.

Adductor magnus muscle   FIG. 9.34
(ad-duk´tor mag´nus)

Origin
Edge of the entire ramus of the pubis and the ischium and ischial tuberosity

Insertion
Whole length of the linea aspera, inner condyloid ridge, and adductor tubercle

Action
Adduction of the hip

External rotation as the hip adducts

Palpation
Medial aspect of thigh from ischial tuberosity to adductor tubercle with resisted adduction from abducted position

Innervation
Anterior: obturator nerve (L2–L4)

Posterior: sciatic nerve (L4–L5, S1–S3)

Application, strengthening, and flexibility

The adductor magnus muscle is used in the breaststroke kick in swimming or in horseback riding. Since the adductor muscles (adductor magnus, adductor longus, adductor brevis, and gracilis muscles) are not heavily used in ordinary movement, some prescribed activity for them should be provided. Some modern exercise equipment is engineered to provide resistance for hip adduction movement. Hip adduction exercises such as those described for the adductor brevis and the adductor longus may be used for strengthening the adductor magnus as well. The adductor magnus is stretched in the same manner as the adductor brevis and adductor longus.

O, Edge of entire ramus of the pubis and the ischium and ischial tuberosity

I, Whole length of linea aspera, inner condyloid ridge and adductor tubercle

External rotation

Adduction

Adductor magnus m.

FIG. 9.34 ● Adductor magnus muscle, posterior view. *O*, Origin; *I*, insertion.

Pectineus muscle FIG. 9.35

(pek-tin´e-us)

Origin

Space 1 inch wide on the front of the pubis just above the crest

Insertion

Rough line leading from the lesser trochanter down to the linea aspera

Action

Flexion of the hip
Adduction of the hip
Internal rotation of the hip

Palpation

Difficult to palpate; anterior aspect of hip approximately 1.5 inches below center of inguinal ligament with active hip flexion/extension of supine subject, immediately medial to iliopsoas

Innervation

Femoral nerve (L2–L4)

Application, strengthening, and flexibility

As the pectineus contracts, it also tends to rotate the pelvis anteriorly. The abdominal muscles pulling up on the pelvis in front prevent this tilting action.

The pectineus muscle is exercised together with the iliopsoas muscle in leg raising and lowering. Hip flexion exercises and hip adduction exercises against resistance may be used for strengthening this muscle.

The pectineus is stretched by fully abducting the extended and externally rotated hip.

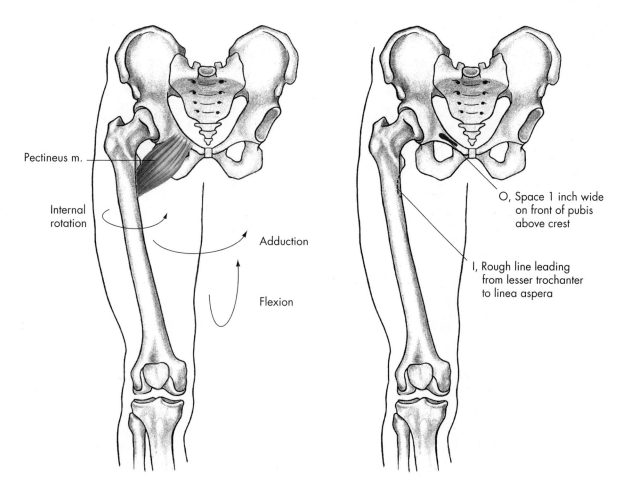

Pectineus m.

Internal rotation

Adduction

Flexion

O, Space 1 inch wide on front of pubis above crest

I, Rough line leading from lesser trochanter to linea aspera

FIG. 9.35 ● Pectineus muscle, anterior view. *O*, Origin; *I*, insertion.

Gracilis muscle FIG. 9.36

(gras´-il-is)

Origin

Anteromedial edge of the descending ramus of the pubis

Insertion

Anterior medial surface of the tibia just below the condyle

Action

Adduction of the hip
Flexion of the knee
Internal rotation of the hip

Palpation

A thin tendon on anteromedial thigh with knee flexion and resisted adduction

Innervation

Obturator nerve (L2–L4)

Application, strengthening, and flexibility

The gracilis muscle performs the same function as the other adductors, but adds some weak assistance to knee flexion.

The adductor muscles as a group (adductor magnus, adductor longus, adductor brevis, and gracilis) are called into action in horseback riding and in doing the breaststroke kick in swimming. Proper development of the adductor group prevents soreness after participation in these sports. The gracilis is strengthened with the same exercises as described for the other hip adductors. The gracilis may be stretched in a manner similar to the adductors, except that the knee must be extended.

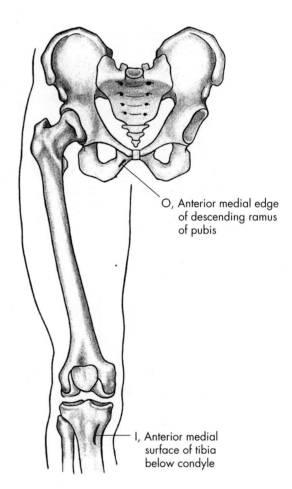

FIG. 9.36 ● Gracilis muscle, anterior view. *O*, Origin; *I*, insertion.

Web sites

Anatomy & Physiology Tutorials:

www.gwc.maricopa.edu/class/bio201/index.htm

Radiologic Anatomy Browser:

**radlinux1.usuf1.usuhs.mil/rad/iong/
index.html**

This site has numerous radiological views of the musculoskeletal system.

University of Arkansas Medical School Gross Anatomy for Medical Students:

**anatomy.uams.edu/htmlpages/anatomyhtml/
gross.html**

Dissections, anatomy tables, atlas images, links, etc.

Loyola University Medical Center: Structure of the Human Body:

**www.meddean.luc.edu/lumen/MedEd/
GrossAnatomy/GA.html**

An excellent site with many slides, dissections, tutorials, etc., for the study of human anatomy.

Wheeless's Textbook of Orthopaedics:

www.ortho-u.net/

This site has an extensive index of links to the fractures, joints, muscles, nerves, trauma, medications, medical topics, and lab tests, as well as links to orthopedic journals and other orthopedic and medical news.

Premiere Medical Search Engine:

www.medsite.com

This site allows the reader to enter any medical condition and it will search the net to find relevant articles.

Virtual Hospital:

www.vh.org

Numerous slides, patient information, etc.

Dynamic Human version 2.0 CD-ROM: The Visual Guide to Anatomy & Physiology:

www.mhhe.com/biosci/ap/dynamichuman2/

Web site that accompanies this CD-ROM.

Worksheet exercises

As an aid to learning, for in-class or out-of-class assignments, or for testing, tear-out worksheets are found at the end of the text (pp. 333 and 334).

Anterior skeletal worksheet (no. 1)

Draw and label on the worksheet the anterior hip joint and pelvic girdle muscles.

Posterior skeletal worksheet (no. 2)

Draw and label on the worksheet the anterior hip joint and pelvic girdle muscles.

Laboratory and review exercises

1. Locate the following parts of the pelvic girdle and hip joint on a human skeleton and on a subject:
   a. Skeleton
      1. Ilium
      2. Ischium
      3. Pubis
      4. Symphysis pubis
      5. Acetabulum
      6. Rami (ascending and descending)
      7. Obturator foramen
      8. Ischial tuberosity
      9. Anterior superior iliac spine
      10. Greater trochanter
      11. Lesser trochanter
   b. Subject
      1. Crest of ilium
      2. Anterior superior iliac spine
      3. Ischial tuberosity
      4. Greater trochanter
2. How and where can the following muscles be palpated on a human subject?
   a. Gracilis
   b. Sartorius
   c. Gluteus maximus
   d. Gluteus medius
   e. Gluteus minimus
   f. Biceps femoris
   g. Rectus femoris
   h. Semimembranosus
   i. Semitendinosus
   j. Adductor magnus
   k. Adductor longus
   l. Adductor brevis

Chapter 9

3. Be prepared to indicate on a human skeleton, using a long rubber band, where each muscle has its origin and insertion.
4. Distinguish between hip flexion and trunk flexion.
5. Demonstrate the movement and list the muscles primarily responsible for the following hip movements:
   a. Flexion
   b. Extension
   c. Adduction
   d. Abduction
   e. External rotation
   f. Internal rotation
6. List the planes in which each of the following hip joint movements occur. List the respective axis of rotation for each movement in each plane.
   a. Flexion
   b. Extension
   c. Adduction
   d. Abduction
   e. External rotation
   f. Internal rotation
7. How is walking different from running in relation to the use of the hip joint muscle actions and the range of motion?
8. How may the walking gait be affected by a weakness in the gluteus medius muscle? Have a laboratory partner demonstrate the gait pattern associated with gluteus medius weakness. What is the name of this dysfunctional gait?
9. How might bilateral iliopsoas tightness affect the posture and movement of the lumbar spine in the standing position? Demonstrate and discuss this effect with a laboratory partner.
10. How might bilateral hamstring tightness affect the posture and movement of the lumbar spine in the standing position? Demonstrate and discuss this effect with a laboratory partner.
11. Fill in the muscle analysis chart below by listing the muscles primarily involved in each movement.
12. Fill in the antagonistic muscle action chart on the next page by listing the muscle(s) or parts of muscles that are antagonistic in their actions to the muscles in the left column.

Muscle analysis chart • Hip joint

Flexion	Extension
Abduction	Adduction
External rotation	Internal rotation

Antagonistic muscle action chart • Hip joint and pelvic girdle

Agonist	Antagonist
Gluteus maximus	
Gluteus medius	
Gluteus minimas	
Biceps femoris	
Semimembranosus/ semitendinosus	
Adductor magnus/ adductor brevis	
Adductor longus	
Gracilis	
Lateral rotators	
Rectus femoris	
Sartorius	
Pectineus	
Iliopsoas	
Tensor fasciae latae	

Chapter

9

References

Field D: *Anatomy: palpation and surface markings,* ed 3, Oxford, 2001, Butterworth-Heinemann.

Hamilton N, Luttgens K: *Kinesiology: scientific basis of human motion,* ed 10, Boston, 2002, McGraw-Hill.

Hislop HJ, Montgomery J: *Daniels and Worthingham's muscle testing: techniques of manual examination,* ed 6, Philadelphia, 1995, Saunders.

Kendall FP, McCreary EK, Provance, PG: *Muscles: testing and function,* ed 4, Baltimore, 1993, Lippincott Williams & Wilkins.

Lindsay DT: *Functional human anatomy,* St. Louis, 1996, Mosby.

Lysholm J, Wikland J: Injuries in runners, *American Journal of Sports Medicine* 15:168, September–October 1986.

Noahes TD, et al: Pelvic stress fractures in long distance runners, *American Journal of Sports Medicine* 13:120, March–April 1985.

Perreira J: Treating the quadriceps contusion, *Scholastic Coach* 57:38, October 1987.

Seeley RR, Stephens TD, Tate P: *Anatomy & physiology,* ed 6, Dubuque, IA, 2003, McGraw-Hill.

Sieg KW, Adams SP: *Illustrated essentials of musculoskeletal anatomy,* ed 2, Gainesville, FL, 1985, Megabooks.

Stone RJ, Stone JA: *Atlas of the skeletal muscles,* 1990, McGraw-Hill Companies Inc., New York.

Thibodeau GA, Patton KT: *Anatomy & physiology,* ed 9, St. Louis, 1993, Mosby.

Van de Graaff KM: *Human anatomy,* ed 6, Dubuque, IA. 2002, WCB McGraw-Hill.

The Knee Joint

Objectives

- To identify on a human skeleton selected bony features of the knee

- To explain the cartilaginous and ligamentous structures of the knee joint

- To draw and label on a skeletal chart muscles and ligaments of the knee joint

- To palpate the superficial knee joint structures and muscles on a human subject

- To demonstrate and palpate with a fellow student all the movements of the knee joint and list their respective planes of motion and axes of rotation

- To name and explain the actions and importance of the quadriceps and hamstring muscles

- To list and organize the muscles that produce the movements of the knee joint and list their antagonists

---

Online Learning Center Resources

Visit *Manual of Structural Kinesiology's* **Online Learning Center** at **www.mhhe.com/floyd15e** for additional information and study material for this chapter, including:

- *Self-grading quizzes*
- *Anatomy flashcards*
- *Animations*

The knee joint is the largest joint in the body and is very complex. It is primarily a hinge joint. The combined functions of weight bearing and locomotion place considerable stress and strain on the knee joint. Powerful knee joint extensor and flexor muscles, combined with a strong ligamentous structure, provide a strong functioning joint in most instances.

Bones   FIG. 10.1

The enlarged femoral condyles articulate on the enlarged condyles of the tibia, somewhat in a horizontal line. Since the femur projects downward at an oblique angle toward the midline, its medial condyle is slightly larger than the lateral condyle.

The top of the medial and lateral tibial condyles, known as the medial and lateral tibial plateaus, serve as receptacles for the femoral condyles. The tibia is the medial bone in the leg and bears much more of the body's weight than the fibula. The fibula serves as the attachment for some very important knee joint structures, although it does not articulate with the femur or patella and is not part of the knee joint.

The patella is a sesamoid (floating) bone contained within the quadriceps muscle group and patellar tendon. Its location allows it to serve the quadriceps in a fashion similar to the work of a pulley by creating an improved angle of pull. This results in a greater mechanical advantage when performing knee extension.

Key bony landmarks of the knee include the superior and inferior poles of the patella, the tibial tuberosity, Gerdy's tubercle, the medial and lateral femoral condyles, the upper anterior medial surface of the tibia, and the head of the fibula.

Anterior view with patella removed

Femur

Lateral condyle of femur

Medial condyle of femur

Posterior cruciate ligament

Anterior cruciate ligament

Lateral meniscus

Medial meniscus

Fibular (lateral) collateral ligament

Tibial (medial) collateral ligament

Gerdy's tubercle

Superior tibiofibular joint

Tibial tuberosity

Fibula

Tibia

Posterior view

Femur

Ligament of Wrisberg

Anterior cruciate ligament

Medial femoral condyle

Lateral femoral condyle

Medial meniscus

Lateral meniscus

Posterior cruciate ligament

Lateral tibial condyle

Tibial (medial) collateral ligament

Fibular (lateral) collateral ligament

Tibial collateral ligament

Superior tibiofibular joint

Tibia

Fibula

Superior view with femur removed

Anterior cruciate ligament

Tibial tuberosity

Medial meniscus

Transverse ligament

Lateral tibial plateau

Medial tibial plateau

Lateral meniscus

Posterior cruciate ligament

Ligament of Wrisberg

FIG. 10.1 ● Ligaments and menisci of the right knee.

Modified from Anthony CP, Kolthoff NJ: *Textbook of anatomy and physiology,* ed 9, St. Louis, 1975, Mosby.

The three vasti muscles of the quadriceps originate on the proximal femur and insert on the superior pole of the patella. From here their insertion is ultimately on the tibial tuberosity by way of the large patella tendon, which runs from the inferior patellar pole to the tibial tuberosity. Gerdy's tubercle, located on the anterolateral aspect of the lateral tibial condyle is the insertion point for the iliotibial tract of the tensor fasciae latae.

The upper anteromedial surface of the tibia just below the medial condyle serves as the insertion for the sartorius, gracilis, and semitendinosus. The semimembranosus inserts posteromedially on the medial tibial condyle. The head of the fibula is the primary location of the biceps femoris insertion, although some of its fibers insert on the lateral tibial condyle. The popliteus origin is located on the lateral aspect of the lateral femoral condyle.

Additionally, the tibial collateral ligament originates on the medial aspect of the upper medial femoral condyle and inserts on the medial surface of the tibia. Laterally, the shorter fibula collateral originates on the lateral femoral condyle very close to the popliteus origin and inserts on the head of the fibula.

Joints   FIGS. 10.1 and 10.2

The knee joint proper, or tibiofemoral joint, is classified as a ginglymus joint because it functions like a hinge. It moves between flexion and extension without side-to-side movement into abduction or adduction. However, it is sometimes referred to as a trochoginglymus joint because of the internal and external rotation movements that can occur during flexion. Some authorities argue that it should be classified as a condyloid or "double condyloid" joint due to its bicondylar structure. The patellofemoral joint is classified as an arthrodial joint due to the gliding nature of the patella on the femoral condyles.

The ligaments provide static stability to the knee joint, and contractions of the quadriceps and hamstrings produce dynamic stability. The surfaces between the femur and tibia are protected by articular cartilage, as is true of all diarthrodial joints. In addition to the articular cartilage covering the ends of the bones, there are specialized cartilages (see Fig. 10.1), known as the menisci, that form cushions between the bones. These menisci are attached to the tibia and deepen the tibial fossa, thereby enhancing stability.

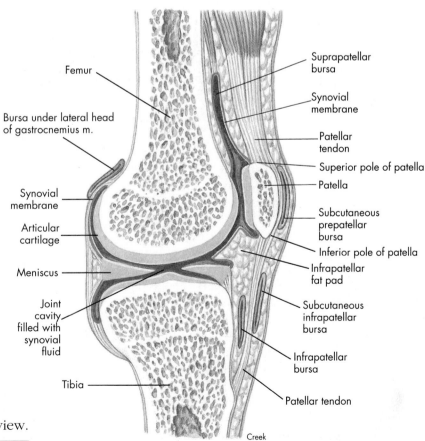

FIG. 10.2 ● Knee joint, sagittal view.

The medial semilunar cartilage or, more technically, the medial meniscus, is located on the medial tibial plateau to form a receptacle for the medial femoral condyle. The lateral semilunar cartilage (lateral meniscus) sits on the lateral tibial plateau to receive the lateral femoral condyle. Both of these menisci are thicker on the outside border and taper down to be very thin on the inside border. They can slip about slightly and are held in place by various small ligaments. The medial meniscus is the larger of the two and has a much more open C appearance than the rather closed C lateral meniscus configuration. Either or both of the menisci may be torn in several different areas from a variety of mechanisms, resulting in varying degrees of severity and problems. These injuries often occur due to the significant compression and shear forces that develop as the knee rotates while flexing or extending during quick directional changes in running.

Two very important ligaments of the knee are the anterior and posterior cruciate, so named because they cross within the knee between the tibia and the femur. These ligaments are vital in respectively maintaining the anterior and posterior stability of the knee joint, as well as the rotatory stability (see Fig. 10.1).

The anterior cruciate ligament (ACL) tear is one of the most common serious injuries to the knee. The mechanism of this injury often involves non-contact rotary forces associated with planting and cutting. Studies have also shown that the ACL may be disrupted in a hyperextension mechanism or solely by a violent contraction of the quadriceps that pulls the tibia forward on the femur. Fortunately, the posterior cruciate ligament (PCL) is not often injured. Injuries of the posterior cruciate usually come about through direct contact with an opponent or with the playing surface.

On the medial side of the knee is the tibial (medial) collateral ligament (MCL) (see Fig. 10.1), which maintains medial stability by resisting valgus forces or preventing the knee joint from being abducted. Injuries to the tibial collateral occur quite commonly, particularly in contact or collision sports in which a teammate or an opponent falls against the lateral aspect of the knee or leg, causing medial opening of the knee joint and stress to the medial ligamentous structures. Its deeper fibers are attached to the medial meniscus, which may be affected with injuries to the ligament.

On the lateral side of the knee, the fibular (lateral) collateral ligament (LCL) joins the fibula and the femur. Injuries to this ligament are infrequent.

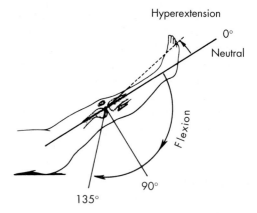

FIG. 10.3 ● Active motion of the knee. Flexion is measured in degrees from the zero starting position, which is an extended straight leg with the athlete either prone or supine. Hyperextension is measured with degrees opposite the zero starting point.

In addition to the other intraarticular ligaments detailed in Fig. 10.1, there are numerous other ligaments not shown that are contiguous with the joint capsule. Generally, these ligaments are of lesser importance and will not be discussed further.*

The knee joint, as shown in Fig. 10.2, is well supplied with synovial fluid from the synovial cavity, which lies under the patella and between the surfaces of the tibia and the femur. Commonly, this synovial cavity is called the "capsule of the knee." Just posterior to the patellar tendon is the infrapatellar fat pad, which is often an insertion point for synovial folds of tissue known as "plica." A plica is an anatomical variant among some individuals that may be irritated or inflamed with injuries or overuse of the knee. More than 10 bursae are located in the knee, some of which are connected to the synovial cavity. Bursae are located where they can absorb shock or prevent friction.

The knee can usually extend to 180 degrees or a straight line, although it is not uncommon for some knees to hyperextend up to 10 degrees or more. When the knee is in full extension, it can move from there to about 140 degrees of flexion. With the knee flexed 30 degrees or more, approximately 30 degrees of internal rotation and 45 degrees of external rotation can occur (Fig. 10.3).

Due to the shape of the medial femoral condyle, the knee must "screw home" to fully extend. As the

---

*More detailed discussion of the knee is found in anatomy texts and athletic training manuals.

knee approaches full extension, the tibia must externally rotate approximately 10 degrees to achieve proper alignment of the tibial and femoral condyles. In full extension, due to the close congruency of the articular surfaces, there is no appreciable rotation of the knee. During initial flexion from a fully extended position, the knee "unlocks" by the tibia rotating internally, to a degree, from its externally rotated position to achieve flexion.

Movements   FIG. 10.4

Flexion and extension of the knee occur in the sagittal plane, whereas internal and external rotation occur in the horizontal plane. The knee will not allow rotation unless it is flexed 20 to 30 degrees or more.

Flexion: bending or decreasing the angle between the femur and lower leg; characterized by the heel moving toward the buttocks

Extension: straightening or increasing the angle between the femur and the lower leg

External rotation: rotary movement of the lower leg laterally away from the midline

Internal rotation: rotary movement of the lower leg medially toward the midline

Muscles   FIG 9.9

Some of the muscles involved in knee joint movements were discussed in Chapter 9 because of their biarticular arrangement with both the hip and knee joints. As a result, they will not be covered again fully in this chapter. The knee joint muscles that have already been addressed are

Knee extensor: rectus femoris
Knee flexors: sartorius, biceps femoris, semitendinosus, semimembranosus, and gracilis

The gastrocnemius muscle, discussed in Chapter 11, also assists minimally with knee flexion.

The muscle group that extends the knee is located in the anterior compartment of the thigh, and is known as the quadriceps. It consists of four muscles: the rectus femoris, the vastus lateralis, the vastus intermedius, and the vastus medialis. The hamstring muscle group is located in the posterior compartment of the thigh and is responsible for knee flexion. The hamstrings consist of three muscles: the semitendinosus, the semimembranosus, and the biceps femoris. The semimembranosus and semitendinosus muscles (medial hamstrings) are assisted by the popliteus in internally rotating the knee, whereas the biceps femoris (lateral hamstring) is responsible for knee external rotation.

Flexion
A

Extension
B

Internal rotation
C

External rotation
D

FIG. 10.4 ● Movements of the knee with prime movers illustrated.

Chapter
10

Two-joint muscles are most effective when either the origin or the insertion is stabilized to prevent movement in the direction of the muscle when it contracts. Additionally, muscles are able to exert greater force when lengthened than when shortened. All of the hamstring muscles, as well as the rectus femoris, sartorius, and gracilis, are biarticular (two-joint) muscles.

As an example, the sartorius muscle becomes a better flexor at the knee when the pelvis is rotated posteriorly and stabilized by the abdominal muscles, thus increasing its total length by moving its origin farther from its insertion. This is exemplified by trying to flex the knee and cross the legs in the sitting position. One usually leans backward to flex the legs at the knees. Again, this is illustrated by kicking a football. The kicker invariably leans well backward to raise and fix the origin of the rectus femoris muscle to make it more effective as an extensor of the leg at the knee. Also, when youngsters hang by the knees, they flex the hips to fix or raise the origin of the hamstrings to make the latter more effective flexors of the knees.

The sartorius, gracilis, and semitendinosus all join together distally to form a tendinous expansion, known as the pes anserinus, which attaches to the anteromedial aspect of the proximal tibia below the level of the tibial tuberosity. This attachment and the line of pull these muscles have posteromedially to the knee enable them to assist with knee flexion, particularly once the knee is flexed and the hip is externally rotated. The medial and lateral heads of the gastrocnemius attach posteriorly on the medial and lateral femoral condyles, respectively. This relationship to the knee provides the gastrocnemius a line of pull to assist with knee flexion.

Knee joint muscles—location

Muscle location closely relates to muscle function with the knee. While viewing the muscles, in Fig. 9.9, correlate them with Table 10.1.

Anterior
  Primarily knee extension
        Rectus femoris*†
        Vastus medialis
        Vastus intermedius
        Vastus lateralis
Posterior
  Primarily knee flexion
        Biceps femoris*†
        Semimembranosus*†
        Semitendinosus*†
        Sartorius*†
        Gracilis*†
        Popliteus
        Gastrocnemius*†

Nerves

The femoral nerve (Fig. 9.18) innervates the knee extensors—rectus femoris, vastus medialis, vastus intermedius, and vastus lateralis. The knee flexors, consisting of the semitendinosus, semimembranosus, biceps femoris (long head), and popliteus are innervated by the tibial division of the sciatic nerve (Fig. 9.20). The biceps femoris short head is supplied by the peroneal nerve (Fig. 11.9).

*Two-joint muscles; hip actions are discussed in Chapter 9 and ankle actions are discussed in Chapter 11.

†Two-joint muscles.

TABLE 10.1 • Agonist muscles of the knee joint

	Muscle	Origin	Insertion	Action	Plane of motion	Palpation	Innervation
Anterior aspect	Rectus femoris	Anterior inferior iliac spine of the ilium and groove (posterior) above the acetabulum	Superior aspect of the patella tendon to the tibial tuberosity	Extension of the knee	Sagittal	Straight down anterior thigh from anterior inferior iliac spine to patella, particularly during resisted hip flexion/knee extension	Femoral nerve (L2–L4)
				Flexion of the hip			
	Vastus intermedius	Upper 2/3 of anterior surface of femur	Upper border of patella and patellar tendon to tibial tuberosity	Extension of the knee	Sagittal	Cannot be palpated; lies under the rectus femoris muscle	Femoral nerve (L2–L4)
	Vastus lateralis (externus)	Intertrochanteric line, anterior and inferior borders of the greater trochanter, gluteal tuberosity, upper half of the linea aspera and entire lateral intermuscular septum	Lateral border of the patella and patellar tendon to the tibial tuberosity	Extension of the knee	Sagittal	Halfway down the anterolateral aspect of the thigh, with extension of the knee, particularly full extension against resistance	Femoral nerve (L2–L4)
	Vastus medialis (internus)	Whole length of linea aspera and medial condyloid ridge	Medial half of upper border of patella and patellar tendon to tibial tuberosity	Extension of the knee	Sagittal	Anterior medial side of the thigh just above the superomedial patella, with extension of the knee, particularly full extension against resistance	Femoral nerve (L2–L4)
Posterior muscles	Biceps femoris	Long head: ischial tuberosity. Short head: lower half of the linea aspera, and lateral condyloid ridge	Head of the fibula and lateral condyle of the tibia	Flexion of the knee	Sagittal	Posterolateral aspect of distal thigh with combined knee flexion and external rotation against resistance	Long head: sciatic nerve—tibial division (S1–S3). Short head: sciatic nerve—peroneal division (L5, S1, S2)
				Extension of the hip			
				External rotation of the knee	Transverse		
				External rotation of the hip			
	Popliteus	Posterior surface of lateral condyle of femur	Upper posterior medial surface of tibia	Internal rotation of the knee	Transverse	With subject sitting, knee flexed 90 degrees, palpate just inferior and anterior to lateral epicondyle, while subject internally rotates knee	Tibial nerve (L5, S1)
				Flexion of the knee	Sagittal		
	Semimembranosus	Ischial tuberosity	Posteromedial surface of the medial tibial condyle	Extension of the hip	Sagittal	Largely covered by other muscles, the tendon can be felt at the posteromedial aspect of the knee with combined knee flexion and internal rotation against resistance	Sciatic nerve—tibial division (L5, S1, S2)
				Flexion of the knee			
				Internal rotation of the hip	Transverse		
				Internal rotation of the knee			
	Semitendinosus	Ischial tuberosity	Upper anterior medial surface of the tibia just below the condyle	Extension of the hip	Sagittal	Posteromedial aspect of distal thigh with combined knee flexion and internal rotation against resistance	Sciatic nerve—tibial division (L5, S1, S2)
				Flexion of the knee			
				Internal rotation of the hip	Transverse		
				Internal rotation of the knee			

Chapter

10

www.mhhe.com/floyd15e   **221**

Quadriceps muscles   FIG. 10.5
(kwod´ri-seps)

The ability to jump is essential in nearly all sports. Individuals who have good jumping ability always have strong quadriceps muscles that extend the leg at the knee. The quadriceps function as a decelerator when it is necessary to decrease speed for changing direction or to prevent falling when landing. This deceleration function is also evident in stopping the body when coming down from a jump. The contraction that occurs in the quadriceps during braking or decelerating actions is eccentric. This eccentric action of the quadriceps controls the slowing of movements initiated in previous phases of the sports skill.

The muscles are the rectus femoris (the only two-joint muscle of the group), vastus lateralis (the largest muscle of the group), vastus intermedius, and vastus medialis. All attach to the patella and by the patellar tendon to the tuberosity of the tibia. All are superficial and palpable, except the vastus intermedius, which is under the rectus femoris. The vertical jump is a simple test that may be used to indicate the strength or power of the quadriceps. This muscle group is generally desired to be 25% to 33% stronger than the hamstring muscle group (knee flexors).

Development of strength and endurance of the quadriceps or "quads" is essential for maintenance of patellofemoral stability, which is often a problem in many physically active individuals. This problem is further perpetuated due to the quads being particularly prone to atrophy when injuries occur. The muscle of the quadriceps may be developed by resisted knee extension activities from a seated position. Performing functional weight-bearing activities such as step-ups or squats is particularly useful for strengthening and endurance.

FIG. 10.5 ● Quadriceps muscle group.

Rectus femoris muscle   FIG. 9.23
(rek´tus fem´o-ris)

Origin

Anterior inferior iliac spine of the ilium and superior margin of the acetabulum

Insertion

Superior aspect of the patella and patellar tendon to the tibial tuberosity

Action

Flexion of the hip
Extension of the knee

Palpation

Straight down anterior thigh from anterior inferior iliac spine to patella, particularly during resisted hip flexion/knee extension

Innervation

Femoral nerve (L2–L4)

Application, strengthening, and flexibility

When the hip is flexed, the rectus femoris becomes shorter, which reduces its effectiveness as an extensor of the knee. The work is then done primarily by the three vasti muscles.

Also see the rectus femoris discussion in Chapter 9, p. 197 (Fig. 9.23).

Vastus lateralis (externus) muscle

FIG. 10.6

(vas´tus lat-er-a´lis)

Origin

Intertrochanteric line, anterior and inferior borders of the greater trochanter, gluteal tuberosity, upper half of the linea aspera and entire lateral intermuscular septum

Insertion

Lateral border of the patella and patellar tendon to the tibial tuberosity

Action

Extension of the knee

Palpation

Halfway down the anterolateral aspect of the thigh, with extension of the knee, particularly full extension against resistance

Innervation

Femoral nerve (L2–L4)

Application, strengthening, and flexibility

All three of the vasti muscles function with the rectus femoris in knee extension. They are typically used in walking and running and must be used to keep the knees straight, as in standing. The vastus lateralis has a slightly superior lateral pull on the patella and, as a result, is occasionally blamed in part for common lateral patellar subluxation and dislocation problems.

The vastus lateralis is strengthened through knee extension activities against resistance. Stretching occurs by pulling the knee into maximum flexion, such as by standing on one leg and pulling the heel of the other leg to the buttocks.

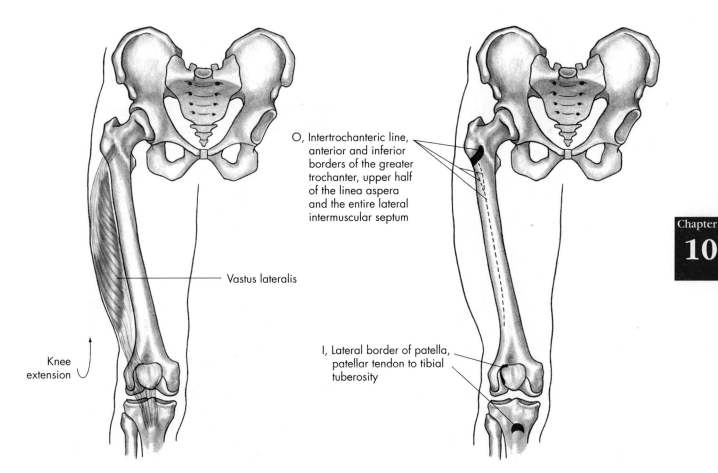

O, Intertrochanteric line, anterior and inferior borders of the greater trochanter, upper half of the linea aspera and the entire lateral intermuscular septum

Vastus lateralis

Knee extension

I, Lateral border of patella, patellar tendon to tibial tuberosity

FIG. 10.6 ● Vastus lateralis muscle, anterior view. *O*, Origin; *I*, insertion.

Vastus intermedius muscle   FIG. 10.7

(vas´tus in´ter-me´di-us)

Origin

Upper two-thirds of the anterior surface of the
femur

Insertion

Upper border of the patella and patellar tendon to
the tibial tuberosity

Action

Extension of the knee

Palpation

Cannot be palpated; lies under the rectus femoris
muscle

Innervation

Femoral nerve (L2–L4)

Application, strengthening, and flexibility

The three vasti muscles all contract in knee extension. They are used together with the rectus femoris
in running, jumping, hopping, skipping, and walking. The vasti muscles are primarily responsible
for extending the knee while the hip is flexed or
being flexed. Thus, in doing a knee bend with the
trunk bent forward at the hip, the vasti are exercised with little involvement of the rectus femoris.
These natural activities mentioned develop the
quadriceps.

Squats with a barbell of varying weights on the
shoulders, depending on strength, are an excellent exercise for developing the quadriceps if
done properly. Caution should be used, along
with strict attention to proper technique, to avoid
injuries to the knees and lower back. Leg press
exercises and knee extensions with weight machines are other good exercises. Full knee flexion
stretches all of the quadriceps musculature.

Vastus intermedius m.

Knee extension

O, Upper two-thirds
of anterior surface
of femur

I, Upper border of patella
and the patellar tendon
to tibial tuberosity

FIG. 10.7 ● Vastus intermedius muscle, anterior view. *O*, Origin; *I*, insertion.

Vastus medialis (internus) muscle

FIG. 10.8

(vas´tus me-di-a´lis)

Origin

Whole length of the linea aspera and the medial
condyloid ridge

Insertion

Medial half of the upper border of the patella and
patellar tendon to the tibial tuberosity

Action

Extension of the knee

Palpation

Anterior medial side of the thigh just above the
superomedial patella, with extension of the knee,
particularly full extension against resistance

Innervation

Femoral nerve (L2–L4)

Application, strengthening, and flexibility

The vastus medialis is thought to be very important in maintaining patellofemoral stability because of the oblique attachment of its distal fibers
to the superior medial patella. This portion of the
vastus medialis is referred to as the vastus medialis
obliquus (VMO). The vastus medialis is strengthened similarly to the other quadriceps muscles by
squats, knee extensions, and leg presses, but the
VMO is not really emphasized until the last 10 to
20 degrees of knee extension. Full knee flexion
stretches all of the quadriceps muscles.

Vastus medialis

Knee
extension

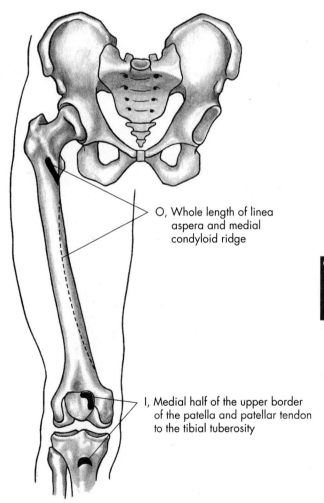

O, Whole length of linea
aspera and medial
condyloid ridge

I, Medial half of the upper border
of the patella and patellar tendon
to the tibial tuberosity

Chapter
10

FIG. 10.8 ● Vastus medialis muscle, anterior view. *O*, Origin; *I*, insertion.

Hamstring muscles FIG. 10.9

The hamstring muscle group, consisting of the biceps femoris, semimembranosus, and semitendinosus, is covered in complete detail in Chapter 9, but further discussion is included here because of its importance in knee function.

Muscle strains involving the hamstrings are very common in football and other sports that require explosive running. This muscle group is often referred to as the "running muscle" because of its function in acceleration. The hamstring muscles are antagonists to the quadriceps muscles at the knee and are named for their cordlike attachments at the knee. All of the hamstring muscles originate on the ischial tuberosity of the pelvic bone. The semitendinosus and semimembranosus insert on the anteromedial and posteromedial side of the tibia, respectively. The biceps femoris inserts on the lateral tibial condyle and head of the fibula—hence the saying "Two to the inside and one to the outside." The second head of the biceps femoris originates on the linea aspera of the femur.

Special exercises to improve the strength and flexibility of this muscle group are important in decreasing knee injuries. Inability to touch the floor with the fingers when the knees are straight is largely a result of a lack of flexibility of the hamstrings. The hamstrings may be strengthened by performing knee or hamstring curls on a knee table against resistance. Additionally, tight or inflexible hamstrings are also contributing factors in painful conditions involving the low back and knee. The flexibility of these muscles may be improved by performing slow, static stretching exercises, such as flexing the hip slowly while maintaining knee extension in a long sitting position.

The hamstrings are primarily knee flexors in addition to serving as hip extensors. Rotation of the knee can occur when it is in a flexed position. Knee rotation is brought about by the hamstring muscles. The biceps femoris externally rotates the lower leg at the knee. The semitendinosus and semimembranosus perform internal rotation. Rotation of the knee permits pivoting movements and change in direction of the body. This rotation of the knee is vital in accommodating to forces developing at the hip or ankle during directional changes in order to make the total movement more functional as well as more fluid in appearance.

Chapter 10

Semitendinosis

(long head)
Biceps femoris
(short head)

Semimembranosus

FIG. 10.9 ● The hamstring muscle group.

Popliteus muscle   FIG. 10.10

(pop´li-te´us)

Origin

Posterior surface of the lateral condyle of the femur

Insertion

Upper posterior medial surface of the tibia

Action

Flexion of the knee

Internal rotation of the flexed knee

Palpation

With subject sitting, knee flexed 90 degrees, palpate just inferior and anterior to lateral epicondyle, while subject internally rotates knee.

Innervation

Tibial nerve (L5, S1)

Application, strengthening, and flexibility

The popliteus muscle is the only true flexor of the leg at the knee. All other flexors are two-joint muscles. The popliteus is vital in providing posterolateral stability to the knee. It assists the medial hamstrings in internal rotation of the lower leg at the knee and is crucial in internally rotating the knee to unlock it from the "screwed home" full extension position.

Hanging from a bar with the legs flexed at the knee strenuously exercises the popliteus muscle. Also, the less strenuous activities of walking and running exercise this muscle. Specific efforts to strengthen this muscle combine knee internal rotation and flexion exercises against resistance. Stretching of the popliteus is difficult but may be done through passive full-knee extension without flexing the hip. Passive maximum external rotation with the knee flexed approximately 20 to 30 degrees also stretches the popliteus.

Flexion

Popliteus m.

Internal rotation

O, Posterior surface of lateral condyle of femur

I, Upper posterior medial surface of tibia

FIG. 10.10 ● Popliteus muscle, posterior view. *O*, Origin; *I*, insertion.

Web sites

Anatomy & Physiology Tutorials:

www.gwc.maricopa.edu/class/bio201/index.htm

Radiologic Anatomy Browser:

radlinux1.usuf1.usuhs.mil/rad/iong/index.html

This site has numerous radiological views of the musculoskeletal system.

University of Arkansas Medical School Gross Anatomy for Medical Students:

anatomy.uams.edu/htmlpages/anatomyhtml/ gross.html

Dissections, anatomy tables, atlas images, links, etc.

Loyola University Medical Center: Structure of the Human Body:

www.meddean.luc.edu/lumen/MedEd/ GrossAnatomy/GA.html

An excellent site with many slides, dissections, tutorials, etc., for the study of human anatomy.

Wheeless's Textbook of Orthopaedics:

www.ortho-u.net/

This site has an extensive index of links to the fractures, joints, muscles, nerves, trauma, medications, medical topics and lab tests, as well as links to orthopedic journals and other orthopedic, and medical news.

Premiere Medical Search Engine:

www.medsite.com

This site allows the reader to enter any medical condition and it will search the net to find relevant articles.

Arthroscopy.Com:

www.arthroscopy.com/sports.htm

Patient information on various musculoskeletal problems of the upper and lower extremity.

Virtual Hospital:

www.vh.org

Numerous slides, patient information, etc.

Dynamic Human version 2.0 CD-ROM: The Visual Guide to Anatomy & Physiology:

www.mhhe.com/biosci/ap/dynamichuman2/

Web site that accompanies this CD-ROM.

Worksheet exercise

As an aid to learning, for in-class or out-of-class assignments, or for testing, a tear-out worksheet is found at the end of the text (p. 335).

Posterior skeletal worksheet (no. 1)

Draw and label on the worksheet the knee joint muscles.

Laboratory and review exercises

1. Locate the following parts of bones on a human skeleton and on a subject:
   a. Skeleton
      1. Head and neck of femur
      2. Greater trochanter
      3. Shaft of femur
      4. Lesser trochanter
      5. Linea aspera
      6. Adductor tubercle
      7. Medial femoral condyle
      8. Lateral femoral condyle
      9. Patella
      10. Fibula head
      11. Medial tibial condyle
      12. Lateral tibial condyle
      13. Tibial tuberosity
      14. Gerdy's tubercle
   b. Subject
      1. Greater trochanter
      2. Adductor tubercle
      3. Medial femoral condyle
      4. Lateral femoral condyle
      5. Patella
      6. Fibula head
      7. Medial tibial condyle
      8. Lateral tibial condyle
      9. Tibial tuberosity
      10. Gerdy's tubercle
2. How and where can the following muscles be palpated on a human subject?
   NOTE: Palpate the previously studied hip joint muscles while they are performing actions at the knee.
   a. Gracilis
   b. Sartorius
   c. Biceps femoris
   d. Semitendinosus
   e. Semimembranosus
   f. Rectus femoris

g. Vastus lateralis

h. Vastus intermedius

i. Vastus medialis

j. Popliteus

3. Be prepared to indicate on a human skeleton, by using a long rubber band, the origin and insertion of the muscles just listed.

4. Demonstrate the following movements and list the muscles primarily responsible for each.
   a. Extension of the leg at the knee
   b. Flexion of the leg at the knee
   c. Internal rotation of the leg at the knee
   d. External rotation of the leg at the knee

5. List the planes in which each of the following movements occurs. List the respective axis of rotation for each movement in each plane.
   a. Extension of the leg at the knee
   b. Flexion of the leg at the knee
   c. Internal rotation of the leg at the knee
   d. External rotation of the leg at the knee

6. With a laboratory partner, determine how and why maintaining the position of full knee extension limits the ability to maximally flex the hip both actively and passively. Does maintaining excessive hip flexion limit your ability to accomplish full knee extension?

7. With a laboratory partner, determine how and why maintaining the position of full knee flexion limits the ability to maximally extend the hip both actively and passively. Does maintaining excessive hip extension limit your ability to accomplish full knee flexion?

8. Compare and contrast the bony, ligamentous, articular, and cartilaginous aspects of the medial knee joint versus the lateral knee joint.

9. Research the acceptability of deep knee-bends and duck-walk activities in a physical education program and report your findings in class.

10. Prepare a report on the knee on one of the following topics: ligamentous injuries, meniscus injuries, joint structure, patellofemoral injuries, knee bracing, quadriceps rehabilitation.

11. Research preventive and rehabilitative exercises to strengthen the knee joint and report your findings in class.

12. Which muscle group about the knee would be most important to develop for an athlete with a torn anterior cruciate ligament and why? A torn posterior cruciate ligament? Why?

13. Fill in the muscle analysis chart below by listing the muscles primarily involved in each joint movement.

14. Fill in the antagonistic muscle action chart on the next page by listing the muscle(s) or parts of muscles that are antagonistic in their actions to the muscles in the left column.

Muscle analysis chart • Knee joint

Flexion	Extension
Internal rotation	External rotation

Antagonistic muscle action chart • Knee joint

Agonist	Antagonist
Biceps femoris	
Semitendinosus	
Semimembranosus	
Rectus femoris	
Vastus lateralis	
Vastus intermedius	
Vastus medialis	
Rectus femoris	
Popliteus	

References

Baker BE, et al: Review of meniscal injury and associated sports, *American Journal of Sports Medicine* 13:1, January–February 1985.

Evans W: Hamstring strength and flexibility development, *Scholastic Coach* 56:42, April 1987.

Field D: *Anatomy: palpation and surface markings,* ed 3, Oxford, 2001, Butterworth-Heinemann.

Garrick JG, Regna RK: Prophylactic knee bracing, *American Journal of Sports Medicine* 15:471, September–October 1987.

Hamilton N, Luttgens K: *Kinesiology: scientific basis of human motion,* ed 10, Boston, 2002, McGraw-Hill.

Kelly DW, et al: Patellar and quadriceps tendon ruptures—jumping knee, *American Journal of Sports Medicine* 12:375, September–October 1984.

Lysholm J, Wikland J: Injuries in runners, *American Journal of Sports Medicine* 15:168, September–October 1986.

Perreira J: Treating the quadriceps contusion, *Scholastic Coach* 57:38, October 1987.

Seeley RR, Stephens TD, Tate P: *Anatomy & physiology,* ed 6, Dubuque, IA, 2003, McGraw-Hill.

Sieg KW, Adams SP: *Illustrated essentials of musculoskeletal anatomy,* ed 2, Gainesville, FL, 1985, Megabooks.

Stone RJ, Stone JA: *Atlas of the skeletal muscles,* 1990. McGraw-Hill Companies, Inc., New York.

Van de Graaff KM: *Human anatomy,* ed 6, Dubuque, IA. 2002, McGraw-Hill.

Wroble RR, et al: Pattern of knee injuries in wrestling, a six-year study, *American Journal of Sports Medicine* 14:55, January–February 1986.

Chapter 11
The Ankle and Foot Joints

Objectives

- To identify on a human skeleton the most important bone features, ligaments, and arches of the ankle and foot

- To draw and label on a skeletal chart the muscles of the ankle and foot

- To demonstrate and palpate with a fellow student the movements of the ankle and foot and list their respective planes of motion and axes of rotation

- To palpate the superficial joint structures and muscles of the ankle and foot on a human subject

- To list and organize the muscles that produce movement of the ankle and foot and list their antagonists

---

Online Learning Center Resources

Visit *Manual of Structural Kinesiology's* **Online Learning Center** at **www.mhhe.com/floyd15e** for additional information and study material for this chapter, including:

- *Self-grading quizzes*
- *Anatomy flashcards*
- *Animations*

The complexity of the foot is evidenced by the 26 bones, 19 large muscles, many small (intrinsic) muscles, and more than 100 ligaments that make up its structure.

Support and propulsion are the two functions of the foot. Proper functioning and adequate development of the muscles of the foot and practice of proper foot mechanics are essential for everyone. In our modern society, foot trouble is one of the most common ailments. Quite often, people develop poor foot mechanics or gait abnormalities secondary to improper shoe wear or other relatively minor problems. Poor foot mechanics early in life inevitably leads to foot discomfort in later years.

Walking and running may be divided into stance and swing phases (Fig. 11.1). The *stance* phase is further divided into three components—heel-strike, midstance, and toe-off. Normally, *heel-strike* is characterized by landing on the heel with the foot in supination, followed immediately by the foot moving into pronation during *midstance* with return to supination prior to and during *toe-off*. The *swing* phase occurs when the foot leaves the ground and the leg moves forward to another point of contact. Problems often arise when the foot is too rigid and does not pronate adequately or when the foot remains in pronation past midstance. Walking differs from running in that one foot is always in contact with the ground, whereas in running there is a point when neither foot is in contact with the ground.

The fitness revolution that has occurred during the past three decades has resulted in great improvements in shoes available for sports and recreational activities. In the past, a pair of sneakers would suffice for most activities. Now there are basketball, baseball, football, jogging, soccer,

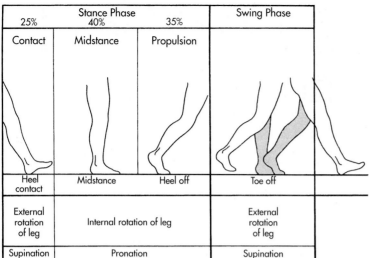

Stance Phase			Swing Phase
25%	40%	35%	
Contact	Midstance	Propulsion	
Heel contact	Midstance	Heel off	Toe off
External rotation of leg	Internal rotation of leg		External rotation of leg
Supination	Pronation		Supination

FIG. 11.1 ● Walking gait cycle.

tennis, walking, and cross-training shoes. Good shoes are important, but there is no substitute for adequate muscular development, strength, and proper foot mechanics.

Bones

Each foot has 26 bones, which collectively form the shape of an arch. They connect with the thigh and the remainder of the body through the fibula and tibia (Figs. 11.2 and 11.3). Body weight is transferred from the tibia to the talus and the calcaneus.

In addition to the talus and calcaneus, there are five other bones in the rear foot and midfoot known as the tarsals. Between the talus and the three cuneiform bones lies the navicular. The cuboid is located between the calcaneus and the fourth and fifth metatarsals. Distal to the tarsals are the five metatarsals, which in turn correspond to each of the five toes. The toes are known as the phalanges. There are three individual bones in each phalange, except for the great toe, which has only two. Each of these bones is known as a phalanx. Finally, there are two sesamoid bones located beneath the first metatarsophalangeal joint and contained within the flexor hallucis longus tendons.

The distal end of the tibia and fibula are enlarged and protrude horizontally and inferiorly. These bony protrusions, known as malleoli, serve as a sort of pulley for the tendons of the muscles that run directly posterior to them. Specifically, the peroneus brevis and peroneus longus are immediately behind the lateral malleolus. The muscles immediately posterior to the medial malleolus

FIG. 11.2 ● Right fibula and tibia.

From Anthony CP, Kolthoff NJ: *Textbook of anatomy and physiology,* ed 9, St. Louis, 1975, Mosby.

Interphalangeal (IP) joint

Phalanxes:
3, Distal
2, Middle
1, Proximal

Forefoot

Metatarsals

Distal interphalangeal (DIP) joints

Proximal interphalangeal (PIP) joints

Metatarsophalangeal (MP) joints

Midfoot

Cuneiforms

Medial
Intermediate
Lateral
Navicular

Transverse tarsal joint

Cuboid

Talus

Subtalar joint

Rearfoot

Calcaneus

FIG. 11.3 ● Right foot, superior view.

Modified from Anthony CP, Kolthoff NJ: *Textbook of anatomy and physiology,* ed 9, St. Louis, 1975, Mosby.

may be remembered by the phrase "Tom, Dick and Harry" with the "T" for the tibialis posterior, the "D" for the flexor digitorum longus, and the "H" for the flexor hallucis longus. This bony arrangement increases the mechanical advantage of these muscles in performing their actions of inversion and eversion. The base of the fifth metatarsal is enlarged and prominent to serve as an attachment point for the peroneus brevis and tertius.

The inner surface of the medial cuneiform and base of the first metatarsal provide insertion points for the tibialis anterior, while the undersurface of the same bones serves as the insertion for the peroneus longus. The tibialis posterior has multiple insertions on the lower inner surfaces of the navicular, cuneiform, and second through fifth metatarsal bases. The tops and undersurfaces of the bases of the second through fifth distal phalanxes are the insertion points for the extensor digitorum longus and the flexor digitorum longus, respectively. Similarly, the top and undersurface of the base of the first distal phalanx provide insertions for the extensor hallucis longus and flexor hallucis longus, respectively.

The posterior surface of the calcaneus is very prominent and serves as the attachment point for the Achilles tendon of the gastrocnemius-soleus complex.

Chapter
11

Joints

The tibia and fibula form the tibiofibular joint, a syndesmotic amphiarthrodial joint (see Fig. 11.2). The bones are joined at both the proximal and distal tibiofibular joints. In addition to the ligaments supporting both of these joints, there is a strong, dense interosseus membrane between the shafts of these two bones. Although only minimal movement is possible between these bones, the distal joint does become sprained occasionally in heavy contact sports such as football. This injury, a sprain of the syndesmosis joint, is commonly referred to as a high ankle sprain and primarily involves the anterior inferior tibiofibular ligament. Secondarily, and with more severe injuries, the posterior tibiofibular ligament, interosseus ligament, and interosseus membrane may be involved.

The ankle joint, technically known as the talocrural joint, is a hinge or ginglymus-type joint (Fig. 11.4). Specifically, it is the joint made up of the talus, the distal tibia, and the distal fibula. The ankle joint allows approximately 50 degrees of plantar flexion and 15 to 20 degrees of dorsiflexion (Fig. 11.5). Greater range of dorsiflexion, particularly in weight bearing, is possible when the knee is flexed, which reduces the tension of the biarticular gastrocnemius muscle. The fibula rotates on its axis 3 to 5 degrees externally with dorsiflexion of the ankle and 3 to 5 degrees internally during plantar flexion. The syndesmosis joint widens by approximately 1 to 2 millimeters during full dorsiflexion.

Inversion and eversion, although commonly thought to be ankle joint movements, technically occur in the subtalar and transverse tarsal joints. These joints, classified as gliding or arthrodial, combine to allow approximately 20 to 30 degrees of inversion and 5 to 15 degrees of eversion. There is minimal movement within the remainder of the intertarsal and tarsometatarsal arthrodial joints.

The phalanges join the metatarsals to form the metatarsophalangeal joints, which are classified as condyloid-type joints. The metatarsophalangeal (MP) joint of the great toe flexes 45 degrees and extends 70 degrees, whereas the interphalangeal (IP) joint can flex from 0 degrees of full extension to 90 degrees of flexion. The MP joints of the four lesser toes allow approximately 40 degrees of flexion and 40 degrees of extension. The MP joints also abduct and adduct minimally. The proximal interphalangeal (PIP) joints in the lesser toes flex from 0 degrees of extension to 35 degrees of flexion. The distal interphalangeal (DIP) joints flex 60 degrees and extend 30 degrees. There is much variation from joint to joint and from person to person in all of these joints.

Ankle sprains are one of the most common injuries among physically active people. Sprains involve the stretching or tearing of one or more ligaments. There are far too many ligaments in the foot and ankle to discuss in this text, but a few of the ankle ligaments are shown in Fig. 11.4. Far and away the most common ankle sprain results from excessive inversion, which causes damage to the lateral ligamentous structures, primarily the anterior talofibular ligament and the calcaneofibular ligament. Excessive eversion forces causing injury to the deltoid ligament on the medial aspect of the ankle occur less commonly.

Ligaments in the foot and the ankle maintain the position of an arch. All 26 bones in the foot are connected with ligaments. This brief discussion is focused on the longitudinal and transverse arches.

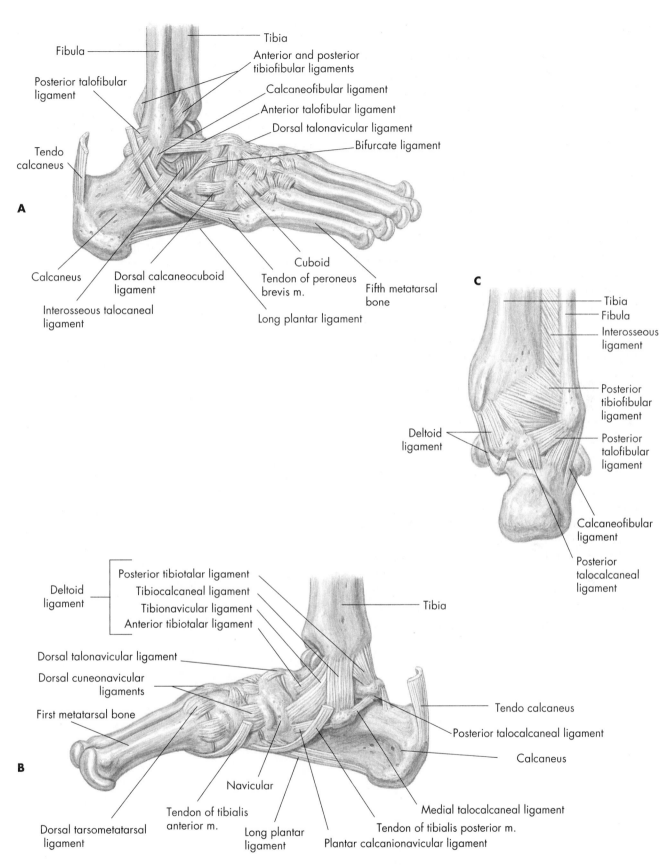

FIG. 11.4 ● Right ankle joint. **A,** Lateral view; **B,** medial view; **C,** posterior view.

Modified from Van De Graaff KM: *Human anatomy,* ed 6, 2002, McGraw-Hill Companies Inc., New York.

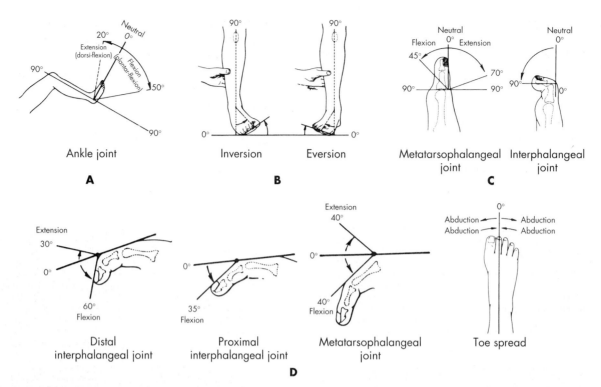

FIG. 11.5 ● Active motion of the ankle, foot, and toes. **A,** Dorsiflexion and plantar flexion are measured in degrees from the right-angle neutral position or in percentages of motion as compared to the opposite ankle; **B,** Inversion and eversion are normally estimated in degrees or expressed in percentages as compared to the opposite foot; **C,** Flexion and extension of the great toe; **D,** ROM for the lateral four toes.

There are two longitudinal arches (Fig. 11.6). The medial longitudinal arch is located on the medial side of the foot and extends from the calcaneus bone to the talus, the navicular, the three cuneiforms, and the proximal ends of the three medial metatarsals. The lateral longitudinal arch is located on the lateral side of the foot and extends from the calcaneus to the cuboid and proximal ends of the fourth and fifth metatarsals. Individual long arches can be high, medium, or low, but a low arch is not necessarily a weak arch.

The transverse arch (see Fig. 11.6) extends across the foot from one metatarsal bone to the other.

Cuneiform bones
Cuboid bone
Talus
Calcaneus
Navicular bone
Transverse arch
Longitudinal arch
First metatarsal bone
Phalanges of big toe

A

Creek

FIG. 11.6 ● Longitudinal and transverse arches. **A,** A medial view of the right foot showing both arches, and **B,** a transverse view through the bases of the metatarsal bones showing a portion of the transverse arch.

Bases of metatarsal bones
Transverse arch

B

Movements FIG. 11.7

Dorsiflexion (flexion): dorsal flexion; movement of the top of the ankle and foot toward the anterior tibia bone

Plantar flexion (extension): movement of the ankle and foot away from the tibia

Eversion: turning the ankle and foot outward; abduction, away from the midline; weight is on the medial edge of the foot

Inversion: turning the ankle and foot inward; adduction, toward the midline; weight is on the lateral edge of the foot

Toe flexion: movement of the toes toward the plantar surface of the foot

Toe extension: movement of the toes away from the plantar surface of the foot

Pronation: a combination of ankle dorsiflexion, subtalar eversion, and forefoot abduction (toe-out)

Supination: a combination of ankle plantar flexion, subtalar inversion, and forefoot adduction (toe-in)

A

Dorsiflexion

B

Plantar flexion

C

Transverse tarsal and subtalar eversion

D

Transverse tarsal and subtalar inversion

E

Flexion of the toes

FIG. 11.7 ● Movements of the ankle and foot (continued next page).

Extension of the toes

Pronation

Supination

FIG. 11.7 (continued) • Movements of the ankle and foot.

Ankle and foot muscles   FIG. 11.8 &
FIG. 11.9

The large number of muscles in the ankle and foot may be easier to learn if grouped according to location and function. In general, the muscles located on the anterior aspect of the ankle and foot are the dorsal flexors. Those on the posterior aspect are plantar flexors. Specifically, the gastrocnemius and the soleus collectively are known as the triceps surae, due to their three heads, which join together to the Achilles tendon. Muscles that are evertors are located more to the lateral side, whereas the invertors are located medially.

The lower leg is divided into four compartments, each containing specific muscles (Fig. 11.9). Tightly surrounding and binding each compartment is a dense fascia, which facilitates venous return and prevents excessive swelling of the muscles during exercise. The anterior compartment contains the dorsiflexor group, consisting of the tibialis anterior, peroneus tertius, extensor digitorum longus, and extensor hallucis longus. The lateral compartment contains the peroneus longus and peroneus brevis—the two most powerful evertors. The posterior compartment is divided into deep and superficial compartments. The gastrocnemius, soleus, and plantaris are located in the superficial posterior compartment, while the deep posterior compartment is composed of the flexor digitorum longus, flexor hallucis longus,

popliteus, and tibialis posterior. All of the muscles of the superficial posterior compartment are primarily plantar flexors. The plantaris, absent in some humans, is a vestigial biarticular muscle that contributes minimally to ankle plantar flexion. The deep posterior compartment muscles, except for the popliteus, are plantar flexors but also function as invertors.

Due to heavy demands placed on the musculature of the legs in the running activities of most sports, both acute and chronic injuries are common. "Shin splints" is a common term used to describe a painful condition of the leg that is often associated with running activities. This condition is not a specific diagnosis but, rather, is attributed to a number of specific musculotendinous injuries. Most often the tibialis posterior, medial soleus, or anterior tibialis is involved, but the extensor digitorum longus may also be involved. Shin splints may be prevented in part by stretching the plantar flexors and strengthening the dorsiflexors.

Additionally, painful cramps caused by acute muscle spasm in the gastrocnemius and soleus occur somewhat commonly and may be relieved through active and passive dorsiflexion. Also, a very disabling injury involves the complete rupture of the strong Achilles tendon, which connects these two plantar flexors to the calcaneus.

NOTE: A number of the ankle and foot muscles are capable of helping produce more than one movement.

Chapter
11

Labels in image A (lateral view):
- Biceps femoris
- Vastus lateralis
- Iliotibial tract
- Plantaris
- Common fibular nerve
- Head of fibula
- Lateral head of gastrocnemius
- Peroneus longus
- Soleus
- Tibialis anterior
- Extensor digitorum longus
- Peroneus brevis
- Extensor hallucis longus
- Tendo calcaneus
- Peroneus tertius
- Lateral malleolus

A

Labels in image B (medial view):
- Sartorius
- Tendon of gracilis
- Patella
- Tendon of semimembranosus
- Tendon of semitendinosus
- Medial head of gastrocnemius
- Tibia
- Tibialis anterior
- Soleus
- Tendo calcaneus
- Tendon of plantaris
- Tibialis posterior
- Flexor digitorum longus
- Inferior extensor retinaculum
- Flexor hallucis longus
- Flexor retinaculum
- Abductor hallucis (cut)

Creek

B

FIG. 11.8 ● Lower leg, ankle, and foot muscles. **A,** Lateral view; **B,** medial view (continued next page).

C

D

FIG. 11.8 (continued) ● Lower leg, ankle, and foot muscles. **C,** Anterior view; **D,** deep posterior view.

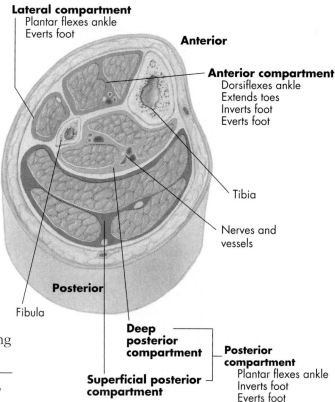

Lateral compartment
Plantar flexes ankle
Everts foot

Anterior

Anterior compartment
Dorsiflexes ankle
Extends toes
Inverts foot
Everts foot

Tibia

Nerves and vessels

Posterior

Fibula

Deep posterior compartment

Superficial posterior compartment

Posterior compartment
Plantar flexes ankle
Inverts foot
Everts foot

FIG. 11.9 ● Cross-section of the leg, demonstrating the muscular compartments.

From Seeley RR, Stephens TD, Tate P: *Anatomy and physiology,* ed 3, St. Louis, 1995, Mosby.

Ankle and foot muscles by function

Plantar flexors
    Gastrocnemius
    Flexor digitorum longus
    Flexor hallucis longus
    Peroneus (fibularis) longus
    Peroneus (fibularis) brevis
    Plantaris
    Soleus
    Tibialis posterior
Evertors
    Peroneus (fibularis) longus
    Peroneus (fibularis) brevis
    Peroneus (fibularis) tertius
    Extensor digitorum longus
Dorsiflexors
    Tibialis anterior
    Peroneus (fibularis) tertius
    Extensor digitorum longus (extensor of the lesser toes)
    Extensor hallucis longus (extensor of the great toe)
Invertors
    Tibialis anterior
    Tibialis posterior
    Flexor digitorum longus (flexor of the lesser toes)
    Flexor hallucis longus (flexor of the great toe)

Ankle and foot muscles by compartment

Anterior compartment
    Tibialis anterior
    Extensor hallucis longus
    Extensor digitorum longus
    Peroneus (fibularis) tertius
Lateral compartment
    Peroneus (fibularis) longus
    Peroneus (fibularis) brevis
Deep posterior compartment
    Flexor digitorum longus
    Flexor hallucis longus
    Tibialis posterior
Superficial posterior compartment
    Gastrocnemius (medial head)
    Gastrocnemius (lateral head)
    Soleus
    While viewing the muscles in Figs. 11.8 and 11.9 correlate them with Table 11.1.

Chapter

11

TABLE 11.1 • Agonist muscles of the ankle and foot joints

	Muscle	Origin	Insertion	Action	Plane of motion	Palpation	Innervation
Superficial posterior compartment	Gastrocnemius	Medial head: Posterior surface of the medial femoral condyle Lateral head: Posterior surface of the lateral femoral condyle	Posterior surface of the calcaneus (Achilles tendon)	Plantar flexion of the ankle	Sagittal	Upper one-half of posterior aspect of the lower leg	Tibial nerve (S1, S2)
				Flexion of the knee			
	Soleus	Posterior surface of the proximal fibula and proximal two-thirds of the posterior tibial surface	Posterior surface of the calcaneus (Achilles tendon)	Plantar flexion of the ankle	Sagittal	Posteriorly under the gastrocnemius muscle on the medial and lateral side of the lower leg, particularly while standing with knee flexed and slightly plantarflexing ankle	Tibial nerve (S1, S2)
Deep posterior compartment	Tibialis posterior	Posterior surface of the upper half of the interosseus membrane and the adjacent surfaces of the tibia and fibula	Lower inner surfaces of the navicular and cuneiform bones and bases of the 2nd, 3rd, 4th, and 5th metatarsal bones	Inversion of the foot	Frontal	The tendon may be palpated immediately behind the medial malleolus with inversion and plantar flexion	Tibial nerve (L5, S1)
				Plantar flexion of the ankle	Sagittal		
	Flexor digitorum longus	Middle third of the posterior surface of the tibia	Base of the distal phalanx of each of the four lesser toes	Flexion of the four lesser toes	Sagittal	The tendon may be palpated immediately posterior to the medial malleolus and tibialis posterior and immediately anterior with flexion of the lesser toes	Tibial nerve (L5, S1)
				Plantar flexion of the ankle			
				Inversion of the foot	Frontal		
	Flexor hallucis longus	Middle two-thirds of the posterior surface of the fibula	Base of the distal phalanx of the big toe; under surface	Flexion of the great toe	Sagittal	Anteromedial to the Achilles tendon near the heel	Tibial nerve (L5, S1, S2)
				Inversion of the foot	Frontal		
				Plantar flexion of the ankle	Sagittal		

Chapter **11**

TABLE 11.1 (continued) • Agonist muscles of the ankle and foot joints

	Muscle	Origin	Insertion	Action	Plane of motion	Palpation	Innervation
Lateral compartment	Peroneus longus	Head and upper two-thirds of the lateral surface of the fibula	Under surfaces of the medial cuneiform and 1st metatarsal bone	Eversion of the foot	Frontal	Upper lateral side of the tibia; just posterolateral from the tibialis anterior and extensor digitorum longus	Superficial peroneal nerve (L4, L5, S1)
				Plantar flexion of the ankle	Sagittal		
	Peroneus brevis	Lower two-thirds of the lateral surface of the fibula	Tuberosity of the 5th metatarsal bone	Eversion of the foot	Frontal	Tendon of the muscle at the proximal end of the fifth metatarsal	Superficial peroneal nerve (L4, L5, S1)
				Plantar flexion of the ankle	Sagittal		
Anterior compartment	Peroneus tertius	Distal third of the anterior fibula	Base of the 5th metatarsal	Dorsal flexion of the ankle	Sagittal	Lateral to the extensor digitorum longus tendon on the anterolateral aspect of the foot down to the medial side of the base of the fifth metatarsal	Deep peroneal nerve (L4, L5, S1)
				Eversion of the foot	Frontal		
	Extensor digitorum longus	Lateral condyle of the tibia, head of the fibula, and upper two-thirds of the anterior surface of the fibula	Tops of the middle and distal phalanges of the lesser four toes	Extension of the lesser toes	Sagittal	Second muscle to the lateral side of the anterior tibial border; upper lateral side of the tibia between the tibialis anterior medially and the fibula laterally; divides into 4 tendons just distal to anterior ankle	Deep peroneal nerve (L4, L5, S1)
				Dorsiflexion of the ankle			
				Eversion of the foot	Frontal		
	Extensor hallucis longus	Middle two-thirds of the medial surface of the anterior fibula	Base of the distal phalanx of the great toe	Dorsiflexion of the ankle	Sagittal	From the dorsal aspect of the great toe to just lateral of the tibialis anterior at the anterior ankle joint	Deep peroneal nerve (L4, L5, S1)
				Extension of the great toe			
				Weak inversion of the foot	Frontal		
	Tibialis anterior	Upper two-thirds of the lateral surface of the tibia	Inner surface of the medial cuneiform and the base of the 1st metatarsal bone	Dorsal flexion of the ankle	Sagittal	First muscle to the lateral side of the anterior tibial border, particularly palpable with full active ankle dorsiflexion	Deep peroneal nerve (L4, L5, S1)
				Inversion of the foot	Frontal		

Chapter

11

Nerves

As described in Chapter 9, the sciatic nerve originates from the sacral plexus and becomes the tibial nerve and peroneal nerve. The tibial division of the sciatic nerve (Fig. 9.20) continues down to the posterior aspect of the lower leg to innervate the gastrocnemius (medial head), soleus, tibialis posterior, flexor digitorum longus, and flexor hallucis longus. Just before reaching the ankle the tibial nerve branches to become the medial and lateral plantar nerves, which innervate the intrinsic muscles of the foot. The medial plantar nerve innervates the abductor hallucis, flexor hallucis brevis, first lumbricale, and the flexor digitorum brevis. The lateral plantar nerve supplies the adductor hallucis, quadratus plantae, lumbricales (2, 4, and 4), dorsal interossei, plantar interossei, abductor digiti minimi, and the flexor digiti minimi.

The peroneal or fibular nerve (Fig. 11.10) divides just below the head of the fibula to become the superficial and deep peroneal nerve. The superficial branch innervates the peroneus longus and peroneus brevis, while the deep branch innervates the tibialis anterior, extensor digitorum longus, extensor hallucis longus, peroneus tertius, and extensor digitorum brevis.

FIG. 11.10 ● Muscular and cutaneous distribution of the peroneal (fibular) nerve.

L4
L5
S1
S2

Peroneal (fibular) nerve

Short head of biceps femoris m.

Tibialis anterior m.

Peroneus longus m.

Extensor digitorum longus m.

Superficial peroneal (fibular) nerve

Peroneus brevis m.

Deep peroneal (fibular) nerve

Extensor hallucis longus m.

Peroneus tertius m.

Extensor digitorum brevis m.

Extensor hallucis brevis m.

Creek

Gastrocnemius muscle   FIG. 11.11

(gas-trok-ne´mi-us)

Origin

Medial head: posterior surface of the medial femoral
  condyle
Lateral head: posterior surface of the lateral femoral
  condyle

Insertion

Posterior surface of the calcaneus (Achilles tendon)

Action

Plantar flexion of the ankle
Flexion of the knee

Palpation

Easiest muscle in the lower extremity to palpate;
  upper one-half posterior aspect of the lower leg

Innervation

Tibial nerve (S1, S2)

Application, strengthening, and flexibility

Because the gastrocnemius is a biarticular muscle,
it is more effective as a knee flexor if the ankle is
dorsiflexed and more effective as a plantar flexor
of the foot if the knee is held in extension. This is
observed when one sits too close to the wheel in
driving a car, which significantly shortens the entire muscle, reducing its effectiveness. When the
knees are bent, the muscle becomes an ineffective plantar flexor, and it is more difficult to de-
press the brakes. Running, jumping, hopping, and
skipping exercises all depend significantly on the
gastrocnemius and soleus to propel the body upward and forward. Heel-raising exercises with the
knees in full extension and the toes resting on a
block of wood are an excellent way to strengthen
the muscle through the full range of motion. By
holding a barbell on the shoulders, the resistance
may be increased.

The gastrocnemius may be stretched by standing and placing both palms on a wall about 3 feet
away and leaning into the wall. The feet should
be pointed straight ahead, and the heels should
remain on the floor. The knees should remain
fully extended throughout the exercise to accen-
tuate the stretch on the gastrocnemius.

FIG. 11.11 ● Gastrocnemius muscle, posterior
view. *O*, Origin; *I*, insertion.

Chapter
11

Soleus muscle   FIG. 11.12

(so´le-us)

Origin

Posterior surface of the proximal fibula and proximal two-thirds of the posterior tibial surface

Insertion

Posterior surface of the calcaneus (Achilles tendon)

Action

Plantar flexion of the ankle

Palpation

Posteriorly under the gastrocnemius muscle on the medial and lateral side of the lower leg, particularly while standing with knee flexed and slightly plantarflexing ankle

Innervation

Tibial nerve (S1, S2)

Application, strengthening, and flexibility

The soleus muscle is one of the most important plantar flexors of the ankle. Some anatomists believe that it is nearly as important in this movement as the gastrocnemius. This is especially true when the knee is flexed. When one rises up on the toes, the soleus muscle can plainly be seen on the outside of the lower leg if one has exercised the legs extensively, as in running and walking.

The soleus muscle is used whenever the ankle plantar flexes. Any movement with body weight on the foot with the knee flexed or extended calls it into action. When the knee is flexed slightly, the effect of the gastrocnemius is reduced, thereby placing more work on the soleus. Running, jumping, hopping, skipping, and dancing on the toes are all exercises that depend heavily on the soleus. It may be strengthened through any plantar flexion exercise against resistance, particularly if the knee is flexed slightly to deemphasize the gastrocnemius. Heel-raising exercises as described for the gastrocnemius, except with the knees flexed slightly, are one way to isolate this muscle for strengthening. Resistance may be increased by holding a barbell on the shoulders.

The soleus is stretched in the same manner as is the gastrocnemius, except that the knees must be flexed slightly, which releases the stretch on the gastrocnemius and places it on the soleus. Again, it is important to attempt to keep the heels on the floor.

Soleus m.

O, Proximal two-thirds of posterior surfaces of tibia and fibula

I, Posterior surface of calcaneus

Plantar flexion

FIG. 11.12 ● Soleus muscle, posterior view. *O*, Origin; *I*, insertion.

Peroneus (fibularis) longus muscle

FIG. 11.13

(per-o-ne´us long´gus)

Origin

Head and upper two-thirds of the lateral surface of the fibula

Insertion

Undersurfaces of the medial cuneiform and first metatarsal bones

Action

Eversion of the foot
Plantar flexion of the ankle

Palpation

Upper lateral side of the tibia; just posterolateral from the tibialis anterior and extensor digitorum longus

Innervation

Superficial peroneal nerve (L4–L5, S1)

Application, strengthening, and flexibility

The peroneus longus muscle passes posteroinferiorly to the lateral malleolus and under the foot from the outside to under the inner surface. Because of its line of pull, it is a strong evertor and assists in plantar flexion.

When the peroneus longus muscle is used effectively with the other ankle flexors, it helps bind the transverse arch as it flexes. Developed without the other plantar flexors, it would produce a weak, everted foot. In running, jumping, hopping, and skipping, the foot should be placed so that it is pointing forward to ensure proper development of the group. Walking barefoot or in stocking feet on the inside of the foot (everted position) is the best exercise for this muscle.

Eversion exercises to strengthen this muscle may be performed by turning the sole of the foot outward while resistance is applied in the opposite direction.

The peroneus longus may be stretched by passively taking the foot into extreme inversion and dorsiflexion while the knee is flexed.

Peroneus longus m.

Plantar flexion

Foot eversion

O, Head and upper two-thirds of lateral surface of fibula

I, Undersurfaces of medial cuneiform and first metatarsal bones

FIG. 11.13 ● Peroneus longus muscle, lateral & plantar views. *O*, Origin; *I*, insertion.

Peroneus (fibularis) brevis muscle

FIG. 11.14

(per-o-ne´us bre´vis)

Origin

Lower two-thirds of the lateral surface of the fibula

Insertion

Tuberosity of the fifth metatarsal bone

Action

Eversion of the foot
Plantar flexion of the ankle

Palpation

Tendon of the muscle at the proximal end of the
  fifth metatarsal

Innervation

Superficial peroneal nerve (L4–L5, S1)

Application, strengthening, and flexibility

The peroneus brevis muscle passes posteroinferiorly to the lateral malleolus to pull on the base of the fifth metatarsal. It is a primary evertor of the foot and assists in plantar flexion. In addition, it aids in maintaining the longitudinal arch as it depresses the foot.

The peroneus brevis muscle is exercised with other plantar flexors in the powerful movements of running, jumping, hopping, and skipping. It may be strengthened in a fashion similar to that for the peroneus longus by performing eversion exercises, such as turning the sole of the foot outward against resistance.

The peroneus brevis is stretched in the same manner as the peroneus longus.

FIG. 11.14 ● Peroneus brevis muscle, lateral & plantar views. *O*, Origin; *I*, insertion.

Chapter
11

Peroneus (fibularis) tertius muscle

FIG. 11.15

(per-o-ne´us ter´shi-us)

Origin

Distal third of the anterior fibula

Insertion

Base of the fifth metatarsal

Action

Eversion of the foot
Dorsal flexion of the ankle

Palpation

Lateral to the extensor digitorum longus tendon on
the anterolateral aspect of the foot, down to the
medial side of the base of the fifth metatarsal

Innervation

Deep peroneal nerve (L4–L5, S1)

Application, strengthening, and flexibility

The peroneus tertius, absent in some humans, is a
small muscle that assists in dorsal flexion and
eversion. Some authorities refer to it as the fifth
tendon of the extensor digitorum longus. It may
be strengthened by pulling the foot up toward
the shin against a weight or resistance. Everting
the foot against resistance, such as weighted eversion towel drags, can also be used for strength
development.

The peroneus tertius may be stretched by passively taking the foot into extreme inversion and
plantar flexion.

Peroneus tertius m.

O, Distal third
of anterior fibula

I, Base of
fifth metatarsal

Ankle dorsal flexion

Foot eversion

FIG. 11.15 ● Peroneus tertius muscle,
anterior view. *O*, Origin; *I*, insertion.

Chapter
11

Extensor digitorum longus muscle

FIG. 11.16

(eks-ten´sor dij-i-to´rum long´gus)

Origin

Lateral condyle of the tibia, head of the fibula, and
upper two-thirds of the anterior surface of the
fibula

Insertion

Tops of the middle and distal phalanges of the four
lesser toes

Action

Extension of the four lesser toes
Dorsal flexion of the ankle
Eversion of the foot

Palpation

Second muscle to the lateral side of the anterior tibial border; upper lateral side of the tibia between
the tibialis anterior medially and the fibula laterally;
divides into 4 tendons just distal to anterior ankle

Innervation

Deep peroneal nerve (L4–L5, S1)

Application, strengthening, and flexibility

Strength is necessary in the extensor digitorum
longus muscle to maintain balance between the
plantar and the dorsal flexors.

Action that involves dorsal flexion of the ankle
and extension of the toes against resistance
strengthens both the extensor digitorum longus
and the extensor hallucis longus muscles. This
may be accomplished by manually applying a
downward force on the toes while attempting to
extend them up.

The extensor digitorum longus may be
stretched by passively taking the four lesser toes
into full flexion while the foot is inverted and
plantar flexed.

O, Lateral condyle
of tibia

Extensor digitorum
longus m.

O, Head of fibula,
upper two-thirds
of anterior
surface of fibula

Ankle
dorsal
flexion

Toe extension

Eversion

I, Tops of middle and
distal phalanges
of four lesser toes

FIG. 11.16 ● Extensor digitorum longus muscle,
anterior view. *O*, Origin; *I*, insertion.

Chapter

11

Extensor hallucis longus muscle

FIG. 11.17

(eks-ten´sor hal-u´sis long´gus)

Origin

Middle two-thirds of the medial surface of the anterior fibula

Insertion

Base of the distal phalanx of the great toe

Action

Dorsiflexion of the ankle
Extension of the great toe
Weak inversion of the foot

Palpation

From the dorsal aspect of the great toe to just lateral of the tibialis anterior at the anterior ankle joint

Innervation

Deep peroneal nerve (L4–L5, S1)

Application, strengthening, and flexibility

The three dorsiflexors of the foot—tibialis anterior, extensor digitorum longus, and extensor hallucis longus—may be exercised by attempting to walk on the heels with the ankle flexed dorsally and toes extended. Extension of the great toe, as well as ankle dorsiflexion against resistance, will provide strengthening for this muscle.

The extensor hallucis longus may be stretched by passively taking the great toe into full flexion while the foot is everted and plantar flexed.

Extensor hallucis longus m.

O, Middle two-thirds of medial surface of anterior fibula

Ankle dorsal flexion

Toe extension

I, Top of base of distal phalanx of great toe

FIG. 11.17 ● Extensor hallucis longus muscle, anterior view. *O,* Origin; *I,* insertion.

Tibialis anterior muscle FIG. 11.18

(tib-i-a´lis ant-te´ri-or)

Origin

Upper two-thirds of the lateral surface of the tibia

Insertion

Inner surface of the medial cuneiform and the base of the first metatarsal bone

Action

Dorsal flexion of the ankle
Inversion of the foot

Palpation

First muscle to the lateral side of the anterior tibial border, particularly palpable with fully active ankle dorsiflexion

Innervation

Deep peroneal nerve (L4–L5, S1)

Application, strengthening, and flexibility

By its insertion, the tibialis anterior muscle is in a fine position to hold up the inner margin of the foot. However, as it contracts concentrically, it dorsiflexes the ankle and is used as an antagonist to the plantar flexors of the ankle. The tibialis anterior is forced to contract strongly when a person ice skates or walks on the outside of the foot. It strongly supports the long arch in inversion.

Walking barefoot or in stocking feet on the outside of the foot (inversion) is an excellent exercise for the tibialis anterior muscle.

Turning the sole of the foot to the inside against resistance to perform inversion exercises is one way to strengthen this muscle. Dorsal flexion exercises against resistance may also be used for this purpose.

The tibialis anterior may be stretched by passively taking the foot into extreme eversion and plantar flexion.

O, Upper two-thirds of lateral surface of tibia

Tibialis anterior m.

Ankle dorsal flexion

Foot inversion

I, Inner surface of medial cuneiform, base of the first metatarsal bones

FIG. 11.18 ● Tibialis anterior muscle, anterior view. *O*, Origin; *I*, insertion.

Chapter
11

Tibialis posterior muscle   FIG. 11.19

(tib-i-a´lis pos-te´ri-or)

Origin

Posterior surface of the upper half of the interosseus membrane and adjacent surfaces of the tibia and fibula

Insertion

Lower inner surfaces of the navicular and cuneiform bones and bases of the second, third, fourth, and fifth metatarsal bones

Action

Plantar flexion of the ankle
Inversion of the foot

Palpation

The tendon may be palpated immediately behind the medial malleolus with inversion and plantar flexion

Innervation

Tibial nerve (L5, S1)

Application, strengthening, and flexibility

Passing down the back of the leg, under the medial malleolus, then forward to the navicular and medial cuneiform bones, the tibialis posterior muscle pulls down from the underside and, when contracted concentrically, inverts and the plantar flexes the foot. "Shin splints" is a slang term frequently used to describe an often chronic condition in which the tibialis posterior, tibialis anterior, and extensor digitorum longus muscles are inflamed. This inflammation is usually a tendinitis of one or more of these structures but may be a result of stress fracture, periostitis, tibial stress syndrome, or compartment syndrome. Sprints and long-distance running are common causes, particularly if the athlete has not developed appropriate strength, flexibility, and endurance in the lower-leg musculature.

Use of the tibialis posterior muscle in plantar flexion and inversion gives support to the longitudinal arch of the foot. This muscle is generally strengthened by performing heel raises, as described for the gastrocnemius and soleus, as well as inversion exercises against resistance.

The tibialis posterior may be stretched by passively taking the foot into extreme eversion and dorsiflexion while the knee is flexed.

FIG. 11.19 ● Tibialis posterior muscle, posterior & plantar views. *O*, Origin; *I*, insertion.

O, Posterior surface of upper half of interosseous membrane, adjacent surfaces of tibia and fibula

I, Lower inner surfaces of navicular and cuneiform bones, bases of second, third, fourth, and fifth metatarsal bones

Plantar flexion

Foot inversion

Chapter

11

Flexor digitorum longus muscle

FIG. 11.20

(fleks´or dij-i-to´rum long´gus)

Origin

Middle third of the posterior surface of the tibia

Insertion

Base of the distal phalanx of each of the four lesser
  toes

Action

Flexion of the four lesser toes
Plantar flexion of the ankle
Inversion of the foot

Palpation

The tendon may be palpated immediately posterior
  to the medial malleolus and tibialis posterior and
  immediately anterior to the flexor hallucis longus
  with flexion of the lesser toes.

Innervation

Tibial nerve (L5, S1)

Application, strengthening, and flexibility

Passing down the back of the lower leg under the
medial malleolus and then forward, the flexor
digitorum longus muscle draws the four lesser
toes down into flexion toward the heel as the plantar flexes the ankle. It is very important in helping
other foot muscles maintain the longitudinal arch.
Walking, running, and jumping do not necessarily
call the flexor digitorum longus muscle into action. Some of the weak foot and ankle conditions
result from ineffective use of the flexor digitorum
longus. Walking barefoot with the toes curled
downward toward the heels and with the foot
inverted will exercise this muscle. It may be
strengthened by performing towel grabs against
resistance in which the heel rests on the floor
while the toes extend to grab a flat towel and
then flex to pull the towel under the foot. This
may be repeated numerous times, with a small
weight placed on the opposite end of the towel
for added resistance.

The flexor digitorum longus may be stretched
by passively taking the four lesser toes into extreme extension while the foot is everted and
dorsiflexed. The knee should be flexed.

FIG. 11.20 ● Flexor digitorum longus muscle,
posterior & plantar views. *O*, Origin; *I*, insertion.

Chapter
11

Flexor hallucis longus muscle

FIG. 11.21

(fleks´or hal-u´sis long´gus)

Origin

Middle two-thirds of the posterior surface of the fibula

Insertion

Base of the distal phalanx of the big toe, under the
  surface

Action

Flexion of the great toe
Inversion of the foot
Plantar flexion of the ankle

Palpation

Anteromedial to the Achilles tendon near the heel

Innervation

Tibial nerve (L5, S1–S2)

Application, strengthening, and flexibility

Pulling from the underside of the great toe, the
flexor hallucis longus muscle may work independently of the flexor digitorum longus muscle or
with it. If these two muscles are poorly developed, they cramp easily when they are called on
to do activities to which they are unaccustomed.

These muscles are used effectively in walking
if the toes are used (as they should be) in maintaining balance as each step is taken. Walking
"with the toes" rather than "over" them is an important action for them.

When the gastrocnemius, soleus, tibialis posterior, peroneus longus, peroneus brevis, flexor digitorum longus, flexor digitorum brevis, and flexor
hallucis longus muscles are all used effectively in
walking, the strength of the ankle is evident. If an
ankle and a foot are weak, in most cases it is because of lack of use of all the muscles just mentioned. Running, walking, jumping, hopping, and
skipping provide exercise for this muscle group.
The flexor hallucis longus muscle may be specifically strengthened by performing towel grabs as
described for the flexor digitorum longus.

The flexor hallucis longus may be stretched by
passively taking the great toe into extreme extension while the foot is everted and dorsiflexed.
The knee should be flexed.

FIG. 11.21 ● Flexor hallucis longus muscle,
medial view. *O*, Origin; *I*, insertion.

Flexor hallucis longus m.

O, Middle two-thirds
of posterior
surface of fibula

I, Base of distal
phalanx of large
toe, undersurface

Plantar flexion

Toe flexion

Foot inversion

Intrinsic muscles of the foot FIG. 11.22 & FIG. 11.23

The intrinsic muscles of the foot have their origins and insertions on the bones within the foot (Figs. 11.22 and 11.23). One of these muscles, the extensor digitorum brevis, is found on the dorsum of the foot. The remainder are found in a plantar compartment in four layers on the plantar surface of the foot. The following muscles are found in the four layers:

First (superficial) layer: abductor hallucis, flexor digitorum brevis, abductor digiti minimi (quinti)
Second layer: quadratus plantae, lumbricales (four)
Third layer: flexor hallucis brevis, adductor hallucis, flexor digiti minimi (quinti) brevis
Fourth (deep) layer: dorsal interossei (four), plantar interossei (three)

The intrinsic foot muscles may be grouped by location as well as by the parts of the foot they act. The abductor hallucis, flexor hallucis brevis, and adductor hallucis all insert either medially or laterally on the proximal phalanx of the great toe. The abductor hallucis and flexor hallucis brevis are located somewhat medially, whereas the adductor hallucis is more centrally located beneath the metatarsals.

The quadratus plantae, four lumbricales, four dorsal interossei, three plantar interossei, flexor digitorum brevis, and extensor digitorum brevis are all located somewhat centrally. All are beneath the foot except the extensor digitorum brevis, which is the only intrinsic muscle in the foot located in the dorsal compartment. Although the entire extensor digitorum brevis has its origin on the anterior and lateral calcaneus, some anatomists refer to its first tendon as the extensor hallucis brevis in order to maintain consistency in naming according to function and location.

Located laterally beneath the foot are the abductor digiti minimi and the flexor digiti minimi brevis, which both insert on the lateral aspect of the base of the proximal phalanx of the fifth phalange. Because of these two muscles' insertion and action on the fifth toe, the name "quinti" is sometimes used instead of minimi.

Four muscles act on the great toe. The abductor hallucis is solely responsible for abduction of the great toe, but assists the flexor hallucis brevis in flexing the great toe at the metatarsophalangeal joint. The adductor hallucis is the sole adductor of the great toe, while the extensor digitorum brevis is the only intrinsic extensor of the great toe at the metatarsophalangeal joint.

The four lumbricales are flexors of the second, third, fourth, and fifth phalanges at their metatarsophalangeal joints, while the quadratus plantae are flexors of these phalanges at their distal interphalangeal joints. The three plantar interossei are adductors and flexors of the proximal phalanxes of the third, fourth, and fifth phalanges, while the four dorsal interossei are abductors and flexors of the second, third, and fourth phalanges, also at their metatarsophalangeal joints. The flexor digitorum brevis flexes the middle phalanxes of the second, third, fourth, and fifth phalanges. The extensor digitorum brevis, as previously mentioned, is an extensor of the great toe but also extends the second, third, and fourth phalanges at their metatarsophalangeal joints.

There are two muscles that act solely on the fifth toe. The proximal phalanx of the fifth phalange is abducted by the abductor digiti minimi and is flexed by the flexor digiti minimi brevis.

Refer to Table 11.2 for further details regarding the intrinsic muscles of the foot.

Muscles are developed and maintain their strength only when they are used. One factor in the great increase in weak foot conditions is the lack of exercise to develop these muscles. Walking is one of the best activities for maintaining and developing the many small muscles that help support the arch of the foot. Some authorities advocate walking without shoes or with some of the newer shoes designed to enhance proper mechanics. Additionally, towel exercises such as those described for the flexor digitorum longus and flexor hallucis longus are helpful in strengthening the intrinsic muscles of the foot.

A

Fibrous digital sheaths

Lumbricales

Flexor digiti minimi brevis

Abductor digiti minimi

Plantar interosseous

Tendon of flexor hallucis longus

Flexor hallucis brevis

Flexor digitorum brevis

Abductor hallucis

Plantar aponeurosis (cut)

Calcaneal tuberosity

B

Tendon of flexor digitorum brevis (cut)

Tendon of flexor hallucis longus

Flexor hallucis brevis

Lumbricales

Tendon of flexor digitorum longus

Quadratus plantae

Flexor digiti minimi brevis

Abductor digiti minimi

Flexor digitorum brevis (cut)

Abductor hallucis (cut)

C

Tendon of flexor digitorum brevis (cut)

Plantar interossei

Quadratus plantae (cut)

Tendon of lumbrical (cut)

Tendon of flexor digitorum longus (cut)

Transverse head and

Oblique head of adductor hallucis

Flexor hallucis brevis

Opponens digiti minimi

Tendon of flexor hallucis longus (cut)

Tendon of flexor digitorum longus (cut)

D

Plantar ligaments

Articular capsules

Sesamoid bones

Dorsal interossei

Plantar interossei

Tendon of peroneus longus

Tendon of tibialis posterior

Long plantar ligament

Peroneus brevis tendon

FIG. 11.22 ● The four musculotendinous layers of the plantar aspect of the foot, detailing the intrinsic muscles. **A,** Superficial layer; **B,** second layer; **C,** third layer; **D,** deep layer.

Modified from Van De Graaff KM: *Human anatomy,* ed 4, 1995, McGraw-Hill Companies, Inc., New York.

Chapter

11

Anterior tibial artery and
deep fibular nerve

Superior extensor
retinaculum

Peroneus tertius

Tendon of extensor
digitorum longus

Lateral malleolus

Inferior extensor
retinaculum

Extensor digitorum
brevis

Tendon of peroneus
brevis

Tuberosity of fifth
metatarsal bone

Tendon of peroneus tertius

Abductor digiti minimi

Tendons of extensor
digitorum brevis

Tendons of extensor
digitorum longus

Tendon of tibialis anterior

Medial malleolus

Anterior medial malleolar artery

Tendon of extensor hallucis longus

Dorsalis pedis artery

Deep fibular nerve

Extensor hallucis brevis

Arcuate artery

Abductor hallucis

First dorsal interosseous

Tendon of extensor hallucis
brevis

Extensor expansions

Dorsal digital arteries

Dorsal digital branches of
superficial fibular nerve

Creek

FIG. 11.23 ● Anterior view of dorsum of foot.

TABLE 11.2 • **Intrinsic muscles of the foot**

	Muscle	Origin	Insertion	Action	Palpation	Innervation
Superficial layer	Flexor digitorum brevis	Tuberosity of calcaneus, plantar aponeurosis	Medial and lateral aspects of 2nd, 3rd, 4th, and 5th middle phalanxes	MP and PIP flexion of 2nd, 3rd, 4th, and 5th phalanges	Cannot be palpated	Medial plantar nerve (L4, L5)
	Abductor digiti minimi (quinti)	Tuberosity of calcaneus, plantar aponeurosis	Lateral aspect of 5th proximal phalanx	MP abduction of 5th phalange	Cannot be palpated	Lateral plantar nerve (S1, S2)
	Flexor hallucis brevis	Cuboid, lateral cuneiform	Medial head: medial aspect of 1st proximal phalanx Lateral head: lateral aspect of 1st proximal phalanx	MP flexion of 1st phalange	Cannot be palpated	Medial plantar nerve (L4, L5, S1)
	Abductor hallucis	Tuberosity of calcaneus, flexor retinaculum, plantar aponeurosis	Medial aspect of base of 1st proximal phalanx	MP flexion, abduction of 1st phalanx	On the plantar aspect of the foot from medial tubercle of calcaneus to medial side of great toe proximal phalanx with great toe abduction	Medial plantar nerve (L4, L5)
Second layer	Flexor digiti minimi (quinti) brevis	Base of 5th metatarsal, sheath of peroneus longus tendon	Lateral aspect of base of 5th proximal phalanx	MP flexion of 5th phalange	Cannot be palpated	Lateral plantar nerve (S2, S3)
	Quadratus plantae	Medial head: medial surface of calcaneus Lateral head: Lateral border of inferior surface of calcaneus	Lateral margin of flexor digitorum longus tendon	DIP flexion of 2nd, 3rd, 4th, and 5th phalanges	Cannot be palpated	Lateral plantar nerve (S1, S2)
	Lumbricales (4)	Tendons of flexor digitorum longus	Dorsal surface of 2nd, 3rd, 4th, and 5th proximal phalanxes	MP flexion of 2nd, 3rd, 4th, and 5th phalanges	Cannot be palpated	1st lumbricales: medial plantar nerve (L4, L5) 2nd, 3rd, 4th lumbricales: lateral plantar nerve (S1, S2)

(*continued*)

Chapter
11

TABLE 11.2 (continued) • **Intrinsic muscles of the foot**

	Muscle	Origin	Insertion	Action	Palpation	Innervation
Third layer	Adductor hallucis	Oblique head: 2nd, 3rd, and 4th metatarsals and sheath of peroneus longus tendon Transverse head: plantar metatarsophalangeal ligaments of 3rd, 4th, and 5th phalanges and transverse metatarsal ligaments	Lateral aspect of base of 1st proximal phalanx	MP adduction of 1st phalange	Cannot be palpated	Lateral plantar nerve (S1, S2)
	Plantar interossei (3)	Bases and medial shafts of 3rd, 4th, and 5th metatarsals	Medial aspects of bases of 3rd, 4th, and 5th proximal phalanxes	MP adduction and flexion of 3rd, 4th, and 5th phalanges	Cannot be palpated	Lateral plantar nerve (S1, S2)
Deep layer	Dorsal interossei (4)	Two heads on shafts of adjacent metatarsals	1st interossei: medial aspect of 2nd proximal phalanx 2nd, 3rd, and 4th interossei: lateral aspect of 2nd, 3rd, and 4th proximal phalanxes	MP abduction and flexion of 2nd, 3rd, and 4th phalanges	Cannot be palpated	Lateral plantar nerve (S1, S2)
Dorsal layer	Extensor digitorum brevis	Anterior and lateral calcaneus, lateral talocalcaneal ligament, inferior extensor retinaculum	Base of proximal phalanx of 1st phalange, lateral sides of extensor digitorum longus tendons of 2nd, 3rd, and 4th phalanges	Assists in MP extension of 1st phalanx and extension of middle three phalanges	As a mass anterior to and slightly below lateral malleolus on dorsum of foot	Deep peroneal nerve (L5, S1)

Web sites

Anatomy & Physiology Tutorials:

www.gwc.maricopa.edu/class/bio201/index.htm

Radiologic Anatomy Browser:

radlinux1.usuf1.usuhs.mil/rad/iong/index.html

This site has numerous radiological views of the musculoskeletal system.

University of Arkansas Medical School Gross Anatomy for Medical Students:

anatomy.uams.edu/htmlpages/anatomyhtml/ gross.html

Dissections, anatomy tables, atlas images, links, etc.

Loyola University Medical Center: Structure of the Human Body:

www.meddean.luc.edu/lumen/MedEd/ GrossAnatomy/GA.html

An excellent site with many slides, dissections, tutorials, etc., for the study of human anatomy

Wheeless's Textbook of Orthopaedics:

www.ortho-u.net/

This site has an extensive index of links to the fractures, joints, muscles, nerves, trauma, medications, medical topics, and lab tests, as well as links to orthopedic journals and other orthopedic and medical news.

Foot and Ankle Web Index:

www.footandankle.com

The foot and ankle link library located at this site is very helpful.

American College of Foot and Ankle Surgeons:

www.acfas.org

This site, sponsored by podiatric surgeons and doctors of podiatric medicine (DPM), has information on topics relating to foot health—foot and ankle deformities and injuries; care of the diabetic foot; foot and ankle disorders caused by arthritis, aging, trauma and sports injuries; and congenital deformities and disease.

The University of Texas MD Anderson Cancer Center Multimedia and Learning Resources:

rpiwww.mdacc.tmc.edu/mmlearn/anatomy.html

This site has numerous cadaveric cuts of the foot, knee, hand, arm, and elbow; an interactive ankle; and a rotating foot and ankle.

American Orthopaedic Foot and Ankle Society:

www.aofas.org

Numerous patient education brochures regarding foot and ankle problems are found here.

Premiere Medical Search Engine:

www.medsite.com

This site allows the reader to enter any medical condition and it will search the net to find relevant articles.

Virtual Hospital:

www.vh.org

Numerous slides, patient information, etc.

Dynamic Human version 2.0 CD-ROM: The Visual Guide to Anatomy & Physiology:

www.mhhe.com/biosci/ap/dynamichuman2/

Web site that accompanies this CD-ROM

Worksheet exercise

As an aid to learning, for in-class or out-of-class assignments, or for testing, tear-out worksheets are found at the end of the text (p. 336).

Anterior and posterior skeletal worksheet (no. 1)

Draw and label on the worksheet the following muscles of the ankle and foot:
a. Tibialis anterior
b. Extensor digitorum longus
c. Peroneus longus
d. Peroneus brevis
e. Peroneus tertius
f. Soleus
g. Gastrocnemius
h. Extensor hallucis longus
i. Tibialis posterior
j. Flexor digitorum longus
k. Flexor hallucis longus

Chapter

11

Laboratory and review exercises

1. Locate the following parts of the ankle and foot on a human skeleton and on a subject:
   a. Lateral malleolus
   b. Medial malleolus
   c. Calcaneus
   d. Navicular
   e. Three cuneiform bones
   f. Metatarsal bones
   g. Phalanges
2. How and where can the following muscles be palpated on a human subject?
   a. Tibialis anterior
   b. Extensor digitorum longus
   c. Peroneus longus
   d. Peroneus brevis
   e. Soleus
   f. Gastrocnemius
   g. Extensor hallucis longus
   h. Flexor digitorum longus
   i. Flexor hallucis longus
3. Demonstrate and palpate the following movements:
   a. Plantar flexion
   b. Dorsal flexion
   c. Inversion
   d. Eversion
   e. Flexion of the toes
   f. Extension of the toes
4. List the planes in which each of the following movements occurs. List the respective axis of rotation for each movement in each plane.
   a. Plantar flexion
   b. Dorsal flexion
   c. Inversion
   d. Eversion
   e. Flexion of the toes
   f. Extension of the toes
5. Why are "low arches" and "flat feet" not synonymous terms?
6. Discuss the value of proper footwear in various sports and activities.
7. What are orthotics and how do they function?
8. Research common foot disorders, such as flat feet, ankle injuries, and hammertoes. Report your findings in class.
9. Research the anatomical factors relating to the prevalence of inversion versus eversion ankle sprains and report your findings in class.
10. Report orally or in writing on magazine articles that rate running and walking shoes.
11. Have a laboratory partner raise up on the toes (heel raise) with the knees fully extended and then repeat with the knees flexed approximately 20 degrees. Which exercise position appears to be more difficult to maintain for an extended period of time and why? What are the implications for strengthening these muscles? For stretching these muscles?
12. Fill in the antagonistic muscle action chart on the next page by listing the muscle(s) or parts of muscles that are antagonistic in their actions to the muscles in the left column.
13. Fill in the muscle analysis chart on the next page by listing the muscles primarily involved in each joint movement.

Chapter
11

Antagonistic muscle action chart • Ankle, transverse tarsal and subtalar joints, and toes

Agonist	Antagonist
Gastrocnemius	
Soleus	
Tibialis posterior	
Flexor digitorum longus	
Flexor hallucis longus	
Peroneus longus/ peroneus brevis	
Peroneus tertius	
Tibialis anterior	
Extensor digitorum longus	
Extensor hallucis longus	

Muscle analysis chart • Ankle, transverse tarsal and subtalar joints, and toes

Ankle	
Dorsiflexion	Plantar flexion
Transverse tarsal and subtalar joints	
Eversion	Inversion
Toes	
Flexion	Extension

Chapter

11

References

Astrom M, Arvidson T: Alignment and joint motion in the normal foot, *Journal of Orthopaedic and Sports Physical Therapy* 22:5, November 1995.

Booher JM, Thibodeau GA: *Athletic injury assessment,* ed 4, 2000, McGraw-Hill Companies, Inc., New York.

Coughlin LP, et al: Fracture dislocation of the tarsal navicular: a case report, *American Journal of Sports Medicine* 15:614, November–December 1987.

Dearing M, Ziccardi NJ: Prevention and rehabilitation of ankle injuries, *Athletic Journal* 66:28, November 1985.

Field D: *Anatomy: palpation and surface markings,* ed 3, Oxford, 2001, Butterworth-Heinemann.

Franco AH: Pes cavus and pes planus—analysis and treatment, *Physical Therapy* 67:688, May 1987.

Gench BE, Hinson MM, Harvey PT: *Anatomical kinesiology,* Dubuque, IA, 1995, Eddie Bowers.

Grace P: Prevention and rehabilitation of shin splints, *Scholastic Coach* 57:47, March 1988.

Hamilton N, Luttgens K: *Kinesiology: scientific basis of human motion,* ed 10, Boston, 2002, McGraw-Hill.

Henderson J: Baring the soles, *Runners World* 22:14, November 1987.

Lindsay DT: *Functional human anatomy,* St. Louis, 1996, Mosby.

Robinson M: Feet first, *Coach and Athlete* 44:30, August–September 1981.

Rockar PA: The subtalar joint: anatomy and joint motion, *Journal of Orthopaedic and Sports Physical Therapy* 21:6, June 1995.

Sammarco GJ: Foot and ankle injuries in sports, *American Journal of Sports Medicine* 14:6, November–December 1986.

Seeley RR, Stephens TD, Tate P: *Anatomy & physiology,* ed 6, Dubuque, IA, 2003, McGraw-Hill.

Sieg KW, Adams SP: *Illustrated essentials of musculoskeletal anatomy,* ed 2, Gainesville, FL, 1985, Megabooks.

Stone RJ, Stone JA: *Atlas of the skeletal muscles,* 1990, McGraw-Hill Companies, Inc., New York.

Thibodeau GA, Patton KT: *Anatomy & physiology,* ed 9, St. Louis, 1993, Mosby.

Van de Graaff KM: *Human anatomy,* ed 6, Dubuque, IA, 2002, McGraw-Hill.

Chapter 12

The Trunk and Spinal Column

Objectives

- To identify and differentiate the different types of vertebrae in the spinal column

- To label on a skeletal chart the types of vertebrae and their important features

- To draw and label on a skeletal chart some of the muscles of the trunk and the spinal column

- To demonstrate and palpate with a fellow student the movements of the spine and trunk and list their respective planes of motion and axes of rotation

- To palpate on a human subject some of the muscles of the trunk and spinal column

- To list and organize the muscles that produce the primary movements of the trunk and spinal column and their antagonists

---

Online Learning Center Resources

Visit *Manual of Structural Kinesiology's* Online Learning Center at **www.mhhe.com/floyd15e** for additional information and study material for this chapter, including:

- *Self-grading quizzes*
- *Anatomy flashcards*
- *Animations*

The trunk and spinal column present problems in kinesiology that are not found in the study of other parts of the body. First is the complexity of the vertebral column. It consists of 24 intricate and complex articulating vertebrae. These vertebrae contain the spinal column, with its 31 pairs of spinal nerves. Unquestionably it is the most complex part of the human body other than the brain and the central nervous system.

The anterior portion of the trunk contains the abdominal muscles, which are somewhat different from other muscles in that some sections are linked by fascia and tendinous bands and thus do not attach from bone to bone. In addition, there are many small intrinsic muscles acting on the head, vertebral column, and thorax that assist in spinal stabilization or respiration, depending on their location. These muscles are generally too deep to palpate and consequently will not be given the full attention that the larger superficial muscles will receive in this chapter.

Bones

Vertebral column

The intricate and complex bony structure of the vertebral column consists of 24 articulating vertebrae and nine that are fused together (Fig. 12.1). The column is further divided into the seven cervical (neck) vertebrae, 12 thoracic (chest) vertebrae, and five lumbar (lower back) vertebrae. The sacrum (posterior pelvic girdle) and the coccyx (tail bone) consist of five and four fused vertebrae, respectively. The first two cervical vertebrae are unique in that their shapes allow for extensive rotary movements of the head to the sides, as well as forward and backward. The spine has three normal curves within its movable vertebrae. The

www.mhhe.com/floyd15e **265**

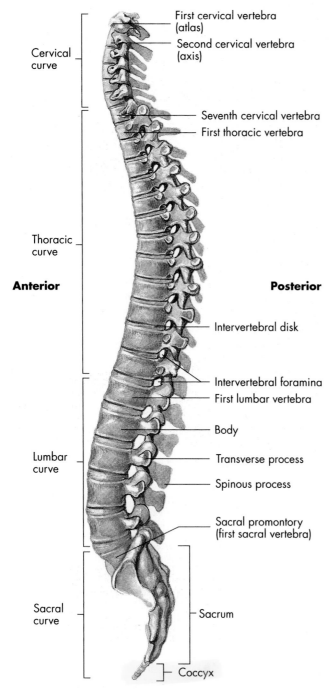

FIG. 12.1 ● Vertebral column.

Cervical curve

First cervical vertebra (atlas)

Second cervical vertebra (axis)

Seventh cervical vertebra
First thoracic vertebra

Thoracic curve

Anterior

Posterior

Intervertebral disk

Intervertebral foramina
First lumbar vertebra

Body

Lumbar curve

Transverse process

Spinous process

Sacral promontory (first sacral vertebra)

Sacral curve

Sacrum

Coccyx

From Seeley, et al: *Anatomy & physiology*, ed 3, St. Louis, 1995, Mosby.

thoracic spine curve is concave anteriorly and convex posteriorly, while the cervical and lumbar curves are concave posteriorly and convex anteriorly. The normal curves of the spine enable it to absorb blows and shocks.

The bones in each region of the spine have slightly different sizes and shapes to allow for

various functions (Fig. 12.2). The vertebrae increase in size from the cervical region to the lumbar region, primarily because they have to support more weight in the lower back than in the neck. The first two cervical vertebrae are known as the atlas and axis, respectively. The vertebrae C2 through L5 have similar architecture: each has a bony block anteriorly, known as the body, a vertebral foramen centrally for the spinal cord to pass through, a transverse process projecting out laterally to each side, and a spinous process projecting posteriorly that is easily palpable.

Undesirable deviations from the normal curvatures occur due to a number of factors. Increased posterior concavity of the lumbar and cervical curves is known as *lordosis,* while increased anterior concavity of the normal thoracic curve is known as *kyphosis.* The lumbar spine may have a reduction of its normal lordotic curve, resulting in a flat-back appearance referred to as *lumbar kyphosis. Scoliosis* refers to lateral curvatures or sideward deviations of the spine.

Thorax

The skeletal foundation of the thorax is formed by 12 pairs of ribs (Fig. 12.3). Seven pairs are true ribs, in that they attach directly to the sternum. Five pairs are considered false ribs. Of these, three pairs attach indirectly to the sternum and two pairs are floating ribs, in that their ends are free. The manubrium, the body of the sternum, and the xiphoid process are the other bones of the thorax. All of the ribs are attached posteriorly to the thoracic vertebrae.

Key bony landmarks for locating the muscles of the neck include the mastoid process, transverse and spinous processes of the cervical spine, spinous processes of the upper four thoracic vertebrae, manubrium of the sternum, and medial clavicle. The spinous and transverse processes of the thoracic spine and the posterior ribs are key areas of attachment for the posterior muscles of the spine. The anterior trunk muscles have attachments on the borders of the lower eight ribs, the costal cartilages of the ribs, the iliac crest, and the pubic crest. The transverse processes of the upper four lumbar vertebrae also serve as points of insertion for the quadratus lumborum, along with the lower border of the twelfth rib.

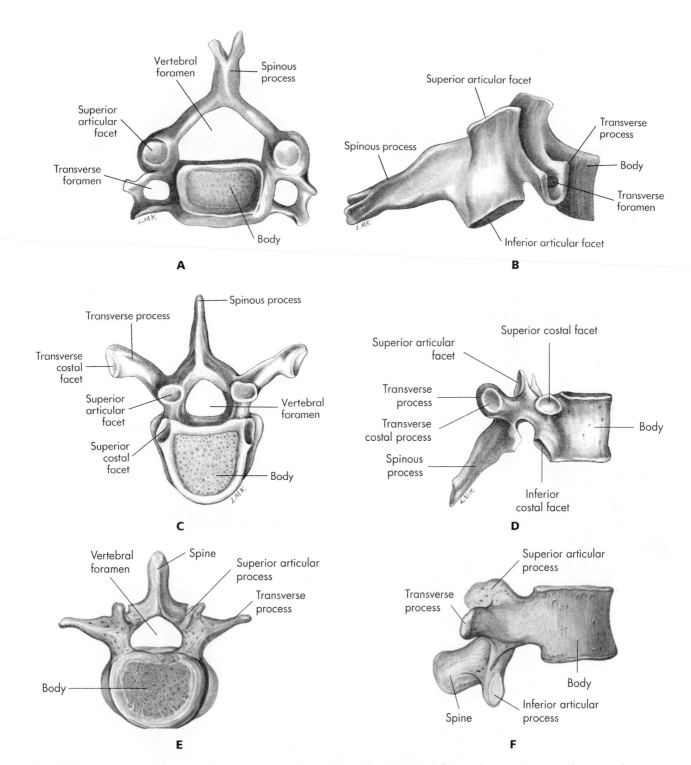

FIG. 12.2 ● Vertebral column. **A,** Typical cervical vertebra viewed from above; **B,** typical cervical vertebra viewed from the side; **C,** typical thoracic vertebra viewed from above; **D,** typical thoracic vertebra viewed from the side; **E,** third lumbar vertebra viewed from above; **F,** third lumbar vertebra viewed from the side.

From Anthony CP, Kolthoff NJ: *Textbook of anatomy and physiology,* ed 9, St. Louis, 1975, Mosby.

Chapter
12

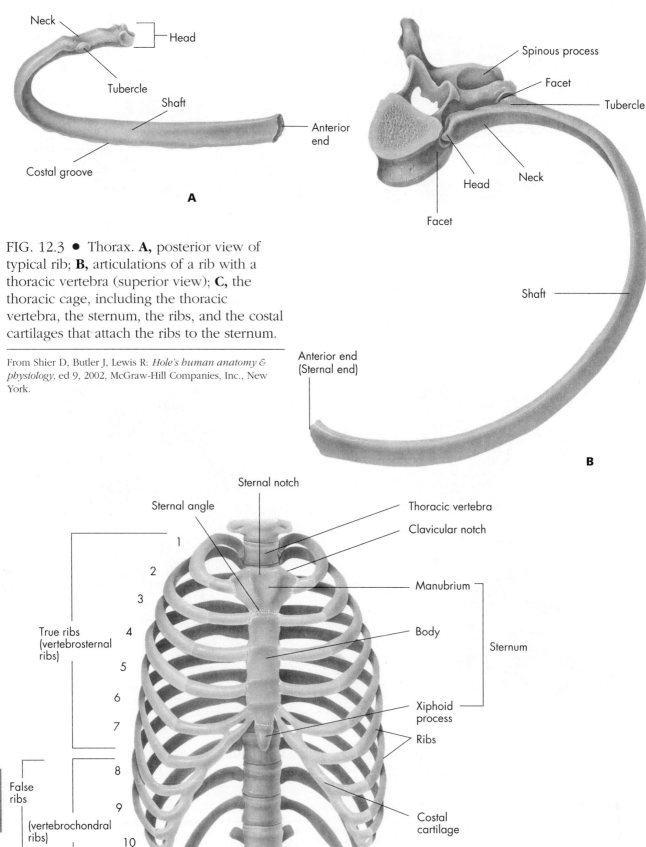

Neck

Head

Tubercle

Shaft

Anterior end

Costal groove

A

FIG. 12.3 ● Thorax. **A,** posterior view of typical rib; **B,** articulations of a rib with a thoracic vertebra (superior view); **C,** the thoracic cage, including the thoracic vertebra, the sternum, the ribs, and the costal cartilages that attach the ribs to the sternum.

From Shier D, Butler J, Lewis R: *Hole's human anatomy & physiology,* ed 9, 2002, McGraw-Hill Companies, Inc., New York.

Spinous process

Facet

Tubercle

Neck

Head

Facet

Shaft

Anterior end (Sternal end)

B

Sternal notch

Sternal angle

Thoracic vertebra

Clavicular notch

1

2

3

True ribs (vertebrosternal ribs)

4

5

6

7

Manubrium

Body

Sternum

Xiphoid process

Ribs

Costal cartilage

False ribs

8

9

(vertebrochondral ribs)

10

11

Floating ribs (vertebral ribs)

12

C

Joints

The first joint in the axial skeleton is the atlanto-occipital joint, formed by the occipital condyles of the skull sitting on the articular fossa of the first vertebra, which allows flexion and extension. The atlas (C1) in turn sits on the axis (C2) to form the atlantoaxial joint (Fig. 12.4, *A*). Except for the atlantoaxial joint, there is not a great deal of movement possible between any two vertebrae. However, the cumulative effect of combining the movement from several adjacent vertebrae allows for substantial movements within a given area. Most of the rotation within the cervical region occurs in the atlantoaxial joint, which is classified as a trochoid or pivot-type joint. The remainder of the vertebral articulations are classified as arthrodial or gliding-type joints because of their limited gliding movements.

Gliding movement occurs between the superior and inferior articular processes that form the facet joints of the vertebrae, as depicted in Figs. 12.2 and 12.4, *B*. Located in between and adhering to the articular cartilage of the vertebral bodies are the intervertebral disks (Fig. 12.4, *C*). These disks are composed of an outer rim of dense fibrocartilage known as the annulus fibrosus and a central gelatinous, pulpy substance known as the nucleus pulposus. This arrangement of compressed elastic material allows compression in all directions, along with torsion. With age, injury, or improper use of the spine, the intervertebral disks become less resilient, resulting in a weakened annulus fibrosus. Substantial weakening combined with compression can result in the nucleus protruding through the annulus, which is known as a herniated nucleus pulposus. Commonly referred to as a herniated or "slipped" disk, this protrusion puts pressure on the spinal nerve root, causing a variety of symptoms, including radiating pain, tingling, numbness, and weakness in the lower extremity (Fig. 12.5).

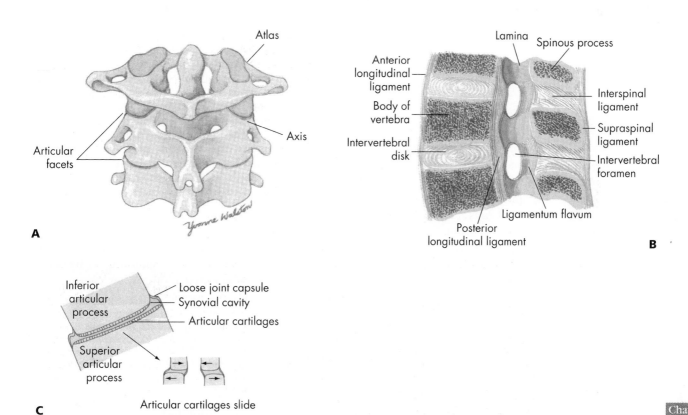

FIG. 12.4 ● Articular facets of vertebrae. **A,** The facets of superior and inferior articular processes articulate between adjacent cervical vertebrae; **B,** Articular cartilages slide back and forth on each other, and the loose articular capsule allows this motion; **C,** Ligaments limit motion between vertebrae, shown in sagittal section through three lumbar vertebrae.

From Lindsay DT: *Functional human anatomy,* St. Louis, 1996, Mosby.

Chapter 12

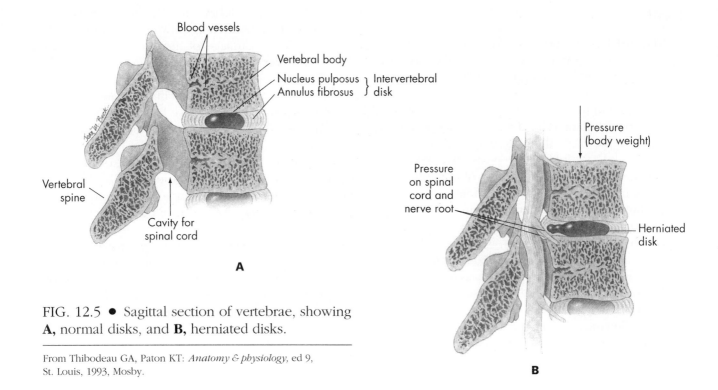

FIG. 12.5 ● Sagittal section of vertebrae, showing **A,** normal disks, and **B,** herniated disks.

From Thibodeau GA, Paton KT: *Anatomy & physiology,* ed 9, St. Louis, 1993, Mosby.

A substantial number of low back problems are caused by improper use of the back over time. These improper mechanics often result in acute strains and muscle spasm of the lumbar extensors and chronic mechanical changes leading to disc herniation. Most problems occur from using the relatively small back muscles to lift objects from a lumbar spine flexed position instead of keeping the lumbar spine in a neutral position while squatting and using the larger, more powerful muscles of the lower extremity. Additionally, our lifestyles chronically place us in lumbar flexion, which over time leads to a gradual loss of lumbar lordosis. This "flat back syndrome" results in increased pressure on the lumbar disc and intermittent or chronic low back pain.

Most of the spinal column movement occurs in the cervical and lumbar regions. There is, of course, some thoracic movement, but it is slight in comparison with that of the neck and low back. In discussing movements of the head, it must be remembered that this movement occurs between the cranium and the first cervical vertebra, as well as within the cervical vertebrae. With the understanding that these motions usually occur together, for simplification purposes this text refers to all movements of the head and neck as cervical movements. Similarly, in discussing trunk movements, lumbar motion terminology is used to describe the combined motion that occurs in both the thoracic and lumbar regions. A closer investigation of specific motion between any two vertebrae is beyond the scope of this text.

The cervical region (Fig. 12.6) can flex 45 degrees and extend 45 degrees. The cervical area laterally flexes 45 degrees and can rotate approximately 60 degrees. The lumbar spine, accounting for most of the trunk movement, (Fig. 12.7) flexes approximately 80 degrees and extends 20 to 30 degrees. Lumbar lateral flexion to each side is usually within 35 degrees, and approximately 45 degrees of rotation occurs to the left and right.

Chapter
12

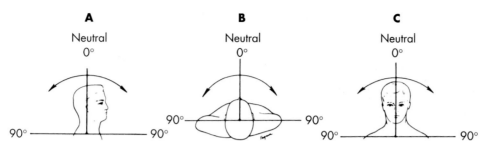

FIG. 12.6 ● Active ROM of the cervical spine. **A,** Flexion and extension. These motions can be estimated in degrees or indicated by the distance the chin lacks from touching the chest; **B,** Rotation can be estimated in degrees or in percentages of motion compared in each direction; **C,** Lateral flexion can be estimated in degrees or indicated by the number of inches the ear lacks from reaching the shoulders.

FIG. 12.7 ● Active ROM of the thoracic and lumbar spine. **A,** Forward flexion. Motion can be estimated in degrees or measurement of fingertips to leg or from floor; **B** and **C,** Flexion tape measuring method; **D,** Hyperextension with the athlete standing; **E,** Hyperextension with the athlete lying prone; **F,** Lateral bending; **G,** Rotation of the spine.

Movements FIG. 12.8

Spinal movements are often preceded by the name given to the region of movement. For example, flexion of the trunk at the lumbar spine is known as lumbar flexion, and extension of the neck is often referred to as cervical extension. Additionally, as was discussed in Chapter 9, the pelvic girdle rotates as a unit due to movement occurring in the hip joints and the lumbar spine. Refer to Table 9.1.

Spinal flexion: anterior movement of the spine; in the cervical region, the head moves toward the chest; in the lumbar region, the thorax moves toward the pelvis

Spinal extension: return from flexion; posterior movement of the spine; in the cervical spine, the head moves away from the chest; in the lumbar spine, the thorax moves away from the pelvis; sometimes referred to as hyperextension

Lateral flexion (left or right): sometimes referred to as side bending; the head moves laterally toward the shoulder, and the thorax moves laterally toward the pelvis

Spinal rotation (left or right): rotary movement of the spine in the horizontal plane; the chin rotates from neutral toward the shoulder, and the thorax rotates to one side

Reduction: return movement from lateral flexion to neutral

Cervical flexion

A

**Cervical extension
(hyperextension)**

B

**Cervical lateral flexion
to the right**

C

**Cervical rotation
to the right**

D

FIG. 12.8 ● Movements of the spine.

Lumbar flexion

E

Lumbar extension (hyperextension)

F

Lumbar lateral flexion to the right

G

Lumbar rotation to the right

H

FIG. 12.8 continued • Movements of the spine.

Trunk and spinal column muscles

The largest muscle in this area is the erector spinae (sacrospinalis), which extends on each side of the spinal column from the pelvic region to the cranium. It is divided into three muscles: the spinalis, the longissimus, and the iliocostalis. From the medial to the lateral side, it has attachments in the lumbar, thoracic, and cervical regions. Thus, the erector spinae group is actually made up of nine muscles. Additionally, the sternocleidomastoid and splenius muscles are large muscles involved in cervical and head movements. Large abdominal muscles involved in lumbar movements include the rectus abdominis, external oblique abdominal, internal oblique abdominal, and quadratus lumborum (Table 12.1)

Numerous small muscles are found in the spinal column region. Many of them originate on one vertebra and insert on the next vertebra. They are important in the functioning of the spine, but knowledge of these muscles is of limited value to most people who use this text. Consequently, discussion will concentrate on the larger muscles primarily involved in trunk and spinal column movements (Table 12.1) and will only briefly address the smaller muscles.

So that the muscles of the trunk and spinal column may be better understood, they may be grouped according to both location and function. It should be noted that some muscles have multiple segments. As a result, one segment of a particular muscle may be located and perform movement in one region, while another segment of the same muscle may be located in another region to perform movements in that region. Many of the muscles of the trunk and spinal column function in moving the spine as well as in aiding respiration. All of the muscles of the thorax are primarily involved in respiration. The abdominal wall muscles are different from other muscles that have been studied. They do not go from bone to bone but attach into an aponeurosis (fascia) around the rectus abdominis area. They are the external oblique abdominal, internal oblique abdominal, and transversus abdominis.

Chapter

12

TABLE 12.1 • Agonist muscles of the spine

	Muscle	Origin	Insertion	Action	Plane of motion	Palpation	Innervation
Anterior neck	Sternocleidomastoid (both sides)	Manubrium of sternum, medial clavicle	Mastoid process	Both sides: flexion of the head and neck	Sagittal	Anterolateral neck, diagonally between the origin and insertion	Spinal accessory (Cr 11, C2–C3)
				Right side: rotation to the left and lateral flexion to the right	Transverse Frontal		
				Left side: rotation to the right and lateral flexion to the left	Transverse Frontal		
Posterior neck	Splenius cervicis	Spinous processes of the 3rd through the 6th thoracic vertebrae	Transverse processes of the first three cervical vertebrae	Both sides: extension of the head and neck	Sagittal	Cannot be palpated	Posterior lateral branches of cervical nerves four through eight (C4–C8)
				Right side: rotation and lateral flexion to the right	Transverse Frontal		
				Left side: rotation and lateral flexion to the left	Transverse Frontal		
	Splenius capitis	Lower half of the ligamentum nuchae and the spinous processes of the 7th cervical and the upper three or four thoracic vertebrae	Mastoid process and occipital bone	Both sides: extension of the head and neck	Sagittal	Cannot be palpated	Posterior lateral branches of cervical nerves four through eight (C4–C8)
				Right side: rotation and lateral flexion to the right	Transverse Frontal		
				Left side: rotation and lateral flexion to the left	Transverse Frontal		
Posterior spine	Erector spinae: Iliocostalis	Thoracolumbar aponeurosis from sacrum, posterior ribs	Posterior ribs, cervical transverse processes	Extension of the spine	Sagittal	Lower lumbar region on either side of the spine	Posterior branches of the spinal nerves
				Lateral flexion of the spine	Frontal		
	Erector spinae: Longissimus	Thoracolumbar aponeurosis from sacrum, lumbar and thoracic transverse processes	Cervical and thoracic transverse processes, mastoid process	Extension of the spine	Sagittal	Lower lumbar region on either side of the spine	Posterior branches of the spinal nerves
				Lateral flexion of the spine	Frontal		
	Erector spinae: Spinalis	Ligamentum nuchae, cervical and thoracic spinous processes	Cervical and thoracic spinous processes, occipital bone	Extension of the spine	Sagittal	Lower lumbar region on either side of the spine	Posterior branches of the spinal nerves
				Lateral flexion of the spine	Frontal		

TABLE 12.1 (continued) • Agonist muscles of the spine

	Muscle	Origin	Insertion	Action	Plane of motion	Palpation	Innervation
Anterior trunk	Rectus abdominis	Crest of pubis	Cartilage of 5th, 6th, and 7th ribs and xiphoid process	Both sides: lumbar flexion	Sagittal	Anteromedial surface of the abdomen, between the rib cage and the pubic bone	Intercostal nerves (T7–T12)
				Right side: lateral flexion to the right	Frontal		
				Left side: lateral flexion to the left	Frontal		
	External oblique abdominal	Borders of lower eight ribs at side of chest dovetailing with serratus anterior	Anterior half of crest of ilium, inguinal ligament, crest of pubis, and fascia of rectus abdominis at lower front	Both sides: lumbar flexion	Sagittal	Lateral side of the abdomen, either left or right	Intercostal nerves (T8–T12), iliohypo-gastric nerve (T12, L1), and ilioinguinal nerve (L1)
				Right side: lumbar lateral flexion to the right and rotation to the left	Frontal Transverse		
				Left side: lumbar lateral flexion to the left and rotation to the right	Frontal Transverse		
	Internal oblique abdominal	Upper half of inguinal ligament, anterior 2/3 of crest of ilium, and lumbar fascia	Costal cartilage of 8th, 9th, and 10th ribs and linea alba	Both sides: lumbar flexion	Sagittal	Palpated on the lateral side of the abdomen when the external oblique is relaxed	Intercostal nerves (T8–T12), iliohypo-gastric nerve (T12, L1), and ilioinguinal nerve (L1)
				Right side: lumbar lateral flexion and rotation to the right	Frontal Transverse		
				Left side: lumbar lateral flexion and rotation to the left	Frontal Transverse		
	Transversus abdominis	Outer 1/3 of the inguinal ligament Inner rim of the iliac crest Inner surface of the cartilage of the lower six ribs Lumbar fascia	Crest of the pubis and the iliopectineal line Abdominal aponeurosis to the linea alba	Forced expiration by pulling the abdominal wall inward	Transverse	Cannot be palpated	Intercostal nerves (T7–T12), iliohypo-gastric nerve (T12, L1), and ilioinguinal nerve (L1)
Lateral lumbar	Quadratus lumborum	Posterior inner lip of the iliac crest	Approximately 1/2 the length of the lower border of the 12th rib and the transverse process of the upper four lumbar vertebrae	Lateral flexion to the side on which it is located Stabilizes the pelvis and lumbar spine	Frontal	For all practical purposes, it is impossible to palpate except on an extremely thin individual	Branches of T12, L1 nerves

Chapter
12

Muscles that move the head

Anterior
  Rectus capitis anterior
  Longus capitis
Posterior
  Longissimus capitis
  Obliquus capitis superior
  Obliquus capitis inferior
  Rectus capitis posterior—major and minor
  Trapezius, superior fibers
  Splenius capitis
  Semispinalis capitis
Lateral
  Rectus capitis lateralis
  Sternocleidomastoid

Muscles of the vertebral column

Superficial
  Erector spinae (sacrospinalis)
      Spinalis—capitis, cervicis, thoracis
      Longissimus—capitis, cervicis, thoracis
      Iliocostalis—cervicis, thoracis, lumborum
  Splenius cervicis
Deep
  Longus colli—superior oblique, inferior oblique, vertical
  Interspinales—entire spinal column
  Intertransversales—entire spinal column
  Multifidus—entire spinal column
  Psoas minor
  Rotatores—entire spinal column
  Semispinalis—cervicis, thoracis

Muscles of the thorax

Diaphragm
Intercostalis—external, internal
Levator costarum
Subcostales
Scalenus—anterior, medius, posterior
Serratus posterior—superior, inferior
Transversus thoracis

Muscles of the abdominal wall

Rectus abdominis
External oblique abdominal (obliquus externus abdominis)
Internal oblique abdominal (obliquus internus abdominis)
Transverse abdominis (transversus abdominis)
Quadratus lumborum

Nerves

Cranial nerve 11 and the spinal nerves of C2 and C3 innervate the sternocleidomastoid. The posterior lateral branches of C4 through C8 innervate the splenius muscles. The entire erector spinae group is supplied by the posterior branches of the spinal nerves, whereas the intercostal nerves of T7 through T12 innervate the rectus abdominis. Both the internal and external oblique abdominal muscles receive innervation from the intercostal nerves (T8–T12), the iliohypogastric nerve (T12, L1), and the ilioinguinal nerve (L1). The same innervation is provided to the transverse abdominis, except that innervation begins with the T7 intercostal nerve. Branches from T12 and L1 supply the quadratus lumborum. Review Figures 2.6, 4.6, 4.7, and 9.16.

Chapter
12

Muscles that move the head

All muscles featured here originate on the cervical vertebrae and insert on the occipital bone of the skull, as implied by their "capitis" name (Figs. 12.9 and 12.10; Table 12.2). Three muscles make up the anterior vertebral muscles—the

FIG. 12.9 ● Anterior muscles of the neck.

Modified from Lindsay DT: *Functional human anatomy,* St. Louis, 1996, Mosby.

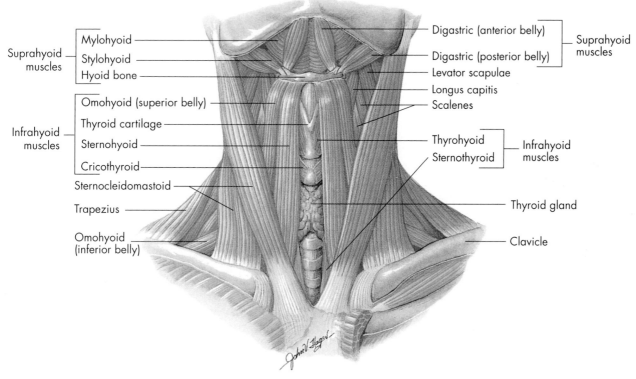

FIG. 12.10 ● Deep muscles of the posterior neck and upper back regions.

Modified from Van De Graaff KM: *Human anatomy,* ed 4, 1995, McGraw-Hill Companies, Inc., New York.

Chapter

12

TABLE 12.2 • Muscles that move the head

Muscle	Origin	Insertion	Action	Innervation
Rectus capitis anterior	Anterior surface of lateral mass of atlas	Basilar part of occipital bone anterior to foramen magnum	Flexion of head and stabilization of atlanto-occipital joint	C1–C3
Rectus capitis lateralis	Superior surface of transverse processes of atlas	Jugular process of occipital bone	Lateral flexion of head and stabilization of atlantooccipital joint	C1–C3
Rectus capitis posterior (major)	Spinous process of axis	Lateral portion of inferior nuchal line of occipital bone	Extension and rotation of head to ipsilateral side	Posterior rami of C1
Rectus capitis posterior (minor)	Spinous process of atlas	Medial portion of inferior nuchal line of occipital bone	Extension of head	Posterior rami of C1
Longus capitis	Transverse processes of C3–C6	Basilar part of occipital bone	Flexes head and cervical spine	C1–C3
Obliquus capitis superior	Transverse process of atlas	Occipital bone between inferior and superior nuchal line	Extension and lateral flexion of head	Posterior rami of C1
Obliquus capitis inferior	Spinous process of axis	Transverse process of atlas	Rotation of atlas	Posterior rami of C1
Semispinalis capitis	Transverse processes of C4–T7	Occipital bone, between superior and inferior nuchal lines	Extension and contralateral rotation of head	Posterior primary divisions on spinal nerves

longus capitis, the rectus capitis anterior, and the rectus capitis lateralis. All are flexors of the head and upper cervical spine. The rectus capitis lateralis laterally flexes the head, in addition to assisting the rectus capitis anterior in stabilizing the atlantooccipital joint.

The rectus capitis posterior major and minor, obliquus capitis superior and inferior, and semispinalis capitis are located posteriorly. All are extensors of the head, except the obliquus capitis inferior, which rotates the atlas. The obliquus capitis superior assists the rectus capitis lateralis

in lateral flexion of the head. In addition to extension, the rectus capitis posterior major is responsible for rotation of the head to the ipsilateral side. It is assisted by the semispinalis capitis, which rotates the head to the contralateral side. The splenius capitis and the sternocleidomastoid (Table 12.1) are much larger and more powerful in moving the head and cervical spine, and will be covered in detail on the following pages. The remaining muscles that act on the cervical spine are addressed with the muscles of the vertebral column.

Chapter
12

Sternocleidomastoid muscle FIG. 12.11

(ster´no-kli-do-mas-toyd)

Origin

Manubrium of the sternum
Medial clavicle

Insertion

Mastoid process

Action

Both sides: flexion of the head and neck

Right side: rotation to the left and lateral flexion to the right

Left side: rotation to the right and lateral flexion to the left

Palpation

Anterolateral side of the neck, diagonally between the origin and insertion

Innervation

Spinal accessory nerve (Cr11, C2–C3)

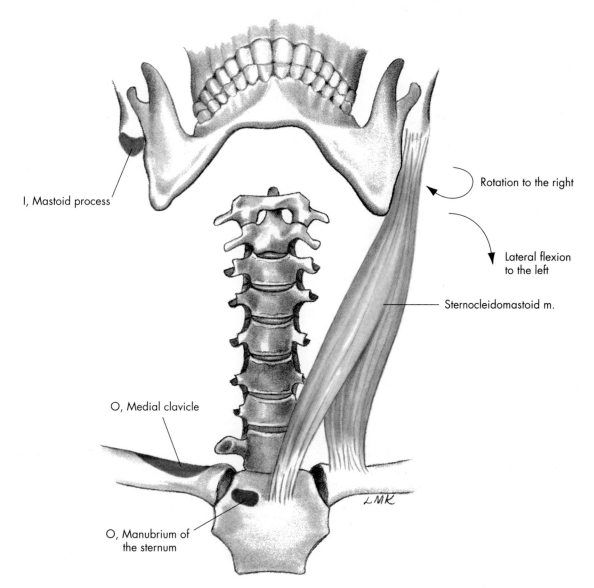

I, Mastoid process

Rotation to the right

Lateral flexion to the left

Sternocleidomastoid m.

O, Medial clavicle

O, Manubrium of the sternum

LMK

FIG. 12.11 ● Sternocleidomastoid muscle, anterior view. *O,* Origin; *I,* insertion (continued on next page).

Chapter
12

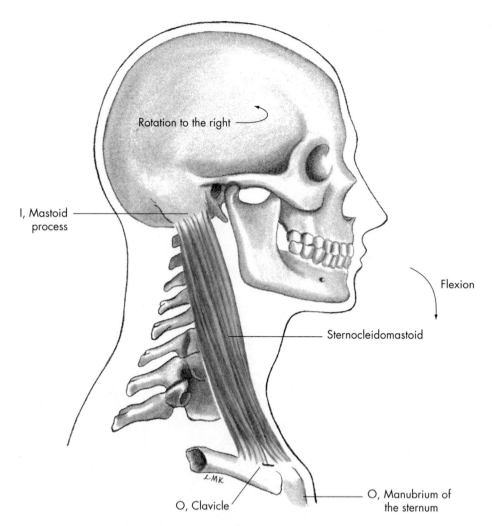

Rotation to the right

I, Mastoid
process

Flexion

Sternocleidomastoid

LMK

O, Clavicle

O, Manubrium of
the sternum

FIG. 12.11 continued ● Sternocleidomastoid muscle, lateral view. *O*, Origin; *I*, insertion.

Application, strengthening, and flexibility

The sternocleidomastoid is primarily responsible for flexion and rotation of the head and neck. One side of this muscle may be easily visualized and palpated when rotating the head to the opposite side.

The sternocleidomastoid is easily worked for strength development by placing the hands on the forehead to apply force posteriorly while using these muscles to pull the head forward into flexion. The hand may also be used on one side of the jaw to apply rotary force in the opposite direction while the sternocleidomastoid is contracting concentrically to rotate the head in the direction of the hand.

Cervical hyperextension provides some bilateral stretching of the sternocleidomastoid. Each side may be stretched individually. The right side is stretched by moving into left lateral flexion and right cervical rotation combined with extension. The opposite movements in extension stretch the left side.

Splenius muscles (cervicis, capitis)

FIG. 12.12

(sple´ni-us) (ser´vi-sis) (kap´i-tis)

Origin

Splenius cervicis: spinous processes of the third through the sixth thoracic vertebrae

Splenius capitis: lower half of the ligamentum nuchae and spinous processes of the seventh cervical and the upper three or four thoracic vertebrae

Insertion

Splenius cervicis: transverse processes of the first three cervical vertebrae

Splenius capitis: mastoid process and occipital bone

Action

Both sides: extension of the head and neck

Right side: rotation and lateral flexion to the right

Left side: rotation and lateral flexion to the left

Palpation

Cannot be palpated

Innervation

Posterior lateral branches of cervical nerves four through eight (C4–C8)

Application, strengthening, and flexibility

Any movement of the head and neck into extension, particularly extension and rotation, would bring the splenius muscle strongly into play, together with the erector spinae and the upper trapezius muscles. Tone in the splenius muscle tends to hold the head and neck in proper posture position.

A good exercise for the splenius muscle is to lace the fingers behind the head with the muscle in flexion and then to slowly contract the posterior head and neck muscles to move the head and neck into full extension. This exercise may also be performed by using a towel or a partner for resistance.

The entire splenius may be stretched with maximal flexion of the head and cervical spine. The right side can be stretched through combined movements of left rotation, left lateral flexion, and flexion. The same movements to the right side apply stretch to the left side.

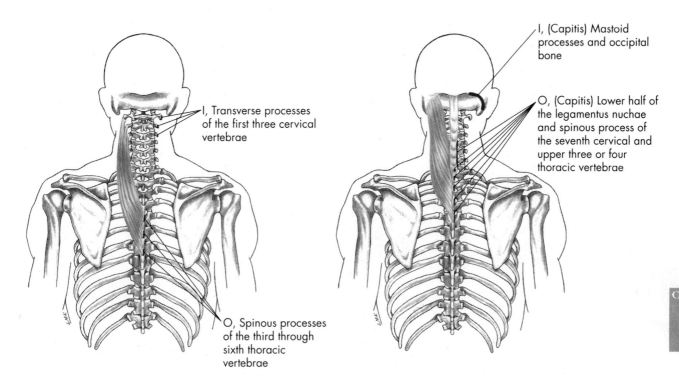

I, Transverse processes of the first three cervical vertebrae

O, Spinous processes of the third through sixth thoracic vertebrae

I, (Capitis) Mastoid processes and occipital bone

O, (Capitis) Lower half of the legamentus nuchae and spinous process of the seventh cervical and upper three or four thoracic vertebrae

FIG. 12.12 ● Splenius muscles (cervicis on the left, capititis on the right), posterior view. *O*, Origin; *I*, insertion.

Muscles of the vertebral column

In the cervical area, the longus colli muscles are located anteriorly and flex the cervical and upper thoracic vertebrae. Posteriorly, the erector spinae group, the transversospinalis group, the interspinal-intertransverse group, and the splenius all run vertically parallel to the spinal column (Fig. 12.13 and Table 12.3). This location enables them to extend the spine as well as assist in rotation and lateral flexion. The splenius and erector spinae group are addressed in detail elsewhere in this chapter. The transversospinalis group consists of the semispinalis, multifidus, and rotatores muscles. These muscles all originate on the transverse processes of their respective vertebrae and generally run

posteriorly to attach to the spinous processes on the vertebrae just above their vertebrae of origin. All are extensors of the spine and contract to rotate their respective vertebrae to the contralateral side. The interspinal-intertransverse group lies deep to the rotatores and consists of the interspinales and the intertransversarii muscles. As a group, they laterally flex and extend but do not rotate the vertebrae. The interspinales are extensors that connect from the spinous process of one vertebra to the spinous process of the adjacent vertebra. The intertransversarii muscles flex the vertebral column laterally by connecting to the transverse processes of adjacent vertebrae.

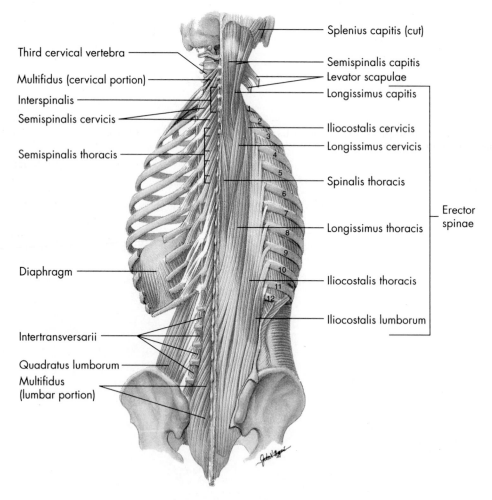

FIG. 12.13 ● Deep back muscles, posterior view. **Right,** the erector spinae group of muscles is demonstrated. **Left,** these muscles have been removed to reveal the deeper back muscles.

Modified from Seeley RR, Stephens TD, Tate P: *Anatomy & physiology,* ed 6, Dubuque, IA, 2003, McGraw-Hill.

Chapter
12

TABLE 12.3 • Muscles of the vertebral column

Muscle	Origin	Insertion	Action	Innervation
Longus colli (superior oblique)	Transverse processes of C3–C5	Anterior arch of atlas	Flexion of cervical spine	C2–C7
Longus colli (inferior oblique)	Bodies of T1–T3	Transverse processes of C5–C6	Flexion of cervical spine	C2–C7
Longus colli (vertical)	Bodies of C5–C7 and T1–T3	Anterior surface of bodies of C2–C4	Flexion of cervical spine	C2–C7
Interspinalis	Spinous process of each vertebra	Spinous process of next vertebra	Extension of spinal column	Posterior primary ramus of spinal nerves
Intertransversarii	Tubercles of transverse processes of each vertebra	Tubercles of transverse processes of next vertebra	Lateral flexion of spinal column	Anterior primary ramus of spinal nerves
Multifidus	Sacrum, iliac spine, transverse processes of lumbar, thoracic, and lower four cervical vertebra	Spinous processes of 2nd, 3rd, or 4th vertebra above origin	Extension and contralateral rotation of spinal column	Posterior primary ramus of spinal nerves
Rotatores	Transverse process of each vertebra	Base of spinous process of next vertebra above	Extension and contralateral rotation of spinal column	Posterior primary ramus of spinal nerves
Semispinalis cervicis	Transverse processes of T1–T5 or 6	Spinous processes from C2–C5	Extension and contralateral rotation of vertebral column	All divisions, posterior primary ramus of spinal nerves
Semispinalis thoracis	Transverse processes of T6–T10	Spinous processes of C6–C7 and T1–T4	Extension and contralateral rotation of vertebral column	Posterior primary ramus of spinal nerves

Chapter
12

Muscles of the thorax

The thoracic muscles are involved almost entirely in respiration (Fig. 12.14). During quiet rest, the diaphragm is responsible for breathing movements. As it contracts and flattens, the thoracic volume is increased and air is inspired to equalize the pressure. When larger amounts of air are needed, such as during exercise, the other thoracic muscles take on a more significant role in inspiration. The scalene muscles elevate the first two ribs to increase the thoracic volume. Further expansion of the chest is accomplished by the external intercostals. Additional muscles of inspiration are the levator costarum and the serratus posterior. Forced expiration occurs with contraction of the internal intercostals, transversus thoracis, and subcostales. All of these muscles are detailed in Table 12.4.

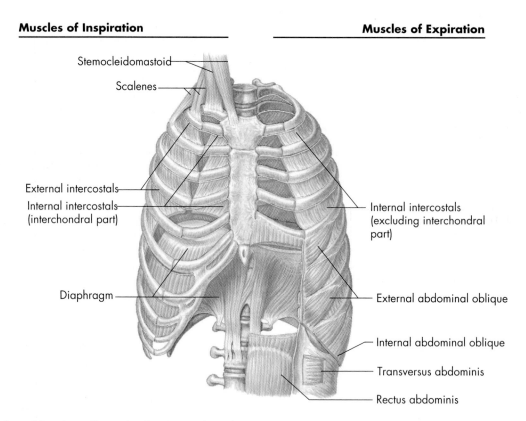

Muscles of Inspiration

Muscles of Expiration

Sternocleidomastoid
Scalenes
External intercostals
Internal intercostals (interchondral part)
Diaphragm

Internal intercostals (excluding interchondral part)
External abdominal oblique
Internal abdominal oblique
Transversus abdominis
Rectus abdominis

FIG. 12.14 ● Muscles of respiration, anterior view.

Modified from Van De Graaff KM: *Human anatomy,* ed 4, 1995, McGraw-Hill Companies, Inc., New York.

TABLE 12.4 • **Muscles of the thorax**

Muscle	Origin	Insertion	Action	Innervation
Diaphragm	Circumference of thoracic inlet from xiphoid process, costal cartilages 6–12, and lumbar vertebrae	Central tendon of diaphragm	Depresses and draws central tendon forward in inhalation, reduces pressure in thoracic cavity, and increases pressure in abdominal cavity	Phrenic nerve (C3–C5)
Internal intercostals	Longitudinal ridge on inner surface of ribs and costal cartilages	Superior border of next rib below	Elevates costal cartilages of ribs 1–4 during inhalation, depresses all ribs in exhalation	Intercostal branches of T1–T11
External intercostals	Inferior border of ribs	Superior border of next rib below	Elevates ribs	Intercostal branches of T1–T11
Levator costarum	Ends of transverse processes of C7, T2–T12	Outer surface of angle of next rib below origin	Elevates ribs, lateral flexion of thoracic spine	Intercostal nerves
Subcostales	Inner surface of each rib near its angle	Medially on the inner surface of 2nd or 3rd rib below	Draws the ventral part of the ribs downward, decreasing the volume of the thoracic cavity	Intercostal nerves
Scalenus anterior	Transverse processes of C3–C6	Inner border and upper surface of 1st rib	Elevates 1st rib, flexion, lateral flexion, and contralateral rotation of cervical spine	Ventral rami of C5–C6 sometimes C4
Scalenus medius	Transverse processes of C2–C7	Superior surface of 1st rib	Elevates 1st rib, flexion, lateral flexion, and contralateral rotation of cervical spine	Ventral rami of C3–C8
Scalenus posterior	Transverse processes of C5–C7	Outer surface of 2nd rib	Elevates 2nd rib, flexion, lateral flexion, and slight contralateral rotation of cervical spine	Ventral rami of C6–C8
Serratus posterior (superior)	Ligamentum nuchae, spinous processes of C7, T1, and T2 or T3	Superior borders lateral to angles of ribs 2–5	Elevates upper ribs	Branches from anterior primary rami of T1–T4
Serratus posterior (inferior)	Spinous processes of T10–T12 and L1–L3	Inferior borders lateral to angles of ribs 9–12	Counteracts inward pull of diaphragm by drawing last four ribs outward and downward	Branches from anterior primary rami of T9–T12
Transversus thoracis	Inner surface of sternum and xiphoid process, sternal ends of costal cartilages of ribs 3–6	Inner surfaces and inferior borders of costal cartilages 3–6	Depresses ribs	Intercostal branches of T3–T6

Erector spinae muscles* (sacrospinalis)

FIG. 12.15 and FIG. 12.16

(e-rek´tor spi´ne) (sa´kro-spi-na´lis)

Iliocostalis

(il´i-o-kos-ta´lis): lateral layer

Longissimus

(lon-jis´i-mus): middle layer

Spinalis

(spi-na´lis): medial layer

---

*This muscle group includes the iliocostalis, the longissimus dorsi, the spinalis dorsi, and divisions of these muscles in the lumbar, thoracic, and cervical sections of the spinal column.

Origin

Iliocostalis: thoracolumbar aponeurosis from sacrum, posterior ribs

Longissimus: thoracolumbar aponeurosis from sacrum, lumbar and thoracic transverse processes

Spinalis: ligamentum nuchae, cervical and thoracic spinous processes.

Insertion

Iliocostalis: posterior ribs, cervical transverse processes

Longissimus: cervical and thoracic transverse processes, mastoid process

Spinalis: cervical and thoracic spinous processes, occipital bone

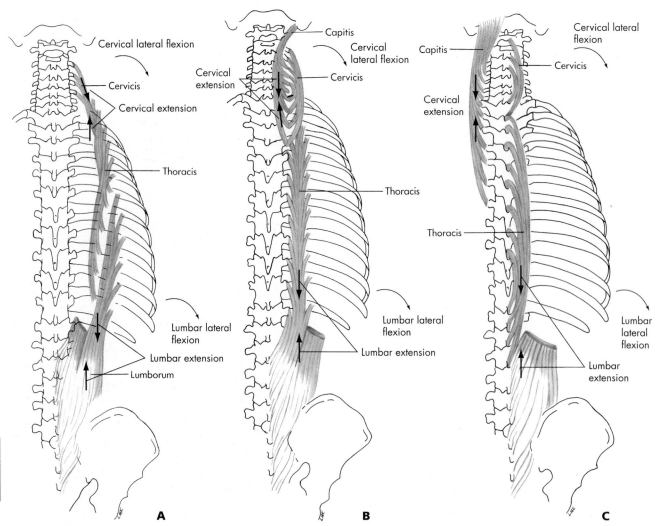

FIG. 12.15 ● Erector spinae (sacrospinalis) muscle, posterior view. **A,** Iliocostalis; **B,** longissimus; **C,** spinalis.

Action
Extension and lateral flexion of the spine

Palpation
Lower lumbar region on either side of the spine

Innervation
Posterior branches of the spinal nerves

Application, strengthening, and flexibility

The erector spinae muscle functions best when the pelvis is posteriorly rotated. This lowers the origin of the erector spinae and makes it more effective in keeping the spine straight. As the spine is held straight, the ribs are raised, thus fixing the chest high and consequently making the abdominal muscles more effective in holding the pelvis up in front and flattening the abdominal wall.

An exercise known as the "dead lift," employing a barbell, uses the erector spinae in extending the spine. In this exercise, the subject bends over, keeping the arms and legs straight; picks up the barbell; and returns to a standing position. In performing this type of exercise, it is very important to always use correct technique to avoid back injuries. Voluntary static contraction of the erector spinae in the standing position would provide a mild exercise and improve body posture.

The erector spinae and its various divisions may be strengthened through numerous forms of back extension exercises. These are usually done in a prone or face-down position in which the spine is already in some state of flexion. The subject then uses these muscles to move part or all of the spine toward extension against gravity. A weight may be held in the hands behind the head to increase resistance.

Maximal hyperflexion of the entire spine stretches the erector spinae muscle group. Stretch may be isolated to specific segments through specific movements. Maximal flexion of the head and cervical spine stretches the capitis and cervical segments. Flexion combined with lateral flexion to one side accentuates the stretch on the contralateral side. Thoracic and lumbar flexion places the stretch primarily on the thoracis and lumborum segments.

Splenius longus (cut)
Longissimus capitis
Semispinalis capitis (cut)
Longissimus cervicis
Iliocostalis cervicis
Semispinalis capitis
Spinalis capitis
Splenius capitis
Spinalis cervicis
Iliocostalis thoracis
Spinalis thoracis
Iliocostalis lumborum
Longissimus thoracis

FIG. 12.16 ● Muscles of the back and the neck help move the head (posterior view) and hold the torso erect. The splenius capitis and semispinalis have been removed on the left to show underlying muscles.

Chapter 12

Muscles of the abdominal wall

FIGS. 12.17, 12.18, 12.19

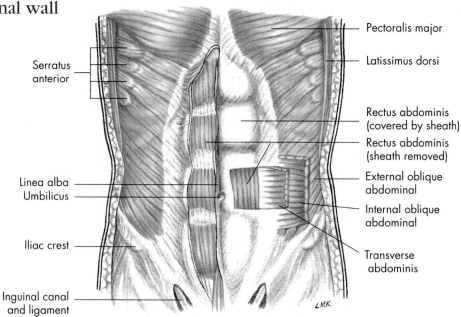

FIG. 12.17 ● Muscles of the abdomen. External oblique and rectus abdominis. The fibrous sheath around the rectus has been removed on the right side to show the muscle within.

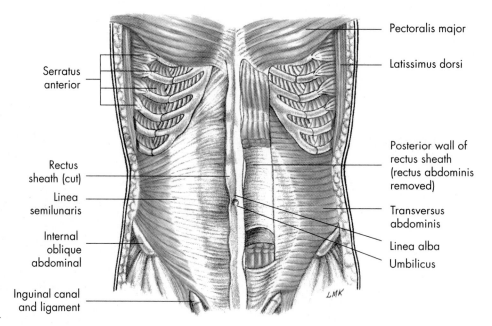

FIG. 12.18 ● Muscles of the abdomen. The external oblique has been removed on the right to reveal the internal oblique. The external and internal obliques have been removed on the left to reveal the transversus abdominis. The rectus abdominis has been cut to reveal the posterior rectus sheath.

FIG. 12.19 ● Abdominal wall. The unique arrangement of the four abdominal muscles with their fascial attachment in and around the rectus abdominis muscle is shown. With no bones for attachments, these muscles can be adequately maintained through exercise.

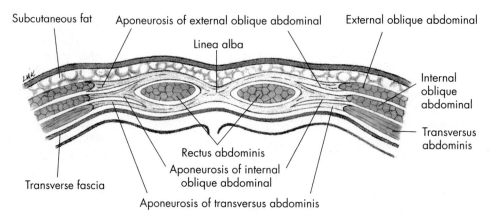

Rectus abdominis muscle FIG. 12.20

(rek´tus ab-dom´i-nis)

Origin

Crest of the pubis

Insertion

Cartilage of the fifth, sixth, and seventh ribs and the xiphoid process

Action

Both sides: lumbar flexion
Right side: lateral flexion to the right
Left side: lateral flexion to the left

Palpation

Anteromedial surface of the abdomen, between the rib cage and the pubic bone

Innervation

Intercostal nerves (T7–T12)

Application, strengthening, and flexibility

The rectus abdominis muscle controls the tilt of the pelvis and the consequent curvature of the lower spine. By rotating the pelvis posteriorly, the rectus abdominis flattens the lower back, making the erector spinae muscle more effective as an extensor of the spine and the hip flexors (the iliopsoas muscle, particularly) more effective in raising the legs.

In a relatively lean person with well-developed abdominals, three distinct sets of lines or depressions may be noted. Each represents an area of tendinous connective tissue connecting or supporting the abdominal arrangement of muscles in lieu of bony attachments. Running vertically from the xiphoid process through the umbilicus to the pubis is the *linea alba.* It divides each rectus abdominis and serves as its medial border. Lateral to each rectus abdominis is the *linea semilunaris,* a crescent, or moon-shaped, line running vertically. This line represents the aponeurosis connecting the lateral border of the rectus abdominis and the medial border of the external and internal abdominal obliques. The *tendinous inscriptions* are horizontal indentations that transect the rectus abdominis at three or more locations, giving the muscle its segmented appearance. Refer to Fig. 12.17.

There are several exercises for the abdominal muscles, such as bent-knee sit-ups, crunches, and isometric contractions. Bent-knee sit-ups with the arms folded across the chest are considered by many to be a safe and efficient exercise. Crunches are also considered to be even more effective for isolating the work to the abdominals. Both of these exercises shorten the iliopsoas muscle and other hip flexors, thus reducing their ability to generate force. Twisting to the left and right brings the oblique muscles into more active contraction. In all of the above exercises, it is important to use proper technique, which involves gradually moving to the up position until the lumbar spine is actively flexed maximally and then slowly returning to the beginning position. Jerking movements using momentum should be avoided. Movement continued beyond full lumbar flexion only exercises the hip flexors, which is not usually an objective. Even though all of these exercises may be helpful in strengthening the abdominals, careful analysis should occur before deciding which are indicated in the presence of various injuries and problems of the low back.

The rectus abdominis is stretched by simultaneously hyperextending both the lumbar and thoracic spine. Extending the hips assists in this process by accentuating the anterior rotation of the pelvis to hyperextend the lumbar spine.

FIG. 12.20 ● Rectus abdominis muscle, anterior view. *O,* Origin; *I,* insertion.

External oblique abdominal muscle

FIG. 12.21

(ek-stur´nel o-bleek´ ab-dom´i-nel)

Origin

Borders of the lower eight ribs at the side of the
chest, dovetailing with the serratus anterior muscle*

Insertion

Anterior half of the crest of the ilium, the inguinal
ligament, the crest of the pubis, and the fascia of
the rectus abdominis muscle at the lower front

Action

Both sides: lumbar flexion
Right side: lumbar lateral flexion to the right and
rotation to the left
Left side: lumbar lateral flexion to the left and
rotation to the right

Palpation

Lateral side of the abdomen, either left or right

---

*Sometimes the origin and insertion are reversed in anatomy books.
This is the result of different interpretations of which bony structure
is the more movable. The insertion is considered the most movable
part of a muscle.

Innervation

Intercostal nerves (T8–T12), iliohypogastric nerve
(T12, L1), and ilioinguinal nerve (L1)

Application, strengthening, and flexibility

Working on each side of the abdomen, the external oblique abdominal muscles aid in rotating the
trunk when working independently of each other.
Working together, they aid the rectus abdominis
muscle in its described action. The left external
oblique abdominal muscle contracts strongly during sit-ups when the trunk rotates to the right, as
in touching the left elbow to the right knee. Rotating to the left brings the right external oblique
into action.

Each side of the external oblique must be
stretched individually. The right side is stretched by
moving into extreme left lateral flexion combined
with extension, or by extreme lumbar rotation to
the right combined with extension. The opposite
movements in extension stretch the left side.

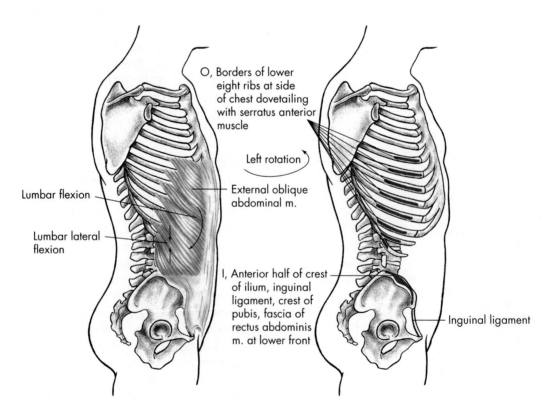

FIG. 12.21 ● External oblique abdominal muscle, lateral view. *O*, Origin; *I*, insertion.

Internal oblique abdominal muscle

FIG. 12.22

(in-ter´nel o-bleek ab-dom´i-nel)

Origin

Upper half of the inguinal ligament, anterior two-
thirds of the crest of the ilium, and lumbar fascia

Insertion

Costal cartilages of the eighth, ninth, and tenth ribs
and the linea alba

Action

Both sides: lumbar flexion
Right side: lumbar lateral flexion and rotation to the
right
Left side: lumbar lateral flexion and rotation to the left

Palpation

Palpated on the lateral side of the abdomen when
the external oblique is relaxed

Innervation

Intercostal nerves (T8–T12), iliohypogastric nerve
(T12, L1), and ilioinguinal nerve (L1)

Application, strengthening, and flexibility

The internal oblique abdominal muscles run diagonally in the direction opposite to that of the external obliques. The left internal oblique rotates to
the left, and the right internal oblique rotates to
the right.

In touching the left elbow to the right knee in
crunches, the left external oblique and the right
internal oblique abdominal muscles rotate at the
same time, assisting the rectus abdominis muscle
in flexing the trunk to make the completion of the
movement possible. In rotary movements, the internal oblique and the external oblique on opposite sides from each other always work together.

Like the external oblique, each side of the internal oblique must be stretched individually. The
right side is stretched by moving into extreme left
lateral flexion and extreme left lumbar rotation
combined with extension. The same movements
to the right combined with extension stretch the
left side.

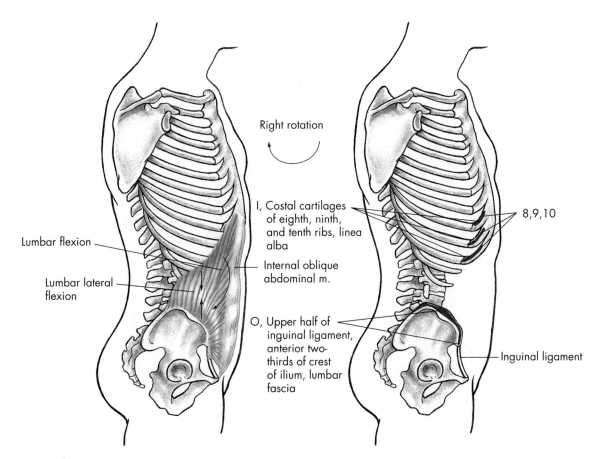

FIG. 12.22 ● Internal oblique abdominal muscle, lateral view. *O*, Origin; *I*, insertion.

Transversus abdominis muscle

FIG. 12.23

(trans-vurs´us ab-dom´i-nis)

Origin

Outer third of the inguinal ligament
Inner rim of the iliac crest
Inner surface of the cartilage of the lower six ribs
Lumbar fascia

Insertion

Crest of the pubis and the iliopectineal line
Abdominal aponeurosis to the linea alba

Action

Forced expiration by pulling the abdominal wall
 inward

Palpation

Cannot be palpated

Innervation

Intercostal nerves (T7–T12), iliohypogastric nerve
 (T12, L1), and ilioinguinal nerve (L1)

Application, strengthening, and flexibility

The transversus abdominis is the chief muscle of forced expiration and is effective—together with the rectus abdominis, the external oblique abdominal, and the internal oblique abdominal muscles—in helping hold the abdomen flat. This abdominal flattening and forced expulsion of the abdominal contents is the only action of this muscle.

The transversus abdominis muscle is exercised effectively by attempting to draw the abdominal contents back toward the spine. This may be done isometrically in the supine position or while standing. A maximal inspiration held in the abdomen applies stretch.

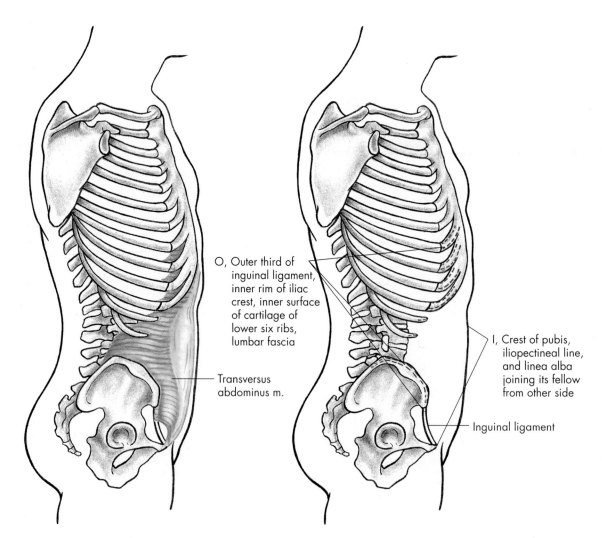

O, Outer third of inguinal ligament, inner rim of iliac crest, inner surface of cartilage of lower six ribs, lumbar fascia

Transversus abdominus m.

I, Crest of pubis, iliopectineal line, and linea alba joining its fellow from other side

Inguinal ligament

FIG. 12.23 ● Transversus abdominis muscle, lateral view. *O,* Origin; *I,* insertion.

Chapter
12

Quadratus lumborum muscle FIG. 12.24

(kwad-ra´tus lum-bo´rum)

Origin

Posterior inner lip of the iliac crest

Insertion

Approximately one-half the length of the lower
border of the twelfth rib and the transverse process
of the upper four lumbar vertebrae

Action

Lateral flexion to the side on which it is located
Stabilizes the pelvis and lumbar spine

Palpation

For all practical purposes, impossible to palpate,
except on an extremely thin individual

Innervation

Branches of T12, L1 nerves

Application, strengthening, and flexibility

The quadratus lumborum is important in lumbar
lateral flexion and in elevating the pelvis on the
same side in the standing position. Trunk rotation
and lateral flexion movements against resistance
are good exercises for development of this muscle. The position of the body relative to gravity
may be changed to increase resistance on this and
other trunk and abdominal muscles. Left lumbar
lateral flexion stretches the right quadratus lumborum and vice versa.

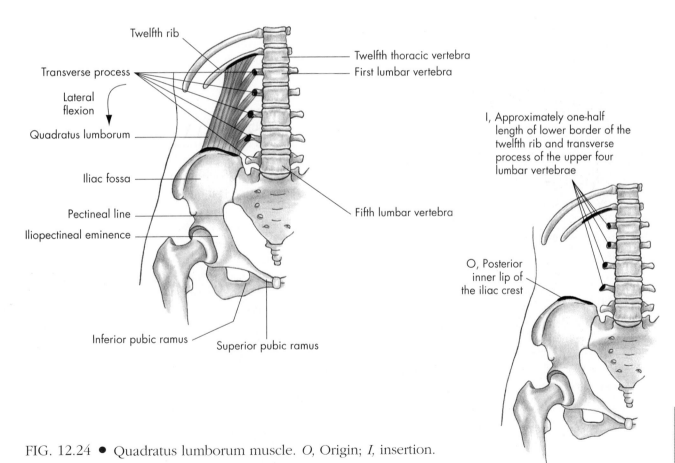

FIG. 12.24 ● Quadratus lumborum muscle. *O,* Origin; *I,* insertion.

Web sites

Anatomy & Physiology Tutorials:

www.gwc.maricopa.edu/class/bio201/index.htm

Radiologic Anatomy Browser:

radlinux1.usuf1.usuhs.mil/rad/iong/index.html

This site has numerous radiological views of the musculoskeletal system.

Loyola University Medical Center: Structure of the Human Body:

www.meddean.luc.edu/lumen/MedEd/GrossAnatomy/GA.html

An excellent site with many slides, dissections, tutorials, etc., for the study of human anatomy

University of Arkansas Medical School Gross Anatomy for Medical Students:

anatomy.uams.edu/htmlpages/anatomyhtml/gross.html

Dissections, anatomy tables, atlas images, links, etc.

Wheeless's Textbook of Orthopaedics:

www.ortho-u.net/

This site has an extensive index of links to the fractures, joints, muscles, nerves, trauma, medications, medical topics, and lab tests, as well as links to orthopedic journals and other orthopedic and medical news.

Premiere Medical Search Engine:

www.medsite.com

This site allows the reader to enter any medical condition and it will search the net to find relevant articles.

Virtual Hospital:

www.vh.org

Numerous slides, patient information, etc.

Dynamic Human version 2.0 CD-ROM: The Visual Guide to Anatomy & Physiology:

www.mhhe.com/biosci/ap/dynamichuman2/

Web site that accompanies this CD-ROM

Worksheet exercises

As an aid to learning, for in-class or out-of-class assignments, or for testing, tear-out worksheets are found at the end of the text (pp. 337 and 338).

Anterior skeletal worksheet (no. 1)

Draw and label the following muscles on the skeletal chart:
a. Rectus abdominis
b. External oblique abdominal
c. Internal oblique abdominal

Posterior skeletal worksheet (no. 2)

Draw and label the following muscles on the skeletal chart:
a. Erector spinae
b. Quadratus lumborum
c. Splenius—cervicis and capitis

Laboratory and review exercises

1. Locate the following parts of the spine on a human skeleton and on a human subject:
   a. Cervical vertebrae
   b. Thoracic vertebrae
   c. Lumbar vertebrae
   d. Spinous processes
   e. Transverse processes
   f. Sacrum
   g. Manubrium
   h. Xiphoid process
   i. Sternum
   j. Rib cage (various ribs)
2. How and where can the following muscles be palpated on a human subject?
   a. Rectus abdominis
   b. External oblique abdominal
   c. Internal oblique abdominal
   d. Erector spinae
   e. Sternocleidomastoid
3. List the planes in which each of the following movements occurs. List the respective axis of rotation for each movement in each plane.
   a. Cervical flexion
   b. Cervical extension
   c. Cervical rotation
   d. Cervical lateral flexion
   e. Lumbar flexion
   f. Lumbar extension
   g. Lumbar rotation
   h. Lumbar lateral flexion
4. Contrast crunches, bent-knee sit-ups, and straight-leg sit-ups. Does having a partner to hold the feet make a difference in the ability to do the bent-knee and straight-leg sit-ups? If so, why?
5. Have a laboratory partner stand and assume a position exhibiting good posture. What motions in each region of the spine does gravity

attempt to produce? Which muscles are responsible for counteracting these motions against the pull of gravity?

6. Compare and contrast the spinal curves of a laboratory partner sitting erect with those of one sitting slouched in a chair. Which muscles are responsible for maintaining good sitting posture?

7. Which exercise is better for the development of the abdominal muscles—leg lifts or sit-ups? Analyze each one in regard to the activity of the abdominal muscles. Defend your answer.

8. Why is good abdominal muscular development so important? Why is this area so frequently neglected?

9. Why are weak abdominal muscles frequently blamed for lower back pain?

10. Prepare an oral or a written report on abdominal or back injuries found in the literature.

11. Fill in the muscle analysis chart below by listing the muscles primarily involved in each movement.

12. Fill in the antagonistic muscle action chart on the next page by listing the muscle(s) or parts of muscles that are antagonistic in their actions to the muscles in the left column.

Muscle analysis chart • Cervical and lumbar spine

Cervical spine	
Flexion	Extension
Lateral flexion right	Rotation right
Lateral flexion left	Rotation left
Lumbar spine	
Flexion	Extension
Lateral flexion right	Rotation right
Lateral flexion left	Rotation left

Antagonistic muscle action chart • Cervical and lumbar spine

Agonist	Antagonist
Splenius capitis	
Splenius cervicis	
Sternocleidomastoid	
Erector spinae	
Rectus abdominis	
External oblique abdominal	
Internal oblique abdominal	
Quadratus lumborum	

References

Clarkson HM, Gilewich GB: *Musculoskeletal assessment: joint range of motion and manual muscle strength,* Baltimore, 1989, Williams & Wilkins.

Day AL: Observation on the treatment of lumbar disc disease in college football players, *American Journal of Sports Medicine,* 15:275, January–February 1987.

Field D: *Anatomy: palpation and surface markings,* ed 3, Oxford, 2001, Butterworth-Heinemann.

Gench BE, Hinson MM, Harvey PT: *Anatomical kinesiology,* Dubuque, IA, 1995, Eddie Bowers.

Hamilton N, Luttgens K: *Kinesiology: scientific basis of human motion,* ed 10, Boston, 2002, McGraw-Hill.

Hislop HJ, Montgomery J: *Daniels and Worthingham's muscle testing: techniques of manual examination,* ed 6, Philadelphia, 1995, Saunders.

Holden DL, Jackson DW: Stress fractures of ribs in female rowers, *American Journal of Sports Medicine,* 13:277, July–August 1987.

Lindsay DT: *Functional human anatomy,* St. Louis, 1996, Mosby.

Martens MA, et al: Adductor tendonitis and muscular abdominis tendopathy, *American Journal of Sports Medicine,* 15:353, July–August 1987.

Marymont JV: Exercise-related stress reaction of the sacroiliac joint, an unusual cause of low back pain in athletes, *American Journal of Sports Medicine,* 14:320, July–August 1986.

National Strength and Conditioning Association; Baechle TR, Earle RW: *Essentials of strength training and conditioning,* ed 2, Champaign, IL, 2000, Human Kinetics.

Perry JF, Rohe DA, Garcia AO: *The kinesiology workbook,* Philadelphia, 1992, Davis.

Rasch PJ: *Kinesiology and applied anatomy,* ed 7, Philadelphia, 1989, Lea & Febiger.

Seeley RR, Stephens TD, Tate P: *Anatomy & physiology,* ed 6, Dubuque, IA, 2003, McGraw-Hill.

Sieg KW, Adams SP: *Illustrated essentials of musculoskeletal anatomy,* ed 2, Gainesville, FL, 1985, Megabooks.

Stone RJ, Stone JA: *Atlas of the skeletal muscles,* 1990, McGraw-Hill Companies, Inc., New York.

Thibodeau GA, Patton KT: *Anatomy & physiology,* ed 9, St. Louis, 1993, Mosby.

Van de Graaff KM: *Human anatomy,* ed 6, Dubuque, IA, 2002, McGraw-Hill.

Chapter 12

Muscular Analysis of Trunk and Lower Extremity Exercises

Objectives

- To understand various conditioning principles and how to apply them to strengthening major muscle groups

- To apply the concept of the kinetic chain to the lower extremity

- To analyze an exercise for the types of contractions occurring in specific muscles to create major joint movements

- To discuss the various types of exercise equipment used in developing muscular strength and endurance

- To learn to analyze and prescribe exercises to strengthen all major muscle groups

---

Online Learning Center Resources

Visit *Manual of Structural Kinesiology's* Online Learning Center at **www.mhhe.com/floyd15e** for additional information and study material for this chapter, including:

- *Self-grading quizzes*
- *Anatomy flashcards*
- *Animations*

Chapter 8 presented an introduction to the analysis of exercise and activities. That chapter included only the analysis of the muscles previously studied in the upper extremity region.

Since that chapter, all the other joints and large muscle groups of the human body have been considered. The exercises and activities found in this chapter concentrate more on the muscles in the trunk and lower extremity.

Strength, endurance, and flexibility of the muscles of the lower extremity, trunk, and abdominal sections are also very important in skillful physical performance and body maintenance.

The type of contraction is determined by whether the muscle is lengthening or shortening during the movement. However, muscles may shorten or lengthen in the absence of a contraction through passive movement caused by other contracting muscles, momentum, gravity, or external forces such as manual assistance and exercise machines.

A concentric contraction is a shortening contraction of the muscles against gravity or resistance, whereas an eccentric contraction is a contraction in which the muscle lengthens under tension to control the joints moving with gravity or resistance.

Contraction against gravity is also quite evident in the lower extremities.

The quadriceps muscle group contracts eccentrically when the body slowly lowers in a weight-bearing movement through lower extremity action. The quadriceps functions as a decelerator to knee joint flexion in weight-bearing movements by contracting eccentrically to prevent too rapid a downward movement. One can easily demonstrate this fact by palpating this muscle group when slowly moving from a standing position to a half-squat.

Almost as much work is done in this type of contraction as in concentric contractions.

In this example involving the quadriceps, the slow descent is eccentric, and the ascent from the squatted position is concentric. If the descent were under no muscular control, it would be at the same speed as gravity and the muscle lengthening would be passive. That is, the movement and change in length of the muscle would be caused by gravity and not by active muscular contractions.

In recent years, more and more muscle educators on all levels have been emphasizing the development of muscle groups through resistance training and circuit-training activities. Athletes and nonathletes, both male and female, need to have overall muscular development.

Sport participation does not ensure sufficient development of muscle groups. Also, more and more emphasis has been placed on mechanical kinesiology in physical education and athletic skill teaching. This is desirable and can help bring about more skillful performance. However, one must remember that mechanical principles will be of little or no value to performers without adequate strength and endurance of their muscular system, which is developed through planned exercises and activities. In the fitness and health revolution of recent years, a much greater emphasis has been placed on exercises and activities that improve the physical fitness, strength, endurance, and flexibility of participants. This chapter will continue the practice of analyzing the muscles through simple exercises that began in Chapter 8. When these techniques are mastered, the individual is ready to analyze and prescribe exercises and activities for muscular strength and endurance needed in sport activities and for healthful living.

Conditioning considerations

Overload principle

A basic physiological principle of exercise is the overload principle. It states that, within appropriate parameters, a muscle or muscle group increases in strength in direct proportion to the overload placed on it. While it is beyond the scope of this text to fully explain specific applications of the overload principle for each component of physical fitness, some general concepts will be mentioned. To improve the strength and functioning of major muscles, educators need to apply this principle to every large muscle group in the body,

progressively throughout each year, at all age levels. In actual practice, the amount of overload applied varies significantly based on several factors. For example, an untrained person beginning a strength training program will usually make significant gains in the amount of weight he or she is able to lift in the first few weeks of the exercise program. Most of this increased ability is due to a refinement of neuromuscular function, rather than an actual increase in muscle tissue strength. Similarly, a well-trained person will see relatively minor improvements in the amount of weight that can be lifted over a much longer period of time. Therefore, the amount and rate of progressive overload are extremely variable and must be adjusted to match the specific needs of the individual's exercise objectives. Overload is not always progressively increased. In certain periods of conditioning, the overload should actually be prescriptively reduced or increased to improve the total results of the entire program. Overload may be modified by changing any one or a combination of three exercise variables—*frequency, intensity,* and *duration.* Increasing the speed of doing the exercise, the number of repetitions, the weight, and more bouts of exercise are all ways to modify these variables and apply this principle.

SAID principle

The SAID (**S**pecific **A**daptations to **I**mposed **De**mands) principle should be considered in all aspects of physiological conditioning and training. This principle, which states that the body will gradually, over time, adapt very specifically to the various stresses and overloads to which it is subjected, is applicable in every form of muscle training, as well as to the other systems of the body. For example, if an individual were to undergo several weeks of strength-training exercises for a particular joint through a limited range of motion, the specific muscles involved in performing the strengthening exercises would improve primarily in the ability to move against increased resistance through the specific range of motion used. There would be, in most cases, minimal strength gains beyond the range of motion used in the training. Additionally, other components of physical fitness—such as flexibility, cardiorespiratory endurance, and muscular endurance—would be enhanced minimally, if at all. In other words, to achieve specific benefits, exercise programs must be specifically designed for the adaptation desired.

It should be recognized that this adaptation may be positive or negative, depending on whether or not the correct techniques are used and stressed in the design and administration of the conditioning program. Inappropriate or excessive demands placed on the body in too short a time span can result in injury. If the demands are too minimal or administered too infrequently over too long a time period, less-than-desired improvement will occur. Conditioning programs and the exercises included in them should be analyzed to determine if they are using the specific muscles for which they were intended in the correct manner.

Specificity

Specificity of exercise strongly relates to the discussion of the SAID principle. The components of physical fitness, such as muscular strength, muscular endurance, and flexibility, are not general body characteristics. They are specific to each body area and muscle group. Therefore, the specific needs of the individual must be addressed when designing an exercise program. Quite often, it will be necessary to analyze an individual's exercise and skill technique to design an exercise program to meet his or her specific needs. Potential exercises to be used in the conditioning program must be analyzed to determine their appropriateness for the individual's specific needs. The goals of the exercise program should be determined regarding specific areas of the body, preferred time to physically peak, and physical fitness needs such as strength, muscular endurance, flexibility, cardiorespiratory endurance, and body composition. After establishing goals, a regimen incorporating the overload variables of frequency, intensity, and duration may be prescribed to include the entire body or specific areas in a manner to address the improvement of the preferred physical fitness components. Regular observation and follow-up exercise analysis is necessary to ensure proper adherence to correct technique.

Muscular development

For years it was thought that a person developed adequate muscular strength, endurance, and flexibility through participation in sport activities. Now the philosophy is that one needs to develop muscular strength, endurance, and flexibility in order to be able to participate safely and effectively in sport activities.

Adequate muscular strength, endurance, and flexibility of the entire body from head to toe should be developed through correct use of the appropriate exercise principles. Individuals responsible for this development need to prescribe exercises that will meet these objectives.

In schools this development should start at an early age and continue throughout the school years. Results of fitness tests reveal the need for considerable improvement in this area. The chin-up (pull-up) test had to be modified because more than 50% of children could not do one chin-up. Sit-ups, the standing long jump, the mile run, and other tests all indicated fitness deficiencies in the children of the United States. Adequate muscular strength and endurance are important in the adult years for the activities of daily living, as well as job-related requirements and recreational needs. Many back problems and other physical ailments could be avoided through proper maintenance of the musculoskeletal system.

The sampling of exercises in this chapter will assist individuals in analyzing and prescribing exercises for overall muscular development of the trunk and lower extremities in all age groups. All muscles listed in the analysis are contracting concentrically unless specifically noted to be contracting isometrically or eccentrically. Chapter 8 includes several exercises for the upper extremities.

Free weight training exercises*

Exercise through the use of weights has become increasingly important as a means of developing and maintaining muscular strength in young people and adults. When this type of exercise is undertaken, a thorough knowledge of the muscles being used is essential so that one group of muscles is not overdeveloped and another underdeveloped.

Most schools have free weights, barbells, and dumbbells available for use by students. Some physical education teachers and coaches recommend that junior and senior high school students have their own barbell set for use at home.

An analysis of several selected weight-training exercises will introduce the muscular analysis of these activities. In these exercises, the only equipment needed is a barbell with weights.

---

*These are only sample weight-training exercises. Students are encouraged to continue the study of muscular analysis of the many other weight-training exercises and activities.

Sit-up, bent knee   FIG. 13.1

Description

The participant lies on the back, forearms crossed and lying across the chest, with the knees flexed approximately 90 degrees and the feet about hip width apart. The hips and knees are flexed in this manner to reduce the length of the hip flexors, thereby reducing their contribution to the sit-up. This positioning will allow more emphasis on the abdominals, as compared with a straight leg sit-up.

The participant curls up to a sitting position, rotates the trunk to the right, touches the left elbow to the left knee, and then returns to the starting position. On the next repetition, the participant should rotate to the left instead of the right for balanced muscular development.

Analysis

This exercise is divided into four phases for analysis: (1) curling phase to sitting-up position, (2) rotating to right phase, (3) return phase to sitting-up position, and (4) return phase to starting position (Table 13.1).

FIG. 13.1 ● Sit-up, bent knee. **A,** Beginning relaxed position; **B,** sitting-up position; **C,** rotated to the right position.

TABLE 13.1 • Sit-up, bent knee

Joint	Curling phase to sitting-up position		Rotating to right phase		Return phase to sitting-up position		Return phase to starting position	
	Action	Agonists	Action	Agonists	Action	Agonists	Action	Agonists
Cervical spine	Flexion	Cervical spine flexors Sternoclei-domastoid	Mainte-nance of cervical flexion	Cervical spine flexors (isometric contraction) Sternoclei-domastoid	Mainte-nance of cer-vical flexion	Cervical spine flexors (isometric contraction) Sternoclei-domastoid	Extension	Cervical spine flexors (eccentric contraction) Sternoclei-domastoid
Trunk	Flexion	Trunk flexors Rectus abdominis External oblique abdominal Internal oblique abdominal	Right lumbar rotation	Right lumbar rotators R) Rectus abdominis L) External oblique abdominal R) Internal oblique abdominal R) Erector spinae	Left lumbar rotation to neutral position	Right lumbar rotators (eccentric contraction) R) Rectus abdominis L) External oblique abdominal R) Internal oblique abdominal R) Erector spinae	Extension	Trunk flexors (eccentric contraction) Rectus abdominis External oblique abdominal Internal oblique abdominal
Hip	Flexion	Hip flexors Iliopsoas Rectus femoris Pectineus	Mainte-nance of hip flexion	Hip flexors (isometric contraction) Iliopsoas Rectus femoris Pectineus	Mainte-nance of hip flexion	Hip flexors (isometric contraction) Iliopsoas Rectus femoris Pectineus	Extension	Hip flexors (eccentric contraction) Iliopsoas Rectus femoris Pectineus

Chapter

13

Alternating prone extensions FIG. 13.2

Description

The participant lies in a prone position, face down, with the shoulders fully flexed in a relaxed position lying in front of the body. The head, upper trunk, right upper extremity, and left lower extremity are raised from the floor. The knees are kept in full extension. Then the participant returns to the starting position. On the next repetition, the head, upper trunk, left upper extremity, and right lower extremity are raised from the floor.

Analysis

This exercise is separated into two phases for analysis: (1) lifting phase to raise the right shoulder off the surface and extend the left lower extremity off the floor and (2) lowering phase to relaxed position (Table 13.2).

A

B

FIG. 13.2 ● Alternating prone extensions. **A,** Beginning relaxed position; **B,** raised position.

TABLE 13.2 • Alternating prone extensions (Superman exercise)

| Joint | Lifting phase to raise upper and lower extremities | | Lowering phase to relaxed position | |
	Action	Agonists	Action	Agonists
Shoulder	Flexion	Shoulder joint flexors Pectoralis major (clavicular head or upper fibers) Deltoid Coracobrachialis Biceps brachii	Extension	Shoulder joint flexors (eccentric contraction) Pectoralis major (clavicular head or upper fibers) Deltoid Coracobrachialis Biceps brachii
Shoulder girdle	Adduction	Shoulder girdle adductors Trapezius Rhomboids	Abduction	Shoulder girdle adductors (eccentric contraction) Trapezius Rhomboids
Trunk	Extension	Trunk extensors Erector spinae Splenius Quadratus lumborum	Flexion (return to neutral relaxed position)	Trunk and cervical spine extensors (eccentric contraction) Erector spinae Splenius Quadratus lumborum
Hip	Extension	Hip extensors Gluteus maximus Semitendinosus Semimembranosus Biceps femoris	Flexion (return to neutral relaxed position)	Hip extensors (eccentric contraction) Gluteus maximus Semitendinosus Semimembranosus Biceps femoris

Squat   FIG. 13.3

Description

The participant places a barbell on the shoulders behind the neck and grasps it with the palms-forward position of the hands. The participant squats down, flexing at the hips while keeping the spine in normal alignment, until the thighs are parallel to the floor. The participant then returns to the starting position. This exercise is commonly performed improperly by allowing the knees to move forward beyond the plane of the feet, which greatly increases the risk of injury. Care should be taken to ensure that the shins remain as vertical as possible during this exercise.

The feet should be parallel, with slight external rotation of the lower extremity. The knees should point over the ankles and feet without going in front, between, or outside of the vertical plane of the feet.

Analysis

This exercise is separated into two phases for analysis: (1) lowering phase to the squatted position and (2) lifting phase to the starting position (Table 13.3). NOTE: It is assumed that no movement will take place in the shoulder joint, shoulder girdle, wrists, hands, and back.

FIG. 13.3 • Squat. **A,** Starting position; **B,** squatted position.

TABLE 13.3 • Squat

Joint	Lowering phase to squatted position			Lifting phase to starting position	
	Action	Agonists		Action	Agonists
Hip	Flexion	Hip extensors (eccentric contraction) Gluteus maximus Semimembranosus Semitendinosus Biceps femoris		Extension	Hip extensors Gluteus maximus Semimembranosus Semitendinosus Biceps femoris
Knee	Flexion	Knee extensors (eccentric contraction) Rectus femoris Vastus medialis Vastus intermedius Vastus lateralis		Extension	Knee extensors Rectus femoris Vastus medialis Vastus intermedius Vastus lateralis
Ankle	Dorsiflexion	Plantar flexors (eccentric contraction) Gastrocnemius Soleus		Plantar flexion	Plantar flexors Gastrocnemius Soleus

Dead lift   FIG. 13.4

Description

The participant begins in hip flexed position, keeping the arms, legs, and back straight, and grasps the barbell on the floor. Then a movement to the standing position is made by extending the hips. This exercise, when done improperly by allowing lumbar flexion, may contribute to low back problems. It is essential that the lumbar extensors be used more as isometric stabilizers of the low back while the hip extensors perform the majority of the lift in this exercise.

Analysis

This exercise is divided into two phases for analysis: (1) lifting phase to the hip extended/knee extended position and (2) lowering phase to the hip flexed/knee flexed starting position (Table 13.4).

A

B

FIG. 13.4 ● Dead lift. **A,** Beginning hip/knee flexed position; **B,** ending hip/knee extendend position.

TABLE 13.4 • Dead lift

| Joint | Lifting phase to hip/knee extended position | | Lowering phase to hip/knee flexed position | |
	Action	Agonists	Action	Agonists
Wrist and hand	Flexion	Wrist and hand flexors (isometric contraction) 　Flexor carpi radialis 　Flexor carpi ulnaris 　Palmaris longus 　Flexor digitorum profundus 　Flexor digitorum superficialis 　Flexor pollicis longus	Flexion	Wrist and hand flexors (isometric contraction) 　Flexor carpi radialis 　Flexor carpi ulnaris 　Palmaris longus 　Flexor digitorum profundus 　Flexor digitorum superficialis 　Flexor pollicis longus
Trunk	Maintenance of extension	Trunk extensors (isometric contraction) 　Erector spinae (sacrospinalis) 　Quadratus lumborum	Maintenance of extension	Trunk extensors (isometric contraction) 　Erector spinae (sacrospinalis) 　Quadratus lumborum
Hip	Extension	Hip extensors 　Gluteus maximus 　Semimembranosus 　Semitendinosus 　Biceps femoris	Flexion	Hip extensors (eccentric contraction) 　Gluteus maximus 　Semimembranosus 　Semitendinosus 　Biceps femoris
Knee	Extension	Knee extensors (quadriceps) 　Rectus femoris 　Vastus medialis 　Vastus intermedius 　Vastus lateralis	Flexion	Knee extensors (quadriceps) (eccentric contraction) 　Rectus femoris 　Vastus medialis 　Vastus intermedius 　Vastus lateralis

Note: Slight movement of the shoulder joint and shoulder girdle is not being analyzed.

Chapter

13

Isometric exercises

An exercise technique called "isometrics" is a type of muscular activity in which there is contraction of muscle groups with little or no muscle shortening. Although not as productive in terms of overall strength gains as isotonics, isometrics are an effective way to build and maintain muscular strength in a limited range of motion.

A few selected isometric exercises are analyzed muscularly to show how they are designed to develop specific muscle groups. Although there are varying approaches to isometrics, most authorities agree that isometric contractions should be held approximately 7 to 10 seconds for a training effect.

Abdominal contraction FIG. 13.5

Description

The participant contracts the muscles in the anterior abdominal region as strongly as possible, with no movement of the trunk or hips. This exercise can be performed in sitting, standing, or supine positions. The longer the contraction in seconds, the more valuable the exercise will be, to a degree.

Analysis

Abdomen
    Contraction
        Rectus abdominis
        External oblique abdominal
        Internal oblique abdominal
        Transversus abdominis

A **B**

FIG. 13.5 ● Abdominal contraction. **A,** Beginning position; **B,** contracted position.

Leg lifter FIG. 13.6

Description

The participant sits on a bench or chair with the knees slightly bent and with the left leg over the right. An attempt to raise the right leg while resisting it with the left leg is conducted.

Analysis*

This exercise involves only a single isometric contraction of the muscles as listed in Table 13.5. Upon completion of the exercise, the position of the legs may be reversed so that right leg is over the left in order to exercise the contralateral muscles.

*When the legs are alternated, the muscles used will be the same muscles, but in the other leg.

A

B

FIG. 13.6 ● Leg lifter. **A,** Beginning relaxed position; **B,** up position.

TABLE 13.5 • Leg lifter

| Joint | Right leg—attempting upward movement | | Left leg—resisting upward movement | |
	Action	Agonists	Action	Agonists
Ankle	Dorsiflexion	Ankle dorsiflexors Tibialis anterior Extensor hallucis longus Extensor digitorum longus Peroneus tertius	Plantar Flexion	Plantar flexors Gastrocenemius Soleus
Knee	Extension	Knee extensors (quadriceps) Rectus femoris Vastus medialis Vastus intermedius Vastus lateralis	Flexion	Knee flexors (hamstrings) Biceps femoris Semitendinosus Semimbranosus
Hip	Flexion	Hip flexors Iliopsoas Rectus femoris Pectineus Sartorius Tensor fasciae latae	Extension	Hip extensors Gluteus maximus Biceps femoris Semitendinosus Semimbranosus

Chapter
13

Total Gym exercise machine

The Total Gym exercise machine* or similar machines by other manufacturers (Fig. 13.7) are used by professional, college, and many high school athletes, as well as thousands of home users. Health clubs, YMCAs, YWCAs, fitness centers, and body gyms have these machines for use by their members. Many similar types of machines are available; these include Cybex Eagle, Universal, Nautilus, Paramount, Olympus, and others. Many of these machines rely on various pulleys, cams, and positions to vary the resistance, as opposed to free weights, which were discussed earlier in this chapter.

All exercise machines come with a list of recommended exercises that can be done by the user. The advantages of these machines are that they may be used individually to perform a wide variety of exercises for many body areas, regardless of the strength level. See Fig. 13.7 for a few of the exercises for the Total Gym.

*Efi medical systems, San Diego, CA.

FIG. 13.7 ● Total Gym exercise machine. **A,** biceps curl; **B,** single-leg hip extension; **C,** pull-up; **D,** incline press; **E,** alternating shoulder punch; **F,** squat; **G,** dip.

Courtesy Efi medical systems, San Diego, CA.

Hip sled FIG. 13.8

Description

The participant lies in a supine position on the floor with the knees and hips flexed in a position close to the chest. The feet are placed on the apparatus plate. The plate is moved upward until the knees and hips are completely extended. Then the participant returns to the starting position.

Analysis

This exercise is divided into two phases for analysis: (1) Pushing phase to the straight leg position and (2) Lowering phase to the starting position (Table 13.6).

A   **B**

FIG. 13.8 ● Hip sled (hip and leg press). **A,** Starting position; **B,** high position.

TABLE 13.6 • Hip sled

Joint	Pushing phase to straight leg position		Lowering phase to starting position	
	Action	Agonists	Action	Agonists
Ankle	Plantar flexion	Ankle plantar flexors Gastrocnemius Soleus	Dorsiflexion	Ankle plantar flexors (eccentric contraction) Gastrocnemius Soleus
Knee	Extension	Knee extensors (quadriceps) Rectus femoris Vastus medialis Vastus intermedius Vastus lateralis	Flexion	Knee extensors (quadriceps) (eccentric contraction) Rectus femoris Vastus medialis Vastus intermedius Vastus lateralis
Hip	Extension	Hip extensors Biceps femoris Semimembranosus Semitendinosus Gluteus maximus	Flexion	Hip extensors (eccentric contraction) Biceps femoris Semimembranosus Semitendinosus Gluteus maximus

Rowing exercise   FIG. 13.9

Description

The participant sits on a movable seat with the knees and hips flexed close to the chest. The arms are reaching forward to grasp a horizontal bar. The legs are extended forcibly as the arms are pulled toward the chest. Then the legs and arms are returned to the starting position.

Analysis

This exercise is divided into two movements for analysis: (1) Arm pull to chest/leg push to extend knees and hip phase and (2) Return phase to the starting position (Table 13.7).

A

B

FIG. 13.9 ● Rowing exercise machine. **A,** Starting position; **B,** movement.

TABLE 13.7 • Rowing exercise

Joint	Arm pull/leg push phase		Return phase to starting position	
	Action	Agonists	Action	Agonists

Foot and ankle	Plantar flexion	Ankle plantarflexors
		  Gastrocnemius
		  Soleus
			Dorsiflexion	Ankle dorsiflexors
				  Tibialis anterior
				  Extensor hallucis longus
				  Extensor digitorum longus
				  Peroneus tertius

Knee	Extension	Quadriceps (knee extensors)
		  Rectus femoris
		  Vastus medialis
		  Vastus intermedius
		  Vastus lateralis
			Flexion	Knee flexors (hamstrings)
				  Biceps femoris
				  Semitendinosus
				  Semimembranosus

Hip	Extension	Hip extensors
		  Gluteus maximus
		  Biceps femoris
		  Semimembranosus
		  Semitendinosus
			Flexion	Hip flexors
				  Iliopsoas
				  Rectus femoris
				  Pectineus

Trunk	Extension	Trunk extensors
		  Erector spinae
			Flexion	Trunk flexors
				  Rectus abdominis
				  Internal oblique abdominal
				  External oblique abdominal

Shoulder girdle	Adduction, downward rotation, and depression	Shoulder girdle adductors, downward rotators, and depressors
		  Trapezius (lower)
		  Rhomboid
		  Pectoralis minor
			Abduction, upward rotation, and elevation	Shoulder girdle adductors, downward rotators, and depressors (eccentric contraction)
				  Trapezius (lower)
				  Rhomboid
				  Pectoralis minor

Shoulder joint	Extension	Shoulder joint extensors
		  Latissimus dorsi
		  Teres major
		  Posterior deltoid
		  Teres minor
		  Infraspinatus
			Flexion	Shoulder joint extensors (eccentric contraction)
				  Latissimus dorsi
				  Teres major
				  Posterior deltoid
				  Teres minor
				  Infraspinatus

Elbow joint	Flexion	Elbow joint flexors
		  Biceps brachii
		  Brachialis
		  Brachioradialis
			Extension	Elbow joint flexors (eccentric contraction)
				  Biceps brachii
				  Brachialis
				  Brachioradialis

Wrist and hand	Flexion	Wrist and hand flexors (isometric contraction)
		  Flexor carpi radialis
		  Flexor carpi ulnaris
		  Palmaris longus
		  Flexor digitorum profundus
		  Flexor digitorum superficialis
		  Flexor pollicis longus
			Flexion	Wrist and hand flexors (isometric contraction)
				  Flexor carpi radialis
				  Flexor carpi ulnaris
				  Palmaris longus
				  Flexor digitorum profundus
				  Flexor digitorum superficialis
				  Flexor pollicis longus

Chapter

13

Web sites

American College of Sports Medicine:

www.acsm.org

Scientific research, education, and practical applications of sports medicine and exercise science to maintain and enhance physical performance, fitness, health, and quality of life

Concept II:

www.concept2.com/index.html

Information on the technique of rowing and the muscles used.

Fitness World:

www.fitnessworld.com

The information at this site is about fitness in general and includes access to *Fitness Management* magazine.

National Council of Strength & Fitness:

www.ncsf.org

Personal Training Certification & Continuing Education for the Fitness Professional

National Strength and Conditioning Association:

www.nsca-lift.org

Information on the profession of strength and conditioning specialists and personal trainers

NSCA Certification Commission:

www.nsca-cc.org

The certifying body for the National Strength and Conditioning Association

President's Council on Physical Fitness and Sports:

www.fitness.gov

Information and links from the U.S. government on fitness

Worksheet exercises

As an aid to learning, for in-class and out-of-class assignments, or for testing, a tear-out worksheet is found at the end of the text (pp. 339).

Skill analysis worksheets (no. 1)

Using the techniques taught in this chapter and in Chapter 8, analyze the joint movements and muscles used in each phase of movement for selected exercises from the Total Gym examples on page 308 and/or from selected sports skills. For each joint, list the initial and subsequent position, the motion and degrees of movement, and the agonists, and denote whether they are contracting concentrically or eccentrically.

Laboratory and review exercises

1. Obtain, describe, and completely analyze five conditioning exercises.
2. Collect, analyze, and evaluate exercises that are found in newspapers and magazines or are observed on television.
3. Prepare a set of exercises that will ensure development of all large muscle groups in the body.
4. Select exercises from exercise books for analysis.
5. Bring to class other typical exercises for members to analyze.
6. Analyze the conditioning exercises given by your physical education teachers, coaches, and athletic trainers.
7. Observe children using playground equipment. Analyze muscularly the activities they are performing.
8. Visit the room on your campus where the free weights and specific or multifunction exercise machines are located. Analyze exercises that can be done with each machine. Compare and contrast similar exercises using different exercise machines and free weights. NOTE: Manufacturers of all types of exercise apparatus have a complete list of exercises that can be performed with their machines. Secure a copy of recommended exercises and muscularly analyze each exercise.
9. Consider a sport (basketball or any other sport) and develop exercises applying the overload principle that would develop all the large muscle groups used in the sport.
10. Lie supine on a table with the knees flexed and hips flexed 90 degrees and the ankles in the neutral 90-degree position. Extend each joint until your knee is fully extended, your hip is flexed only 10 degrees, and your ankle is plantar flexed 10 degrees by performing each of the following movements before proceeding to the next:
    - Full knee extension
    - Hip extension to within 10 degrees of neutral
    - Plantar flexion to 10 degrees

    Analyze the movements and the muscles responsible for each movement at the hip, knee, and ankle.

Chapter
13

11. Now stand with your back and buttocks against a smooth wall and place your feet (shoulder width apart) with approximately 12 inches between your heels and the wall. Maintain your feet in position, with the hips and knees each flexed approximately 90 degrees so that the thighs are parallel to the floor. Keeping your feet in place, slowly slide your back and buttocks up the wall until your buttocks are as far away from the floor as possible without removing your feet from their position on the floor. Analyze the movements and the muscles responsible for each movement at the hip, knee, and ankle.

12. What is the difference between the two exercises in questions #10 and #11? Can you perform #11 one step at a time, as you did #10?

13. Analyze each exercise in the exercise analysis chart below. Use one row for each joint involved that actively moves during the exercise. Do not include joints where there is no active movement or where the joint is maintained in one position isometrically.

Exercise analysis chart

Exercise	Phase	Joint, movement occurring	Force causing movement (muscle or gravity)	Force resisting movement (muscle or gravity)	Functional muscle group, type of contraction
Sit-up, bent knee	Curling phase to sitting-up position				
	Rotating-to-right phase				
	Return phase to sitting-up position				
	Return phase to starting position				
Alternating prone extensions	Lifting phase				
	Lowering phase				

(continued)

Chapter
13

Exercise analysis chart (*continued*)

Exercise	Phase	Joint, movement occurring	Force causing movement (muscle or gravity)	Force resisting movement (muscle or gravity)	Functional muscle group, type of contraction
Squat	Lowering phase				
	Lifting phase				
Dead lift	Lifting phase				
	Lowering phase				
Leg press	Pressing phase				
	Return phase				
Hip sled	Pushing phase				
	Lowering phase				
Rowing exercise	Arm pull/leg push phase				
	Return phase to starting position				

References

Adrian M: Isokinetic exercise, *Training and Conditioning* 1:1, June 1991.

Altug Z, Hoffman JL, Martin JL: *Manual of clinical exercise testing, prescription and rehabilitation,* Norwalk, CT, 1993, Appleton & Lange.

Andrews JR, Harrelson GL: *Physical rehabilitation of the injured athlete,* Philadelphia, 1991, Saunders.

Baitch SP: Aerobic dance injuries, a biomechanical approach, *Journal of Physical Education, Recreation and Dance* 58:57, May–June 1987.

Bouche J: Three essential lifts for high school players, *Scholastic Coach* 56:42, April 1987.

Brzycki M: Rx for a safe productive strength program, *Scholastic Coach* 57:70, September 1987.

Epley B: Getting elementary muscles, *Coach and Athlete* 44:60, November–December 1981.

Fahey TD: *Athletic training: principles and practices,* Mountain View, CA, 1986, Mayfield.

Logan GA, McKinney WC: *Anatomic kinesiology,* ed 3, 1982, McGraw-Hill Companies, Inc., New York.

Matheson O, et al: Stress fractures in athletes, *American Journal of Sports Medicine* 15:46, January–February 1987.

Minton S: Dance dynamics avoiding dance injuries (symposium), *Journal of Physical Education, Recreation and Dance* 58:29, May–June 1987.

Northrip JW, Logan GA, McKinney WC: *Analysis of sport motion: anatomic and biomechanic perspectives,* ed 3, 1983, McGraw-Hill Companies, Inc., New York.

Prentice WE: *Rehabilitation techniques in sports medicine,* ed 3, 1999, McGraw-Hill Companies, Inc., New York.

Schlitz J: The athlete's daily dozen stretches, *Athletic Journal* 66:20, November 1985.

Steindler A: *Kinesiology of the human body,* Springfield, IL, 1970, Charles C Thomas.

Todd J: Strength training for female athletes, *Journal of Physical Education, Recreation and Dance,* 56:38, August 1985.

Torg JS, Vegso JJ, Torg E: *Rehabilitation of athletic injuries: an atlas of therapeutic exercise,* Chicago, 1987, Year Book.

Wirhed R: *Athletic ability and the anatomy of motion,* London, 1984, Wolfe.

Chapter
13

Appendix

Appendix 1

Range of motion for diarthrodial joints of the upper extremity

Joint	Type	Motion	Range
Sternoclavicular	Arthrodial	Protraction	Moves anteriorly 15°
		Retraction	Moves posteriorly 15°
		Elevation	Moves superiorly 45°
		Depression	Moves inferiorly 5°
		Upward rotation	45°
		Downward rotation	5°
Acromioclavicular	Arthrodial	Protraction-retraction	20–30° rotational and gliding motion
		Elevation-depression	20–30° rotational and gliding motion
		Upward rotation–downward rotation	20–30° rotational and gliding motion
Scapulothoracic	Not a true synovial joint; all movement totally dependent on AC and SC joints	Abduction-adduction	25° total range
		Upward rotation–downward rotation	60° total range
		Elevation-depression	55° total range
Glenohumeral	Enarthrodial	Flexion	90°–100°
		Extension	40°–60°
		Abduction	90°–95°
		Adduction	0° prevented by trunk, 75° anterior to trunk
		Internal rotation	70°–90°
		External rotation	70°–90°
		Horizontal abduction	45°
		Horizontal adduction	135°
Elbow	Ginglymus	Extension	0°
		Flexion	145°–150°
Radioulnar	Trochoid	Supination	80°–90°
		Pronation	70°–90°

Range of motion for diarthrodial joints of the upper extremity (*continued*)

Joint	Type	Motion	Range
Wrist	Condyloid	Flexion	70°–90°
		Extension	65°–85°
		Abduction	15°–25°
		Adduction	25°–40°
Thumb carpometacarpal	Sellar	Flexion	15°–45°
		Extension	0°–20°
		Adduction	0°
		Abduction	50°–70°
Thumb metacarpo-phalangeal	Ginglymus	Extension	0°
		Flexion	40°–90°
Thumb interphalangeal	Ginglymus	Flexion	80°–90°
		Extension	0°
2nd, 3rd, 4th, and 5th metacarpo-phalangeal joints	Condyloid	Extension	0°–40°
		Flexion	85°–100°
		Abduction	Variable 10°–40°
		Adduction	Variable 10°–40°
2nd, 3rd, 4th, and 5th proximal interphalangeal joints	Ginglymus	Flexion	90°–120°
		Extension	0°
2nd, 3rd, 4th, and 5th distal interphalangeal joints	Ginglymus	Flexion	80°–90°
		Extension	0°

Appendix 2

Range of motion for diarthrodial joints of the spine and lower extremity

Joint	Type	Motion	Range
Cervical	Arthrodial except atlantoaxial joint, which is trochoid	Flexion	80°
		Extension	20°–30°
		Lateral flexion	35°
		Rotation unilaterally	45°
Lumbar	Arthrodial	Flexion	45°
		Extension	45°
		Lateral flexion	45°
		Rotation unilaterally	60°
Hip	Enarthrodial	Flexion	130°
		Extension	30°
		Abduction	35°
		Adduction	0°–30°
		External rotation	50°
		Internal rotation	45°
Knee *For internal and external rotation to occur, the knee must be flexed approximately 30° or more.*	Ginglymus (trochoginglymus)	Extension	0°
		Flexion	140°
		Internal rotation	30°
		External rotation	45°
Ankle (talocrural)	Ginglymus	Plantar flexion	50°
		Dorsal flexion	15°–20°
Transverse tarsal and subtalar	Arthrodial	Inversion	20°–30°
		Eversion	5°–15°
Great toe metatarsophalangeal	Condyloid	Flexion	45°
		Extension	70°
		Abduction	Variable 5°–25°
		Adduction	Variable 5°–25°
Great toe interphalangeal	Ginglymus	Flexion	90°
		Extension	0°
2nd, 3rd, 4th, and 5th metatarsophalangeal joints	Condyloid	Flexion	40°
		Extension	40°
		Abduction	Variable 5°–25°
		Adduction	Variable 5°–25°
2nd, 3rd, 4th, and 5th proximal interphalangeal joints	Ginglymus	Flexion	35°
		Extension	0°
2nd, 3rd, 4th, and 5th distal interphalangeal joints	Ginglymus	Flexion	60°
		Extension	30°

Appendix 3

Commonly used exercises for strengthening selected muscles

Some exercises may be more or less specific for certain muscles. In some cases, certain exercises are designed to emphasize specific portions of a particular muscle more than other portions. Some exercises may be modified slightly to further emphasize or de-emphasize certain muscles or portions of muscles. In addition to the muscles listed, numerous other muscles in surrounding joints or other parts of the body may be involved by contracting isometrically to maintain appropriate position of the body for the muscles listed to carry out the exercise movement. Appropriate strength and endurance of these stabilizing muscles is essential for correct position and execution of the listed exercises. Finally, these exercises may be documented by different names by different authorities. Illustration and documentation of the proper techniques and indications for these exercises is beyond the scope of this text. Please consult several strength and conditioning texts for further details.

Upper extremity		
Muscle groups	Muscles	Exercise
Scapula abductors	Serratus anterior Pectoralis minor	Front press Dumbbell flys Dumbbell press Bench press Close-grip bench press Incline press Push-ups Incline dumbbell press Pec deck flys Cable crossover flys
Scapula adductors	Rhomboid Trapezius, lower fibers Trapezius, middle fibers	Bent-over lateral raises Pec deck rear delt laterals Seated rows Bent rows T-bar rows Deadlifts Sumo deadlifts
Scapula upward rotators	Serratus anterior Trapezius, lower fibers Trapezius, middle fibers	Dumbbell press Dumbbell flys One-arm dumbbell press Lateral raises Upright rows
Scapula downward rotators	Pectoralis minor Rhomboid	Parallel bar dips Dumbbell pullovers Barbell pullovers Chin-ups Reverse chin-ups Lat pulldowns Back lat pulldowns Close-grip lat pulldowns Straight-arm lat pulldowns One-arm dumbbell rows
Scapula elevators	Rhomboid Levator scapulae Trapezius, upper fibers Trapezius, middle fibers	Upright rows Barbell shrugs Dumbbell shrugs Machine shrugs Deadlifts
Scapula depressors	Pectoralis minor Trapezius, lower fibers	Parallel bar dips

Upper extremity		
Muscle groups	Muscles	Exercise
Shoulder flexors	Deltoid, anterior fibers Deltoid, middle fibers Pectoralis major, clavicular fibers Coracobrachialis	Arm curls Triceps dips One-arm dumbbell press Front raises Low pulley front raises One-dumbbell front raises Barbell front raises
Shoulder extensors	Latissimus dorsi Teres major Triceps brachii, long head Pectoralis major, sternal fibers Deltoid, posterior fibers Infraspinatus Teres minor	Dumbbell pullovers Barbell pullovers Reverse chin-ups Close-grip lat pulldowns Straight-arm lat pulldowns One-arm dumbbell rows
Shoulder abductors	Deltoid – anterior fibers Deltoid – posterior fibers Deltoid – middle fibers Pectoralis major, clavicular fibers Supraspinatus	Back press Front press Dumbbell press One-arm dumbbell press Lateral raises Side-lying lateral raises Low pulley lateral raises Upright rows Nautilus lateral raises Upright rows
Shoulder adductors	Pectoralis major Latissimus dorsi Teres major Subscapularis Coracobrachialis	Triceps dips Parallel bar dips Chin-ups Lat pulldowns Back lat pulldowns
Shoulder internal rotators	Pectoralis major Latissimus dorsi Teres major Subscapularis	Triceps dips Sidelying internal rotations Standing internal rotations at 90 degrees abduction
Shoulder external rotators	Infraspinatus Teres minor	Sidelying external rotations Standing external rotations at 90 degrees abduction

Upper extremity		
Muscle groups	Muscles	Exercise
Shoulder horizontal abductors	Latissimus dorsi Infraspinatus Teres minor Deltoid, middle fibers Deltoid, posterior fibers	Bent-over lateral raises Low pulley bent-over lateral raises Pec deck rear delt laterals Bent rows T-bar rows
Shoulder horizontal adductors	Pectoralis major Coracobrachialis	Dumbbell flys Triceps dips Dumbbell press Bench press Close-grip bench press Incline press Decline press Push-ups Incline dumbbell press Incline dumbbell flys Pec deck flys Cable crossover flys Seated rows
Elbow flexors	Biceps brachii Brachialis Brachioradialis	Arm curls concentration curls Hammer curls Low pulley curls High pulley curls Barbell curls Machine curls Preacher curls Reverse barbell curls Chin-ups Reverse chin-ups Lat pulldowns Back lat pulldowns Close-grip lat pulldowns Seated rows One-arm dumbbell rows Bent rows T-bar rows Upright rows
Elbow extensors	Triceps brachii Triceps brachii, lateral head Triceps brachii, long head Triceps brachii, medial head Anconeus	Barbell pullovers Bench press Close-grip bench press Decline press Dumbbell press Dumbbell pullovers Dumbbell triceps extensions Front press Incline dumbbell press Incline press One-arm dumbbell triceps extensions One-arm reverse pushdowns Parallel bar dips Pushdowns Push-ups Reverse pushdowns Seated dumbbell triceps extensions Seated ez-bar triceps extensions Triceps dips Triceps extensions Triceps kickbacks

Upper extremity		
Muscle groups	Muscles	Exercise
Wrist flexors	Flexor carpi radialis Palmaris longus Flexor carpi ulnaris Flexor digitorum superficialis Flexor digitorum profundus	Wrist curls
Wrist extensors	Extensor carpi radialis longus Extensor carpi radialis brevis Extensor carpi ulnaris	Reverse barbell curls Reverse wrist curls Reverse pushdowns
Fingers flexors	Hand intrinsics Flexor digitorum profundus Flexor digitorum superficialis Flexor pollicis longus	Ball squeezes Putty squeezes Rice bucket grips Wrist curls Deadlifts
Finger extensors	Extensor digitorum Extensor digiti minimi Extensor indicis	Reverse barbell curls Reverse wrist curls Rubber band stretches

Lower extremity		
Muscle groups	Muscles	Exercise
Hip flexors	Rectus femoris Iliopsoas Pectineus Tensor fasciae latae	Crunches Sit-ups Gym ladder sit-ups Calves over bench sit-ups Gym ladder sit-ups Calves over bench sit-ups Incline bench sit-ups Specific bench sit-ups Machine crunches Incline leg raises Leg raises Hanging leg raises
Hip extensors	Gluteus maximus Biceps femoris long head Semitendinosus Semimembranosus	Stiff-legged deadlifts Deadlifts Back extensions Dumbbell squats Squats Front squats Power squats Angled leg press Good mornings Lunges Cable back kicks Machine hip extensions Floor hip extensions Bridging Prone arches
Hip abductors	Gluteus medius Gluteus maximus Tensor fascia latae	Cable hip abductions Standing machine hip abductions Floor hip abductions Seated machine hip abductions

Lower extremity		
Muscle groups	Muscles	Exercise
Hip adductors	Adductor magnus Adductor longus Adductor brevis Gracilis	Sumo deadlifts Power squats Cable adductions Machine adductions
Hip external rotators	Gluteus maximus Piriformis Gamellus superior Gamellus inferior Obturator externus Obturator internus Quadratus femoris	Hip turn outs Body turn aways
Knee extensors	Vastus medialis Vastus intermedius Rectus femoris Vastus lateralis	Leg extensions Deadlifts Sumo deadlifts Dumbbell squats Squats Front squats Angled leg press Power squats Hack squats Lunges
Knee flexors	Semitendinosus Biceps femoris, long head Biceps femoris, short head Semimembranosus Gastrocnemius, lateral head Gastrocnemius, medial head	Standing leg curls Seated leg curls Lying leg curls
Ankle dorsiflexors	Tibialis anterior Extensor hallucis longus Extensor digitorum longus Peroneus tertius	Towel pulls Elastic band pulls
Ankle plantar-flexors	Gastrocnemius, lateral head Soleus Gastrocnemius, medial head	Standing calf raises One-leg toe raises Donkey calf raises Seated calf raises Seated barbell calf raises
Transverse tarsal/ subtalar inversion	Tibialis anterior Tibialis posterior Flexor digitorum longus Flexor hallucis longus	Towel drags Elastic band turn-ins
Transverse tarsal/ subtalar eversion	Extensor digitorum longus Peroneus longus Peroneus brevis Peroneus tertius	Towel drags Elastic band turn-outs
Toe extensors	Extensor hallucis longus Extensor digitorum longus	Towel pulls Elastic band pulls
Toe flexors	Flexor digitorum longus Flexor hallucis longus Foot intrinsics	Towel curls Marble pickups Pencil pickups

Cervical Spine and Trunk		
Muscle groups	Muscles	Exercise
Cervical extensors	Splenius cervicis Splenius capitus Trapezius, upper fibers	Deadlifts Neck extensions
Cervical flexors	Sternocleidomastoid	Chin tucks Sit-ups
Cervical rotators	Sternocleidomastoid Splenius cervicis Splenius capitus	Machine neck rotations
Trunk extensors	Erector spinae	Back extensions Alternating prone extensions Prone arches
Trunk flexors	Rectus abdominis External oblique abdominal Internal oblique abdominal	Deadlifts Crunches Crunch twists Sit-ups Gym ladder sit-ups Calves over bench sit-ups Incline bench sit-ups Specific bench sit-ups High pulley crunches Machine crunches Incline leg raises Leg raises Hanging leg raises
Trunk rotators	External oblique abdominal Internal oblique abdominal	Crunches Crunch twists Sit-up twists Gym ladder sit-ups Calves over bench sit-ups Incline bench sit-ups Specific bench sit-ups High pulley crunches Machine crunches Incline leg raises Leg raises Hanging leg raises Broomstick twists Machine trunk rotations
Trunk lateral flexors	External oblique abdominal Internal oblique abdominal Quadratus lumborum Rectus abdominis	Crunches Crunch twists Sit-ups Gym ladder sit-ups Calves over bench sit-ups Incline bench sit-ups Specific bench sit-ups High pulley crunches Machine crunches Incline leg raises Leg raises Hanging leg raises Broomstick twists Dumbbell side bends Roman chair side bends

Worksheets

Chapter one

Worksheet no. 1

On the posterior skeletal worksheet, list the names of the bones and all of the prominent features of each bone.

Chapter one

Worksheet no. 2

On the anterior skeletal worksheet, list the names of the bones and all of the prominent features of each bone.

Chapter four

Worksheet no. 1

Draw and label on the worksheet the following listed muscles. Indicate the origin and insertion of each muscle with an "O" and an "I," respectively.

a. Trapezius

b. Rhomboid

c. Serratus anterior

d. Levator scapulae

e. Pectoralis minor

Chapter four

Worksheet no. 2

Label and indicate by arrows the following movements of the shoulder girdle. For each motion, list the plane in which it occurs and list the axis of rotation.

a. Adduction

b. Abduction

c. Upward rotation

d. Downward rotation

e. Elevation

f. Depression

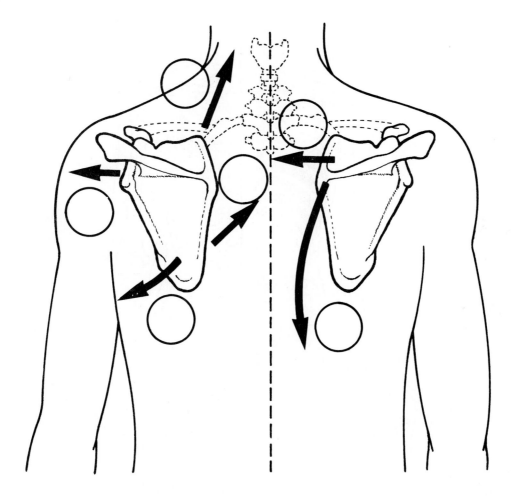

Chapter five

Worksheet no. 1

   Draw and label on the worksheet the following muscles. Indicate the origin
   and insertion of each muscle with an "O" and an "I," respectively.

   a. Deltoid
   b. Supraspinatus
   c. Subscapularis
   d. Teres major
   e. Infraspinatus

   f. Teres minor
   g. Latissimus dorsi
   h. Pectoralis major
   i. Coracobrachialis

Chapter five

Worksheet no. 2

Label and indicate by arrows the following listed movements of the shoulder joint. For each motion, list the plane in which it occurs and list the axis of rotation.

a. Abduction   d. Extension

b. Adduction   e. Horizontal adduction

c. Flexion   f. Horizontal abduction

Chapter six

Worksheet no. 1

Draw and label on the worksheet the following muscles. Indicate the origin and insertion of each muscle with an "O" and an "I," respectively.

a. Biceps brachii
b. Brachioradialis
c. Brachialis
d. Pronator teres

e. Supinator
f. Triceps brachii
g. Anconeus
h. Pronator quadratus

Chapter six

Worksheet no. 2

Label and indicate by arrows the following movements of the elbow and radioulnar joint. For each motion, list the plane in which it occurs and list the axis of rotation.

Elbow
  Flexion
  Extension

Radioulnar joint
  Pronation
  Supination

Chapter seven

Worksheet no. 1

Draw and label on the worksheet the following muscles. Indicate the origin and insertion of each muscle with an "O" and an "I," respectively.

a. Flexor pollicis longus
b. Flexor carpi radialis
c. Flexor carpi ulnaris
d. Extensor digitorum
e. Extensor pollicis longus

f. Extensor pollicis brevis
g. Extensor carpi ulnaris
h. Palmaris longus
i. Extensor carpi radialis longus
j. Extensor carpi radialis brevis

k. Extensor digiti minimi
l. Extensor digitorum indicis
m. Flexor digitorum superficialis
n. Flexor digitorum profundus
o. Abductor pollicis longus

Chapter seven

Worksheet no. 2

Label and indicate by arrows the following movements of the wrist and hands.
For each motion, list the plane in which it occurs and list the axis of rotation.

Wrist and hands
    Extension
    Flexion
    Abduction
    Adduction

Chapter eight

Worksheet no. 1

Analyze this exercise following the procedures explained in this chapter that include joint movements and muscles that produce these movements.

Worksheet no. 2

Analyze this exercise following the procedures explained in this chapter that include joint movements and muscles that produce these movements.

Chapter nine

Worksheet no. 1

Draw and label on the worksheet the anterior hip joint and pelvic girdle muscles. Indicate the origin and insertion of each muscle with an "O" and an "I," respectively.

Chapter nine

Worksheet no. 2

Draw and label on the worksheet the posterior hip and pelvic girdle muscles. Indicate the origin and insertion of each muscle with an "O" and an "I," respectively.

Chapter ten

Worksheet no. 1

Draw and label on the worksheet the knee joint muscles. Indicate the origin and insertion of each muscle with an "O" and an "I," respectively.

Chapter eleven

Worksheet no. 1

Draw and label on the worksheet the following muscles of the ankle and foot. Indicate the origin and insertion of each muscle with an "O" and an "I," respectively.

a. Tibialis anterior   g. Gastrocnemius

b. Extensor digitorum longus   h. Extensor hallucis longus

c. Peroneus longus   i. Tibialis posterior

d. Peroneus brevis   j. Flexor digitorum longus

e. Soleus   k. Flexor hallucis longus

f. Peroneus tertius

Chapter twelve

Worksheet no. 1

Draw and label the following muscles on the skeletal chart. Indicate the origin and insertion of each muscle with an "O" and an "I," respectively.

a. Rectus abdominis

b. External oblique abdominal

c. Internal oblique abdominal

d. Sternocleidomastoid

Chapter twelve

Worksheet no. 2

Draw and label the following muscles on the skeletal chart. Indicate the origin and insertion of each muscle with an "O" and an "I," respectively.

a. Erector spinae

b. Quadratus lumborum

c. Splenius-cervicis and capitis

Chapter thirteen
Worksheet no. 1

Kinesiology skill analysis table

Phase		Toes	TT/ST	Ankle	Knee	Hip	Lumbar	Cervical	Shou G	G-H	Elbow	Wrist	Fingers
	Position												
	Deg/move												
	Agon/con												
	Position												
	Deg/move												
	Agon/con												
	Position												
	Deg/move												
	Agon/con												
	Position												
	Deg/move												
	Agon/con												
	Position												
	Deg/move												
	Agon/con												

Glossary

abduction Lateral movement away from the midline of the trunk, as in raising the arms or legs to the side horizontally.

acceleration The rate of change in velocity.

accessory motion The actual change in relationship between the articular surface of one bone relative to another, characterized as roll, spin, and glide.

active insufficiency Point reached when a muscle becomes shortened to the point that it cannot generate or maintain active tension.

adduction Movement medially toward the midline of the trunk, as in lowering the arms to the side or legs back to the anatomical position.

afferent nerves Nerves that bring impulses from receptors in the skin, joints, muscles, and other peripheral aspects of the body to the central nervous system.

aggregate muscle action Muscles working together in groups rather than independently to achieve given joint motions.

agonist A muscle or muscle group that is described as being primarily responsible for a specific joint movement when contracting.

amphiarthrodial joints Joints that functionally allow only a very slight amount of movement such as synchondrosis (ex. costochondral joint of the ribs with sternum), syndesmosis (ex. distal tibiofibular), and symphysis (ex. symphysis pubis) joints.

amplitude Range of muscle fiber length between maximal and minimal lengthening.

anatomical position The position of reference in which the subject is in the standing position, with feet together and palms of hands facing forward.

angle of pull The angle between the muscle insertion and the bone on which it inserts.

angular displacement The change in location of a rotating body.

angular motion Motion involving rotation around an axis.

antagonist A muscle or muscle group that counteracts or opposes the contraction of another muscle or muscle group.

anteroposterior axis The axis that has the same directional orientation as the sagittal plane of motion and runs from front to back at a right angle to the frontal plane of motion. Also known as the sagittal or AP axis.

appendicular skeleton The appendages, or the upper and lower extremities, and the shoulder and pelvic girdles.

arthrodial joints Joints in which bones glide on each other in limited movement, as in the bones of the wrist (carpal) or the bones of the foot (tarsal).

arthrokinematics Motion between the actual articular surfaces of the bones at a joint.

axial skeleton The skull, vertebral column, ribs, and sternum.

axis of rotation The point in a joint about which a bone moves or turns to accomplish joint motion.

axon An elongated projection that transmits impulses away from the neuron cell body.

balance The ability to control equilibrium, either static or dynamic.

biarticular muscles Those muscles that, from origin to insertion, cross two different joints, allowing them to perform actions at each joint.

biomechanics The study of mechanics as it relates to the functional and anatomical analysis of biological systems, especially humans.

bipennate A type of pennate muscle with fibers running obliquely on both sides from a central tendon, such as the rectus femoris and flexor hallucis longus.

brachial plexus Group of spinal nerves composed of cervical nerves 5 through 8, along with thoracic nerve 1; supplies motor and sensory function to the upper extremity and most of the scapula.

cancellous bone Spongy, porous bone that lies under cortical bone.

cartilaginous joints Joints joined together by hyaline cartilage or fibrocartilage, allowing very slight movement, such as synchondrosis and symphysis.

center of gravity The point at which all of the body's mass and weight are equally balanced or equally distributed in all directions.

central nervous system (CNS) The cerebral cortex, basal ganglia, cerebellum, brain stem, and spinal cord.

cervical plexus Group of spinal nerves composed of cervical nerves 1 through 4; generally responsible for sensory and motor function from the upper part of the shoulders to the back of the head and front of the neck.

circumduction Circular movement of a bone at the joint, as in movement of the hip, shoulder, or trunk around a fixed point. Combination of flexion, extension, abduction, and adduction.

closed kinetic chain When the distal end of an extremity is fixed, preventing movement of any one joint unless predictable movements of the other joints in the extremity occur.

coefficient of friction The ratio between the force needed to overcome friction over the force holding the surfaces together.

concentric contraction A contraction in which there is a shortening of the muscle that causes motion to occur at the joints it crosses.

condyle Large, rounded projection that usually articulates with another bone, such as the medial or lateral condyle of the femur.

condyloid joint Type of joint in which the bones permit movement in two planes without rotation, as in the wrist between the radius and the proximal row of the carpal bones or the second, third, fourth, and fifth metacarpophalangeal joints.

contractility The ability of muscle to contract and develop tension or internal force against resistance when stimulated.

coronal axis Runs from side to side through the body and is at a right angle to the sagittal plane of motion. Also known as the frontal or lateral axis.

cortex Diaphyseal wall of long bones, formed from hard, dense compact bone.

cortical bone Harder, more compact bone that forms the outer bony surface of the diaphysis.

cranial nerves The group of 12 pairs of nerves originating from the undersurface of the brain and exiting from the cranial cavity through skull openings; they supply specific motor and sensory function to the head and face.

crest Prominent, narrow, ridgelike projection of bone, such as the iliac crest of the pelvis.

curvilinear motion Motion along a curved line.

dendrite One or more branching projections from the neuron cell body that transmit impulses to the neuron and cell body.

depression Inferior movement of the shoulder girdle, as in returning to the normal position from a shoulder shrug.

dermatome A defined area of skin supplied by a specific spinal nerve.

diagonal abduction Movement by a limb through a diagonal plane away from the midline of the body.

diagonal adduction Movement by a limb through a diagonal plane toward and across the midline of the body.

diagonal plane A combination of more than one plane. Less than parallel or perpendicular to the sagittal, frontal, or transverse plane. Also known as oblique plane.

diaphysis The long cylindrical portion or shaft of long bones.

diarthrodial joints Freely movable synovial joints containing a joint capsule and hyaline cartilage and lubricated by synovial fluid.

displacement A change in position or location of an object from its original point of reference.

distal Farthest from the midline or point or reference; the fingertips are the most distal part of the upper extremity.

distance The path of movement; refers to the actual sum length of units of measurement traveled.

dorsal flexion (dorsiflexion) Flexion movement of the ankle resulting in the top of foot moving toward the anterior tibia.

dynamic equilibrium Occurs when all of the applied and inertial forces acting on the moving body are in balance, resulting in movement with unchanging speed or direction.

dynamics The study of mechanics involving systems in motion with acceleration.

eccentric contraction A contraction in which the muscle lengthens in an attempt to control the motion occurring at the joints which it crosses, characterized by the force of gravity or applied resistance being greater than the contractile force.

eccentric force Force that is applied in a direction not in line with the center of rotation of an object with a fixed axis. In objects without a fixed axis, it is an applied force that is not in line with the object's center of gravity.

efferent nerves Nerves that carry impulses to the outlying regions of the body from the central nervous system.

elasticity The ability of muscle to return to its original length following stretching.

electromyography (EMG) A method utilizing either surface electrodes or fine wire/needle electrodes to detect the action potentials of muscles and provide an electronic readout of the contraction intensity and duration.

elevation Superior movement of the shoulder girdle, as in shrugging the shoulders.

enarthrodial joint Type of joint which permits movement in all planes, as in the shoulder (glenohumeral) and hip joints.

endosteum Dense, fibrous membrane covering the inside of the cortex of long bones.

epicondyle Projection located above a condyle, such as the medial or lateral epicondyle of the humerus.

epiphyseal plate Thin cartilage plate separating the diaphysis and epiphysis during bony growth; commonly referred to as growth plate.

epiphysis The end of a long bone, usually enlarged and shaped to join the epiphysis of an adjacent bone, formed from cancellous or trabecular bone.

equilibrium State of zero acceleration in which there is no change in the speed or direction of the body.

eversion Turning of the sole of the foot outward or laterally, as in standing with the weight on the inner edge of the foot.

extensibility The ability of muscle to be stretched back to its original length following contraction.

extension Straightening movement resulting in an increase of the angle in a joint by moving bones apart, as when the hand moves away from shoulder during extension of the elbow joint.

external rotation Rotary movement around the longitudinal axis of a bone away from the midline of the body. Also known as rotation laterally, outward rotation, and lateral rotation.

extrinsic muscles Muscles that arise or originate outside of (proximal to) the body part on which they act.

facet Small flat or shallow bony articular surface such as the articular facet of a vertebra.

fascia Fibrous membrane covering, supporting, connecting, and separating muscles.

fibrous joints Joints joined together by connective tissue fibers and generally immovable, such as gomphosis sutures, and syndesmosis.

first-class lever A lever in which the axis (fulcrum) is between the force and the resistance, as in the extension of the elbow joint.

flat muscles A type of parallel muscle that is usually thin and broad, with fibers originating from broad, fibrous, sheet-like aponeuroses such as the rectus abdominus and external oblique.

flexion Movement of the bones toward each other at a joint by decreasing the angle, as in moving the hand toward the shoulder during elbow flexion.

follow-through phase Phase that begins immediately after the climax of the movement phase, in order to bring about negative acceleration of the involved limb or body segment; often referred to as the deceleration phase. The velocity of the body segment progressively decreases, usually over a wide range of motion.

foramen Rounded hole or opening in bone, such as the foramen magnum in the base of the skull.

force The product of mass times acceleration.

force arm The perpendicular distance between the location of force application and the axis. The shortest distance from the axis of rotation to the line of action of the force. Also known as the *moment arm* or *torque arm.*

fossa Hollow, depression, or flattened surface of bone, such as the supraspinatus fossa or iliac fossa.

fovea Very small pit or depression in bone, such as the fovea capitis of the femur.

friction Force that results from the resistance between the surfaces of two objects moving upon one another.

frontal plane Plane that bisects the body laterally from side to side, dividing it into front and back halves. Also known as the lateral or coronal plane.

fundamental position Reference position essentially the same as the anatomical position, except that the arms are at the sides and facing the body.

fusiform muscles A type of parallel muscle with fibers shaped together like a spindle with a central belly that tapers to tendons on each end, such as the brachialis and the biceps brachii.

gaster The central, fleshy, contractile portion of the muscle that generally increases in diameter as the muscle contracts.

ginglymus joint Type of joint which permits a wide range of movement in only one plane, as in the elbow, ankle, and knee joints.

glide (slide) (translation) A type of accessory motion characterized by a specific point on one articulating surface coming in contact with a series of points on another surface.

Golgi tendon organ (GTO) A proprioceptor, sensitive to both muscle tension and active contraction, found in the tendon close to the muscle tendon junction.

gomphosis A type of immovable articulation, as of a tooth inserted into its bony socket.

goniometer Instrument used to measure joint angles or compare the changes in joint angles.

ground reaction force The force of the surface reacting to the force placed on it, as in the reaction force between the body and the ground when running across a surface.

hamstrings A common name given to the group of posterior thigh muscles: biceps femoris, semitendinosus, and semimembranosus.

head Prominent, rounded projection of the proximal end of a bone, usually articulating, such as the humeral or femoral head.

horizontal abduction Movement of the humerus in the horizontal plane away from the midline of the body.

horizontal adduction Movement of the humerus in the horizontal plane toward the midline of the body.

hyaline cartilage Articular cartilage covers the end of bones at diarthrodial joints to provide a cushioning effect and reduce friction during movement.

inertia Resistance to action or change; resistance to acceleration or deceleration. Inertia is the tendency for the current state of motion to be maintained, regardless of whether the body segment is moving at a particular velocity or is motionless.

innervation The supplying of a muscle, organ, or body part with nerves.

insertion The distal attachment or point of attachment of a muscle farthest from the midline or center of the body, generally considered the most movable part.

internal rotation Rotary movement around the longitudinal axis of a bone toward the midline of the body. Also known as rotation medially, inward rotation, and medial rotation.

interneurons Central or connecting neurons that conduct impulses from sensory neurons to motor neurons.

intrinsic muscles Muscles that are entirely contained within a specified body part; usually refers to the small, deep muscles found in the foot and hand.

inversion Turning of the sole of the foot inward or medially, as in standing with the weight on the outer edge of the foot.

irritability The property of muscle being sensitive or responsive to chemical, electrical, or mechanical stimuli.

isokinetic Type of dynamic exercise usually using concentric and/or eccentric muscle contractions in which the speed (or velocity) of movement is constant and muscular contraction (usually maximal contraction) occurs throughout the movement.

isometric contraction A type of contraction with little or no shortening of the muscle resulting in no appreciable change in the joint angle.

isotonic Contraction occurring in which there is either shortening or lengthening in the muscle under tension; also known as a dynamic contraction, and classified as being either concentric or eccentric.

joint capsule Sleevelike covering of ligamentous tissue surrounding diarthrodial joints.

joint cavity The area inside the joint capsule of diarthrodial or synovial joints.

kinematics The description of motion, including consideration of time, displacement, velocity, acceleration, and space factors of a system's motion.

kinesiology The science of movement, which includes anatomical (structural) and biomechanical (mechanical) aspects of movement.

kinesthesia The awareness of the position and movement of the body in space; sense that provides awareness of bodily position, weight, or movement of the muscles, tendons, and joints.

kinetics   The study of forces associated with the motion of a body.

kinetic friction   The amount of friction occurring between two objects that are sliding upon one another.

Krause's end bulbs   A proprioceptor sensitive to touch and thermal changes found in the skin, subcutaneous tissue, lip and eyelid mucosa, and external genitals.

kyphosis   Increased anterior concavity of the normal thoracic curve. The lumbar spine may have a reduction of its normal lordotic curve, resulting in a flat-back appearance referred to as lumbar kyphosis.

lateral axis   Axis that has the same directional orientation as the frontal plane of motion and runs from side to side at a right angle to the sagittal plane of motion. Also known as the frontal or coronal axis.

lateral epicondylitis   A common problem quite frequently associated with gripping and lifting activities that usually involves the extensor digitorum muscle near its origin on the lateral epicondyle; commonly known as tennis elbow.

lateral flexion   Movement of the head and/or trunk laterally away from the midline; abduction of spine.

lever   A rigid bar (bone) that moves about an axis.

ligament   A type of tough connective tissue that attaches bone to bone to provide static stability to joints.

line   Ridge of bone less prominent than a crest, such as the linea aspera of the femur.

linear displacement   The distance that a system moves in a straight line.

linear motion   Motion along a line; also referred to as translatory motion.

lordosis   Increased posterior concavity of the lumbar and cervical curves.

lumbar plexus   Group of spinal nerves composed of L1 through L4 and some fibers from T12, generally responsible for motor and sensory function of the lower abdomen and the anterior and medial portions of the lower extremity.

mass   The amount of matter in a body.

meatus   Tubelike passage within a bone, such as the external auditory meatus of the temporal bone.

mechanics   The study of physical actions of forces; can be subdivided into statics and dynamics.

medial epicondylitis   An elbow problem associated with the medial wrist flexor and pronator group near their origin on the medial epicondyle; frequently referred to as golfer's elbow.

medullary cavity   Marrow cavity between the walls of the diaphysis, containing yellow or fatty marrow.

Meissner's corpuscles   A proprioceptor sensitive to fine touch and vibration found in the skin.

momentum   The quality of motion, which is equal to mass times velocity.

motor neurons   Neurons that transmit impulses away from the brain and spinal cord to muscle and glandular tissue.

movement phase   The action part of a skill, sometimes known as the acceleration, action, motion, or contact phase. Phase

in which the summation of force is generated directly to the ball, sport object, or opponent, and is usually characterized by near-maximal concentric activity in the involved muscles.

multipennate muscle   A type of pennate muscle that has several tendons with fibers running diagonally between them, such as the deltoid.

muscle spindle   A proprioceptor sensitive to stretch and the rate of stretch that is concentrated primarily in the muscle belly between the fibers.

myotome   A muscle or group of muscles supplied by a specific spinal nerve.

neuron   Nerve cell that is the basic functional unit of the nervous system responsible for generating and transmitting impulses.

neutralizers   Muscles that counteract or neutralize the action of other muscles to prevent undesirable movements; referred to as neutralizing, they contract to resist specific actions of other muscles.

open kinetic chain   When the distal end of an extremity is not fixed to any surface, allowing any one joint in the extremity to move or function separately without necessitating movement of other joints in the extremity.

opposition   Diagonal movement of the thumb across the palmar surface of the hand to make contact with the fingers.

origin   The proximal attachment or point of attachment of a muscle closest to the midline or center of the body, generally considered the least movable part.

osteoblasts   Specialized cells that form new bone.

osteoclasts   Specialized cells that resorb new bone.

osteokinematic motion   Motion of the bones relative to the three cardinal planes, resulting from physiological movements.

Pacinian corpuscles   A proprioceptor sensitive to pressure and vibration found in the subcutaneous, submucosa, subserous tissues around joints, external genitals, and mammary glands.

palmar flexion   Flexion movement of the wrist in the sagittal plane with the volar or anterior side of the hand moving toward the anterior side of the forearm.

palpation   Using the sense of touch to feel or examine a muscle or other tissue.

parallel muscles   Muscles that have their fibers arranged parallel to the length of the muscle, such as flat, fusiform, strap, radiate, or sphincter muscles.

passive insufficiency   State reached when an opposing muscle becomes stretched to the point where it can no longer lengthen and allow movement.

pennate muscles   Muscles that have their fibers arranged obliquely to their tendons in a manner similar to a feather, such as unipennate, bipennate, and multipennate muscles.

periosteum   The dense, fibrous membrane covering the outer surface of the diaphysis.

peripheral nervous system (PNS)   Portion of the nervous system containing the sensory and motor divisions of all the nerves throughout the body except those found in the central nervous system.

physiological movement Normal movements of joints such as flexion, extension, abduction, adduction, and rotation, accomplished by bones moving through planes of motion about an axis of rotation at the joint.

plane of motion An imaginary two-dimensional surface through which a limb or body segment is moved.

plantar flexion Extension movement of the ankle, resulting in the foot and/or toes moving away from the body.

preparatory phase Skill analysis phase, often referred to as the cocking or wind-up phase, used to lengthen the appropriate muscles so that they will be in position to generate more force and momentum as they concentrically contract in the next phase.

process Prominent projection of a bone, such as the acromion process of the scapula or the olecranon process of the humerus.

pronation Internally rotating the radius so that it lies diagonally across the ulna, resulting in the palm-down position of the forearm; term also refers to the combined movements of eversion, abduction, and external rotation of the foot and ankle.

proprioception Feedback relative to the tension, length, and contraction state of muscle, the position of the body and limbs, and movements of the joints provided by internal receptors located in the skin, joints, muscles, and tendons.

protraction Forward movement of the shoulder girdle away from the spine; abduction of the scapula.

proximal Nearest to the midline or point of reference; the forearm is proximal to the hand.

quadriceps A common name given to the four muscles of the anterior aspect of the thigh: rectus femoris, vastus medialis, vastus intermedius, and vastus lateralis.

radial deviation (radial flexion) Abduction movement at the wrist of the thumb side of the hand toward the forearm.

radiate muscles A type of parallel muscle with a combined arrangement of flat and fusiform muscle in that they originate on broad aponeuroses and converge onto a tendon such as the pectoralis major or trapezius. Also described sometimes as being triangular, fan-shaped, or convergent.

reciprocal inhibition Activation of the motor units of the agonists, causing a reciprocal neural inhibition of the motor units of the antagonists, which allows them to subsequently lengthen under less tension. Also referred to as reciprocal innervation.

recovery phase Skill analysis phase used after follow-through to regain balance and positioning to be ready for the next sport demand.

rectilinear motion Motion along a straight line.

reduction Return of the spinal column to the anatomic position from lateral flexion; spine adduction.

reposition Diagonal movement of the thumb as it returns to the anatomical position from opposition with the hand and/or fingers.

resistance arm The distance between the axis and the point of resistance application.

retraction Backward movement of the shoulder girdle toward the spine; adduction of the scapula.

roll (rock) A type of accessory motion characterized by a series of points on one articular surface contacting with a series of points on another articular surface.

rolling friction The resistance to an object rolling across a surface, such as a ball rolling across a court or a tire rolling across the ground.

rotation Movement around the axis of a bone, such as the turning inward, outward, downward, or upward of a bone.

rotator cuff Group of muscles intrinsic to the glenohumeral joint, consisting of the subscapularis, supraspinatus, infraspinatus, and teres minor, that is critical in maintaining dynamic stability of the joint.

Ruffini's corpuscles A proprioceptor sensitive to touch and pressure found in the skin, subcutaneous tissue of fingers, and collagenous fibers of the joint capsule.

sacral plexus Group of spinal nerves composed of L4, L5, and S1 through S4, generally responsible for motor and sensory function of the lower back, pelvis, perineum, posterior surface of the thigh and leg, and dorsal and plantar surfaces of the foot.

sagittal plane Plane that bisects the body from front to back, dividing it into right and left symmetrical halves. Also known as the anteroposterior, or AP plane.

scoliosis Lateral curvatures or sideward deviations of the spine.

second-class lever A lever in which the resistance is between the axis (fulcrum) and the force (effort), as in plantar flexing the foot to raise up on the toes.

sellar joints Type of reciprocal reception that is found only in the thumb at the carpometacarpal joint and permits ball-and-socket movement, with the exception of rotation.

sensory neurons Neurons that transmit impulses to the spinal cord and brain from all parts of the body.

sesamoid bones Small bones embedded within the tendon of a musculotendinous unit that provide protection as well as improve the mechanical advantage of musculotendinous units as in the patella.

sinus Cavity or hollow space within a bone, such as the frontal or maxillary sinus.

somatic nerves (voluntary) Afferent nerves, which are under conscious control and carry impulses to skeletal muscles.

speed How fast an object is moving, or the distance an object travels in a specific amount of time.

sphincter muscle A type of parallel muscle that is a technically endless strap muscle with fibers arranged to surround and close openings upon contraction, such as the orbicularis oris. Also referred to as circular muscles.

spin A type of accessory motion characterized by a single point on one articular surface rotating clockwise or counterclockwise about a single point on another articular surface.

spinal cord The common pathway between the central nervous system and the peripheral nervous system.

spinal nerves The group of 31 pairs of nerves that originate from the spinal cord and exit the spinal column on each side through openings between the vertebrae. They run directly to specific anatomical locations, form different plexuses, and eventually become peripheral nerve braches.

spine (spinous process) Sharp, slender projection of a bone, such as the spinous process of a vertebra or spine of the scapula.

stability The resistance to a change in the body's acceleration; the resistance to a disturbance of the body's equilibrium.

stabilizers Muscles that surround the joint or body part and contract to fixate or stabilize the area to enable another limb or body segment to exert force and move; known as fixators, they are essential in establishing a relatively firm base for the more distal joints to work from when carrying out movements.

stance phase Skill analysis phase that allows the athlete to assume a comfortable and balanced body position from which to initiate the sport skill; emphasis is on setting the various joint angles in the correct positions with respect to one another and to the sport surface.

static equilibrium The body at complete rest or motionless.

static friction The amount of friction between two objects that have not yet begun to move.

statics The study of mechanics involving the study of systems that are in a constant state of motion, whether at rest with no motion or moving at a constant velocity without acceleration. Involves all forces acting on the body being in balance, resulting in the body being in equilibrium.

strap muscles A type of parallel muscle with fibers uniform in diameter and arranged with essentially all fibers in a long parallel manner, such as the sartorius.

sulcus (groove) Furrow or groovelike depression on a bone, such as the intertubercular (bicipital) groove of the humerus.

supination Externally rotating the radius to where it lies parallel to the ulna, resulting in the palm-up position of the forearm; term is also used in referring to the combined movements of inversion, adduction, and internal rotation of the foot and ankle.

suture Line of union between bones, such as the sagittal suture between the parietal bones of the skull.

symphysis joint Type of joint separated by a fibrocartilage pad that allows very slight movement between the bones such as the symphysis pubis and the intervertebral discs.

synarthrodial joints Joints which functionally allow no movement such as the suture joints of the cranium and the gomphosis joints of the teeth fitting into the mandible and maxilla.

synchondrosis joint Type of joint separated by a fibro-cartilage that allows very slight movement between the bones such as the costochondral joints of the ribs with the sternum.

syndesmosis joint Type of joint held together by strong ligamentous structures that allow minimal movement between the bones, such as the coracoclavicular joint and the inferior tibiofibular joint.

synergist Muscles that assist in the action of the agonists but are not primarily responsible for the action; known as guiding muscles, they assist in refined movement and rule out undesired motions.

synovial joints Freely movable diarthrodial joints containing a joint capsule and hyaline cartilage and lubricated by synovial fluid.

tendon Fibrous connective tissue, often cordlike in appearance, that connects muscles to bones and other structures.

third-class lever A lever in which the force (effort) is between the axis (fulcrum) and the resistance, as in flexion of the elbow joint.

torque Moment of force. The turning effect of an eccentric force.

transverse plane Plane that divides the body horizontally into superior and inferior halves; also known as horizontal plane.

trochanter A very large bony projection, such as the greater or lesser trochanter of the femur.

trochoidal joint Type of joint with a rotational movement around a long axis, as in rotation of the radius at the radioulnar joint.

tubercle A small, rounded bony projection, such as the greater and lesser tubercles of the humerus.

tuberosity A large, rounded or roughened bony projection, such as the radial tuberosity or tibial tuberosity.

ulnar deviation (ulnar flexion) Adduction movement at the wrist of the little finger side of the hand toward the forearm.

unipennate muscles A type of pennate muscle with fibers that run obliquely from a tendon on one side only, such as the biceps femoris, extensor digitorum longus, and tibialis posterior.

velocity Includes the direction and describes the rate of displacement.

vertical axis Axis that runs straight down through the top of the head and spinal column and is at a right angle to the transverse plane of motion. Also known as the longitudinal or long axis.

visceral nerves (involuntary) Nerves that carry impulses to the heart, smooth muscles, and glands; referred to as the autonomic nervous system.

Illustration credits

CHAPTER 1

1.1, Van de Graff KM: *Human anatomy,* ed 4, Dubuque, IA. 1995, WCB McGraw-Hill; **1.2, 1.10,** Prentice WE: *Arnheim's principles of athletic training,* ed 11; Dubuque, IA, 2003, McGraw-Hill; **1.3, 1.6, 1.7, 1.9,** Booher JM, Thibodeau GA; *Athletic injury assessment,* ed 4, Dubuque, IA, 2000, McGraw-Hill; **1.4,** *Athletic injury assessment,* ed 4, Dubuque, IA, 2000, McGraw-Hill, Shier D, Butler J, Lewis R: *Hole's human anatomy and physiology,* ed 9, Dubuque, IA, 2002, McGraw-Hill; **1.5,** Shier D, Butler J, Lewis R: *Hole's human anatomy and physiology,* ed 9, Dubuque, IA 2002, McGraw-Hill; **1.8,** Seeley R, et al: *Anatomy and physiology,* ed 6, Dubuque, IA, 2003, McGraw-Hill; **1.11,** Lisa Floyd; **1.12, 1.13,** Prentice WE: *Rehabilitation techniques in sports medicine,* ed 3; Dubuque, IA, 1999, McGraw-Hill.

CHAPTER 2

2.1, 2.2, Thibodeau GA: *Anatomy and physiology,* St. Louis, 1987, Mosby; **2.3,** Van de Graff KM: *Human anatomy,* ed 6, Dubuque, IA. 2002, McGraw-Hill; **2.4, 2.5,** Shier D, Butler J, Lewis R: *Hole's human anatomy and physiology,* ed 9, Dubuque, IA, 2002, McGraw-Hill; **2.6,** Booher JM, Thibodeau GA; *Athletic injury assessment,* ed 4, Dubuque, IA, 2000, McGraw-Hill; **2.7, 2.8,** R.T. Floyd; **2.9,** Hall SJ: *Basic biomechanics,* ed 3, Dubuque, IA, 1999, WCB/McGraw-Hill.

CHAPTER 3

3.1, 3.6, Hall SJ: *Basic biomechanics,* ed 3, Dubuque, IA, 1999, WCB/McGraw-Hill; **3.2, 3.3, 3.4,** Booher JM, Thibodeau GA; *Athletic injury assessment,* ed 2, St. Louis, 1989, Mosby, Hall SJ: *Basic biomechanics,* ed 3, Dubuque, IA, 1999, WCB/McGraw-Hill; **3.5, 3.7, 3.11,** R.T. Floyd; **3.8, 3.9, 3.10,** Hamilton N, Luttgens K: *Kinesiology: scientific basis of human motion,* ed 10, New York, 2002.

CHAPTER 4

4.1, 4.2, 4.11, 4.13, Linda Kimbrough; **4.3, 4.4,** Lisa Floyd; **4.5,** Hall SJ: *Basic biomechanics,* ed 3, Dubuque, IA, 1999, WCB/McGraw-Hill; **4.6, 4.7,** Seeley R, et al: *Anatomy and physiology,* ed 6, Dubuque, IA, 2003, McGraw-Hill; **4.8 through 4.10, 4.12** Ernest W. Beck.

CHAPTER 5

5.1 through 5.3, 5.15, 5.16, 5.19 through 5.22, Linda Kimbrough; **5.4,** Booher JM, Thibodeau GA; *Athletic injury assessment,* ed 4, Dubuque, IA, 2000, McGraw-Hill; **5.5,** Lisa Floyd; **5.6, 5.8,** John Hood; **5.7,** Booher JM, Thibodeau GA; *Athletic injury assessment,* ed 2, St. Louis, 1989, Mosby; **5.9, 5.12 through 5.14,** Ernest W. Beck; **5.10, 5.11,** Van de Graff KM: *Human anatomy,* ed 6, Dubuque, IA. 2002, McGraw-Hill; **5.17,** Seeley R, et al: *Anatomy and physiology,* ed 6, Dubuque, IA, 2003, McGraw-Hill; **5.18,** Ernest W. Beck with inserts by Linda Kimbrough.

CHAPTER 6

6.1, 6.2 A, 6.13 through 6.20, Linda Kimbrough; **6.2 B, 6.11, 6.12,** Van de Graff KM: *Human anatomy,* ed 6, Dubuque, IA. 2002, McGraw-Hill; **6.2 C,** Jason McAlexander; **6.3, 6.4,** Booher JM, Thibodeau GA; *Athletic injury assessment,* ed 4, Dubuque, IA, 2000, McGraw-Hill; **6.5, 6.6, 6.8,** Lisa Floyd; **6.7, 6.9,** Thibodeau GA: *Anatomy and physiology,* St. Louis, 1987, Mosby; **6.10 A–B,** Seeley R, et al: *Anatomy and physiology,* ed 6, Dubuque, IA, 2003, McGraw-Hill.

CHAPTER 7

7.1, Anthony CP, Kolthoff NJ: *Textbook of anatomy and physiology,* ed 9, St. Louis, 1975, Mosby; **7.2, 7.11 through 7.25,** Linda Kimbrough; **7.3, 7.10, 7.26,** Van de Graff KM: *Human anatomy,* ed 6, Dubuque, IA. 2002, McGraw-Hill; **7.4 through 7.6, 7.8,** Booher JM, Thibodeau GA; *Athletic injury assessment,* ed 4, Dubuque, IA, 2000, McGraw-Hill; **7.7,** Lisa Floyd; **7.9 A–D,** Seeley R, et al: *Anatomy and physiology,* ed 6, Dubuque, IA, 2003, McGraw-Hill.

CHAPTER 8

8.1, 8.10, R.T. Floyd; **8.2 through 8.6, 8.9,** Lisa Floyd; **8.7 A–C, 8.8 A–B,** Ron Carlberg.

CHAPTER 9

9.1, 9.3 through 9.5, 9.11, 9.21 through 9.36, Linda Kimbrough; **9.2, 9.9,** Anthony CP, Kolthoff NJ: *Textbook of anatomy and physiology,* ed 9, St. Louis, 1975, Mosby; **9.6,** Booher JM, Thibodeau GA; *Athletic injury assessment,* ed 4, Dubuque, IA, 2000, McGraw-Hill; **9.7, A–H, 9.8 A–D,** Lisa Floyd; **9.10,** Ernest W. Beck; **9.12, 9.13, 9.15 through 9.20,** Van de Graff KM: *Human anatomy,* ed 6, Dubuque, IA, 2002, McGraw-Hill; **9.14,** Shier D, Butler J, Lewis R: *Hole's human anatomy and physiology,* ed 9, Dubuque, IA, 2002, McGraw-Hill.

CHAPTER 10

10.1, Anthony CP, Kolthoff NJ: *Textbook of anatomy and physiology,* ed 9, St. Louis, 1975, Mosby; **10.2,** Van de Graff KM: *Human anatomy,* ed 6, Dubuque, IA, 2002, McGraw-Hill; **10.3,** Booher JM, Thibodeau GA; *Athletic injury assessment,* ed 4, Dubuque, IA, 2000, McGraw-Hill; **10.4 A–D,** Lisa Floyd; **10.5 through 10.10,** Linda Kimbrough.

CHAPTER 11

11.1, Prentice WE: *Arnheim's principles of athletic training,* ed 11; Dubuque, IA, 2003, McGraw-Hill; **11.2, 11.3,** Anthony CP, Kolthoff NJ: *Textbook of anatomy and physiology,* ed 9, St. Louis, 1975, Mosby; **11.4, 11.6, 11.8 A–D, 11.10, 11.22, 11.23,** Van de Graff KM: *Human anatomy,* ed 6, Dubuque, IA, 2002, McGraw-Hill; **11.5,** Booher JM, Thibodeau GA; *Athletic injury assessment,* ed 4, Dubuque, IA, 2000, McGraw-Hill; **11.7 A–H,** Lisa Floyd; **11.9,** Seeley R, et al: *Anatomy and physiology,* ed 3, St. Louis, 1995, Mosby; **11.11 through 11.14, 11.16 through 11.21,** Ernest W. Beck; **11.15,** Linda Kimbrough.

CHAPTER 12

12.1, 12.13, Seeley R, et al: *Anatomy and physiology,* ed 6, Dubuque, IA, 2003, McGraw-Hill; **12.2 E–F,** Anthony CP, Kolthoff NJ: *Textbook of anatomy and physiology,* ed 9, St. Louis, 1975, Mosby; **12.2 A–D, 12.11, 12.12, 12.15, 12.17 through 12.19, 12.21 through 12.24,** Linda Kimbrough; **12.3, 12.16,** Shier D, Butler J, Lewis R: *Hole's human anatomy and physiology,* ed 9, Dubuque, IA, 2002, McGraw-Hill; **12.4, 12.9,** Lindsay D: *Functional anatomy,* ed 1, St. Louis, 1996, Mosby, **12.5,** Thibodeau GA, Patton KT: *Anatomy and physiology,* ed 9, St. Louis, 1993, Mosby; **12.6, 12.7,** Booher JM, Thibodeau GA; *Athletic injury assessment,* ed 4, Dubuque, IA, 2000, McGraw-Hill; **12.8 A–H,** Lisa Floyd; **12.10, 12.14,** Van de Graff KM: *Human anatomy,* ed 6, Dubuque, IA, 2002, McGraw-Hill; **12.20,** Ernest W. Beck.

CHAPTER 13

13.1 through 13.6, Lisa Floyd; **13.7,** Efi Medical Systems, San Diego, CA; **13.8, 13.9 A–B,** Ron Carlberg.

Index

body
　machines found in, 44
　of muscle, 27
　of vertebrae, 266, *266*, *267*
bone(s)
　age-related changes in, 8
　calcaneus, *2*, 233, *233*, *235*
　capitate, *7*, 125, *125*
　carpal, *2*, *7*, 125, *126*
　cavities of, 9, *10*
　cervical vertebrae, *2*, 265, 266, *266*, *267*
　clavicle, *2*, 57, *58*, *59*, 77, *82*, 108, 277
　coccyx, *2*, 175, *176*, *177*, 265, *266*
　cuboid, 232, *233*, *235*
　cuneiform, *233*, *233*
　of elbow joint, 103, *104*
　features of, 8, *8*
　femur, *2*, *7*, *8*, 175, *176*, *177*, *183*, 215, *216*, *217*
　fibula, *2*, *176*, *177*, 215, *216*, 232, *232*, *235*, *239*
　flat, *7*, *7*
　of foot, 232–233, *233*
　frontal, *2*
　greater trochanter, *2*, *176*, 177, *177*
　growth of, 8
　hamate, 125, *125*, 126
　of hand, *125*, 125–126
　of hip joint, 175–177, *176*, *177*
　humerus, *2*, 77, 103, *104*
　ilium, *2*, *34*, 175, *176*
　irregular, *7*, *7*
　ischium, *2*, 175, *177*
　of knee, 215–217, *216*
　lesser trochanter, *2*, *176*, 177, *177*
　long, *7*, *7*, 8
　lumbar vertebrae, *2*, *34*, 265, *266*, *267*
　mandible, *2*
　manubrium, *2*, 57, *58*, 266, *268*
　markings of, 9, *10*
　maxilla, *2*
　metacarpal, *2*, *125*, 126
　metatarsal, *2*, 232, *233*, *233*, *235*
　navicular, 232, *233*, *235*
　occipital, *2*
　os coxa, *2*
　parietal, *2*
　patella, *2*, *7*, *176*, *177*, *182*, 215, *217*, *239*
　of pelvic girdle, 175–177, *176*, *177*
　phalanges, *2*, *125*, 126, *127*, 232, *233*
　processes of, 9, *10*
　properties of, 9
　pubic, *185*
　pubis, *2*, 175, *176*, *177*
　of radioulnar joint, 103
　radius, *2*, *7*, 103, *104*, *109*, *125*, *126*, *135*
　ribs, *2*, 266, *268*
　sacrum, *2*, *34*, 175, *176*, *177*, 265, *266*
　scapula, *2*, *7*, 57, *58*, *59*, 77, *83*, 103
　sesamoid, *7*, *7*, *126*, 232, *257*
　shape of, 9
　short, *7*, *7*
　of shoulder girdle, 57
　of shoulder joint, 76–77, *77*
　sternum, *2*, *7*, *82*, 268
　talus, *2*, *7*, 232, *233*
　tarsal, *2*, 232
　temporal, *2*
　thoracic vertebrae, *2*, *34*, 265, *266*, *267*, 268
　of thorax, 266, *268*
　tibia, *2*, *176*, *177*, 215, *216*, *217*, 232, *232*, *235*, *239*, *240*
　types of, *7*, *7*
　ulna, *2*, *7*, 103, *104*, *109*, *125*, *126*, *135*
　of vertebral column, 265–266, *266*, *267*
　of wrist, *125*, 125–126
　zygomatic, *2*
bone marrow, 8
border(s)
　lateral, 57, *58*
　medial, 57, *58*
　superior, *58*
brachial plexus, *34*, *35–36*, 65
brachialis muscle, *23*, 108, *108*, *109*, 110, 112, 114, *114*

brachioradialis muscle, *23*, *24*, 108, *108*, *109*, *110*, 112, 115, *115*, 135
brain stem, 33
bursae, *217*, 218

C

calcaneal tendon (Achilles), *24*, *182*, 232
calcaneal tuberosity, *257*
calcaneocuboid ligament, dorsal, *235*
calcaneofibular ligament, *235*
calcaneus, *2*, 233, *233*, *235*
calcanionavicular ligament, plantar, *235*
calcium carbonate, 9
calcium phosphate, 9
cancellous bone, 8, 9
capitate bone, *7*, 125, *125*
capitulum, *104*
cardinal planes of motion, 5
carpal bones, *2*, *7*, 125, *126*
carpal tunnel, 125–126, 131
carpometacarpal (CMC) joint, *13*, 125, *126*, 127, 317
cartilage(s)
　articular, 8, *8*, 12, *12*, *217*, 269
　costal, *2*, 268
　hyaline, 8, 12
　lateral semilunar, 218
　medial semilunar, 218
　thyroid, 277
cartilaginous joints, 9
cauda equina, *34*
caudal, 3
cavities, of bones, 9, *10*
center of gravity, 53
central nervous system (CNS), 33
cephalic, 3
cerebellum, 33
cerebral cortex, 33
cervical curve, 266, *266*
cervical enlargement, *34*
cervical nerves, 34, *34*
cervical plexus, 34, *34*, *35*, *64*
cervical spine, movements, 270, *271*, *272*, 318
cervical vertebrae, *2*, 265, 266, *266*, *267*
chest press, 165, *165*
chin-up, 89, 113, 157, 166, *166*, *167*, *308*
circular muscles. *See* sphincter muscles
circumduction, 16
clavicle, *2*, 57, *58*, *59*, 77, *82*, 108, 277
clavicular notch, 268
closed kinetic chain, 160
CMC joint. *See* carpometacarpal joint
CNS. *See* central nervous system
coccygeal nerves, 34, *34*
coccygeus muscle, *185*
coccyx, *2*, 175, *176*, *177*, 265, *266*
cocking phase. *See* preparatory phase
coefficient of friction, 53
collagen, 9
collateral ligament, *127*
　fibular, *216*, 217
　tibial, 216, *217*, 218
common fibular nerve, *189*, *239*, *240*
common peroneal nerve, *34*
compact bone, *8*
compression, 54
concentric contraction, 28, *28*, *29*, 297–298
concurrent movement, 40–41
conditioning, 298–299
condyle(s), *10*
　femoral, 215
　　lateral, *2*, *176*, *177*, 215, *216*, 218
　　medial, *2*, *176*, *177*, 215, *216*, 218
　tibial, 215
　　lateral, *176*, 177, *177*, *216*
　　medial, *176*, *177*
condyloid ridge, medial, 103, 126
condyloidal joint, 13, *13*, *14*, 127, 217, 234
conjoined tendon, *82*
conoid ligament, *58*
contractility, of muscles, 26
contraction(s), *28*, *28–30*, *29*, 297–298
　abdominal, 306, *306*
　concentric, 28, *28*, *29*, 297–298

eccentric, 28, *28*, *29*, 158, 297–298
　isometric, 28, *28*, *29*
　isotonic, 28, *28*, *29*
　of quadriceps muscles, 297–298
contralateral, 3
contralateral muscles, 30
conus medullaris, *34*
coracobrachialis muscle, *23*, 81, *82*, *84*, 86, 91, *91*, *109*
coracoclavicular joint, 59
coracoclavicular ligaments, *58*, 59
coracohumeral ligament, 78
coracoid process, *2*, 57, *58*, 77, *77*, *78*
coranoid process, 103, 126
coronal axis, 5, 6, *6*
coronal plane, 5, 6, *6*
coronoid fossa, *104*
coronoid process, *104*
cortex, of bone, 8
cortical bone, 9
costal cartilage, *2*, 268
costoclavicular ligament, *58*, 59
countercurrent movement, 41
cranial nerves, 276
cremaster muscle, *82*
crest, of bone, *10*
cricothyroid muscle, *277*
cruciate ligament
　anterior, *216*, 218
　posterior, *216*, 218
crunches, 289
cuboid bone, 232, *233*, *235*
cuneiform bones, 233, *233*
cuneonavicular ligament, dorsal, *235*
curling exercises, 113, 115, 116, 137, 138, 139
curvilinear motion, 51
cutaneous femoral nerve, posterior, *34*

D

dead lift, 287, 304, *304*, *305*
deep, 4
deep digital flexor tendon, *152*
deep femoral artery, *184*
deep femoral vein, *184*
deep fibular nerve, *258*
deep transverse metacarpal ligament, *127*
deltoid ligament, *235*
deltoid muscle, *23*, *24*, *59*, 81, *82*, *83*, *84*, 86, 87, *87*, *108*, *109*
　anterior, 88
deltoid tuberosity, 77, *77*
dendrites, 35
depression
　of bones, 9, *10*
　of shoulder girdle, 57, 59, *60*, 61, 62
　of shoulder joint, 16
dermatome, 35, *35–36*
deviation
　radial, 17
　ulnar, 17
diagonal abduction, 16, *81*, *85*, 180, *181*
diagonal adduction, 16, 79, *81*, *84*, 180, *181*
diagonal plane, 6
diaphragm, 276, *282*, *284*, *284*, *285*
diaphysis, 8, *8*
diarthrodial joints, 9, 12, *12*, *13*, *14*, 316–318
digastric muscle, *277*
digital arteries, dorsal, *258*
digital sheaths, fibrous, *257*
dip, 116, *308*
DIP joint. *See* distal interphalangeal joint
dips, 89
dislocating component, 39, *40*
displacement, 51
　angular, 51
　linear, 51
distal, *3*, 4
distal interphalangeal (DIP) joint, *125*, *126*, 127, *233*, *234*, 317, 318
distal phalanx, *125*, 126, *127*, *233*, 256
distance, 51
dorsal, 4
dorsal calcaneocuboid ligament, *235*
dorsal cuneonavicular ligament, *235*

opponens pollicis muscle, 134, 136, 152, *152, 153*
opposition, of thumb, 17, *128*, 130, *130, 153*
orbicularis oculi muscle, *23*
orbicularis oris muscle, *23*
origin, of muscle, 27
os coxa, *2*
osteoblasts, 8
osteoclasts, 8
osteokinematic motion, 17
osteology, 6
overhead press, 164, *164*
overload principle, 298
ovoid joint, 13, *14*

P

Pacinian corpuscles, 37, *38*
palmar, 4
palmar aponeurosis, *108, 135*
palmar flexion, 17, 130
palmar interossei muscles, 134, 136, 152, *153*
palmar ligaments, *127*
palmar plates, *152*
palmaris longus muscle, *23, 108*, 131, *131, 132*, 135, *135*, 136, 138, *138, 152*
palmaris longus tendon, *131, 152*
palpation, of muscle, 32
parallel muscles, 25, *26*
parasagittal plane, 5
parietal bone, *2*
passive insufficiency, 41
patella, *2, 7, 176, 177, 182*, 215, *217, 239, 240*
patella tendon reflex, 37
patellar ligament, *240*
patellar tendon, *182, 185, 217, 240*
patellofemoral joint, 217
PCL. *See* posterior cruciate ligament
pectineal line, *176, 177*
pectineus muscle, *23*, 176, *182*, 184, *185*, 186, *186*, 193, 209, *209*
pectoral nerves, 86
pectoralis major muscle, *23, 59*, 81, *82, 84*, 86, 88, *88, 108, 109, 288*
pectoralis minor muscle, 62, *63*, 64, 71, *71*
pelvic girdle, *2*, 175–211
  bones, 175–177, *176, 177*
  joints, *178*, 178–179, *179*
  movements, 179, *180*, 180–181, *181*
  muscles, 182–187, *182–190*, 195–210
  nerves, *191*, 191–194, *192, 193, 194*
pelvic rotation, 178, 179, *180*, 180–181, *181*
pelvis, 6, *177*
pennate muscles, 25–26, *26*
periosteum, 8, *8*
peripheral nervous system (PNS), 33–34
peroneal artery, *240*
peroneal nerve, 220, 244, *244*
  common, *34*
peroneus brevis muscle, *23, 24*, 232, *235*, 238, *239, 240*, 241, *243*, 244, 248, *248*, *257, 258*
peroneus brevis tendon, *235, 257, 258*
peroneus longus muscle, *23, 24, 182*, 233, 238, *239, 240*, 241, *243*, 244, *247, 247, 257*
peroneus longus tendon, *257*
peroneus tertius muscle, 238, *239*, 241, *243*, 244, 249, *249, 258*
peroneus tertius tendon, *258*
phalanges, *2*, 126, *233*
  distal, *125*, 126, *127, 233*
  of foot, 232, 233
  middle, *125*, 126, *127, 233*
  proximal, *125*, 126, *127, 233*
phrenic nerve, *34*
physical activities, laws of, 51–52
physiological movements, 17–19
PIP joint. *See* proximal interphalangeal joint
piriformis muscle, 184, *185, 190*, 194, 202, *202*
pisiform bone, 125, *125*, 126, *152*
pitching, 158–159, *159*
pivot joint, 13, *13, 14*, 106, 269
plane joint, 13, *14*
planes of motion, *5*, 5–6, *6*
plantar aponeurosis, *257*
plantar calcaneonavicular ligament, *235*

plantar flexion, 16
  of ankle, 234, *236*, 237, *237, 242, 243*
plantar interossei muscles, 256, *257, 260*
plantar ligament, long, *235*
plantar ligaments, *257*
plantar nerve, 244
plantaris muscle, *24, 182*, 238, *239, 240*, 241
plantaris tendon, *239*
plica, 218
PNS. *See* peripheral nervous system
popliteal artery, *189, 240*
popliteal vein, *189, 240*
popliteus muscle, 217, 219, 220, *221*, 227, *227*, 238, *240*
posterior, *3, 4*
posterior cruciate ligament (PCL), *216*, 218
posterior cutaneous femoral nerve, *34*
posterior inferior gluteal line, *177*
posterior inferior iliac spine, *177*
posterior interosseous nerve, 112, 136
posterior longitudinal ligament, *269*
posterior pelvic rotation, 180, *181*
posterior sternoclavicular ligament, 59
posterior superior iliac spine, *177*
posterior surface, of scapula, *58*
posterior talocalcaneal ligament, *235*
posterior talofibular ligament, *235*
posterior tibial artery, *240*
posterior tibiofemoral ligament, 234, *235*
posterior tibiofibular ligaments, *235*
posterior tibiotalar ligament, *235*
posterior tilt, of shoulder girdle, 62
posteroinferior, *4*
posterolateral, *4*
posteromedial, *4*
posterosuperior, *4*
preparatory phase, 158, *159*
prepatellar bursa, *217*
primary/prime movers, 30
processes, of bones, 9, *10*
projections, of bones, 9
pronation, 16
  ankle, 237, *238*
  radioulnar, 106, *106*, 107, *107, 110*
pronator quadratus muscle, 108, *110*, 119, *119*, *135, 152*
pronator teres muscle, *23*, 108, *108, 109*, 110, 112, 118, *118, 135*
prone, *4*
prone extensions, alternating, 302, *302*
prone row, 171, *171*
proprioception, 37
proprioceptors, 37
protraction, 17
  of shoulder girdle, 57, 60, *60*
proximal, *3, 4*
proximal interphalangeal (PIP) joint, *125*, 126, *127*, *233*, 234, 317, 318
proximal phalanx, *125*, 126, *127, 233*, 256
psoas major muscle, 184, *185, 186*
psoas minor muscle, 184, *185, 186*, 276
pubic bone, 185
pubic crest, *176, 177*
pubic ramus
  inferior, *176, 177*
  superior, *176, 177*
pubis, *2*, 175, *176*
pubofemoral ligament, 178, *178*
pudendal nerve, *34*
pull
  angle of, 39–40, *40*
  line of, 32–33
pull-up, 157, 166, *166, 167*, 308
pulleys, *50*, 50–51
push-up, 116, 170, *170*
pyramidalis muscle, *82*

Q

quadratus femoris muscle, 184, *190*, 194, 202, *202*
quadratus lumborum muscle, 273, *275*, 276, *282, 293, 293*
quadratus plantae muscle, 256, *257, 259*
quadriceps muscles, *23*, 177, 217, 219, 222, *222*, 297–298

R

radial artery, *152*
radial collateral ligament, 105, *105*
radial deviation, 17, *127*, 129, *129*, 130
radial flexion, 17, 130
radial head, *2, 104*
radial nerve, *34*, 112, *112*, 136
radial notch, *104*
radial tuberosity, *2*, 103, *104*
radiate muscles, 25, *26*
radiocarpal joint, *126*
radiohumeral joint, 105
radioulnar joint, *13*, 103–121, *106, 126*
  bones, 103
  movements, 16, 107, *107*
  muscles, 108, *108, 109*, 110–111, 113–120
  nerves, 112, *112*
  range-of-motion, 316
radius, *2, 7*, 103, *104, 109*, 125, *126, 135*
ramus
  of ischium, *177*
  of pubis, *176, 177*
range-of-motion, 14–15
reaction, law of, 52, *52*, 55
rearfoot, *233*
reciprocal inhibition, 41
reciprocal innervation, 41
recovery phase, 158
rectilinear motion, 51
rectus abdominis muscle, *23, 82*, 273, *275*, 276, *284, 288*, 289, *289*
rectus capitis anterior muscle, 278, *278*
rectus capitis lateralis muscle, 278, *278*
rectus capitis muscle, 276
rectus capitis posterior major muscle, 277, 278, *278*
rectus capitis posterior minor muscle, 277, 278, *278*
rectus capitis posterior muscle, 276
rectus femoris muscle, *23*, 176, *182, 183*, 184, *184, 185, 186, 189*, 193, 197, *197*, 219, 220, *221, 222, 222*
rectus sheath, *23, 288*
red marrow, 8
reduction, 17, 272
reference positions, *3, 3*
reflexes, *35–36*, 37
reposition, of thumb, 17, 130, *130*
resistance, 44, 48, *48*
resistance arm, 48, *48*
respiration, muscles of, 284, *284*
retraction, 17, *60*, 61
  of shoulder girdle, 57
rhomboid major muscle, 69, *69*
rhomboid minor muscle, 69, *69*
rhomboid muscles, 62, *63*, 64, 69, *69*
rhomboideus major muscle, *83, 277*
rhomboideus minor muscle, *277*
rib(s), *2*, 266, *268*
  false (vertebrochondral), 266, *268*
  floating (vertebral), 266, *268*
  true (vertebrosternal), 266, *268*
rib cage, *2*
ridge, lateral, *104*
right lateral pelvic rotation, 180–181, *181*
right transverse pelvic rotation, 181, *181*
roll, 18, *18*, 19, *19*
rolling friction, 53
rope climbing, 89, 97, 113
rotary component, 39, *40*
rotary motion. *See* angular motion
rotation
  ankle, 234
  axes of, *5*, 6, *6*, 44
  cervical, *271, 272*
  downward, 17, 59, *60*, 61, *63*
  external, *15*, 16
    hip, 179, *179*, 180, *181, 186, 187*, 188, *189, 190, 221*
    knee, *188*, 218, 219, *219, 221*
    shoulder, 78, 79, *79, 80, 85*
  head and neck, *274, 278*

tendon(s)—*Cont.*
    extensor digitorum brevis, *258*
    extensor digitorum longus, *182, 258*
    extensor hallucis brevis, *258*
    extensor hallucis longus, *258*
    extensor pollicis brevis, *152*
    extensor pollicis longus, *131*
    flexor carpi radialis, 131, *152*
    flexor carpi ulnaris, *152*
    flexor digitorum brevis, *257*
    flexor digitorum longus, *257*
    flexor digitorum profundus, *152*
    flexor digitorum superficialis, *152*
    flexor hallucis longus, *257*
    flexor pollicis longus, *131, 152*
    gracilis, *239*
    infraspinatus, *78*
    latissimus dorsi, *109*
    lumbrical, *257*
    palmaris longus, *131, 152*
    patellar, *182, 185, 217, 240*
    peroneus brevis, *235, 257, 258*
    peroneus longus, *257*
    peroneus tertius, *258*
    plantaris, *239*
    semimembranosus, *239*
    semitendinosus, *239*
    subscapularis, *78*
    supraspinatus, *78*
    teres minor, *78*
    tibialis anterior, *235, 258*
    tibialis posterior, *235, 240, 257*
tennis elbow, 108
tension, *54*
tensor fasciae latae muscle, *23*, 175, 177, *182, 184, 185, 189*, 198, *198*
teres ligament, 178
teres major muscle, *24*, 81, *83, 85*, 86, 97, *97, 109*
teres minor muscle, *24*, 78, 81, *83, 85*, 86, 92, 96, *96*
teres minor tendon, *78*
tertius muscle, 232
thenar eminence, 152
thigh, regions of, 184–185
third-class levers, 44, *44*, 47, *47*
thoracic cage, *268*
thoracic curve, 266, *266*
thoracic nerves, 34, *34*, 276
thoracic spine, movements, 270, *271*
thoracic vertebrae, *2, 34*, 265, 266, *267, 268*
thoracodorsal nerve, 86
thorax
    bones, 266, *268*
    muscles, 276, 284, *284, 285*
throwing, 54–55
thumb
    bones, 126
    movements, 129–130, *129–130*
    muscles, 152
    opposition, 17
    range-of-motion, *128*, 317
    reposition, 17
thyrohyoid muscle, *277*
thyroid cartilage, *277*
thyroid gland, *277*
tibia, *2, 176, 177*, 215, *216, 217*, 232, *232*, 235, *239, 240*
tibial artery
    anterior, *240, 258*
    posterior, *240*
tibial collateral ligament, *216*, 217, 218
tibial condyle, 215
    lateral, *176, 177, 177*, 215, *216*
    medial, *176, 177*, 215
tibial nerve, *34, 189*, 194, *194*, 220, *240*, 244
tibial plateau
    lateral, *216*, 218
    medial, *216*, 218
tibial tuberosity, *2, 176*, 215, *216, 240*
tibialis anterior muscle, *23, 182*, 233, *235*, 238, *239, 240, 241, 243, 244*, 252, *252, 258*
tibialis anterior tendon, *235, 258*
tibialis posterior muscle, 233, *235*, 238, *239, 240, 241, 242*, 253, *253, 257*
tibialis posterior tendon, *235, 240, 257.*

tibiocalcaneal ligament, *235*
tibiofemoral joint. *See* knee
tibiofemoral ligament
    anterior inferior, 234
    posterior, 234, *235*
tibiofibular joint, 234
    superior, *216*
tibiofibular ligament
    anterior, *235*
    posterior, *235*
tibionavicular ligament, *235*
tibiotalar ligament
    anterior, *235*
    posterior, *235*
tilt
    anterior, 62
    lateral, 61
    medial, 61
    posterior, 61–62
tissue deformation, 54
toe(s), 232
    joints, 234–236, *235, 236*
    movements, 237, *237–238*
    range-of-motion, 234, *236*
toe-off phase, of walking, 231, *232*
torque, *48*, 48–50
torsion, *54*
Total Gym exercise machine, 308, *308*
trabecular bone. *See* cancellous bone
translation. *See* glide
translatory motion. *See* linear motion
transverse arch of foot, 236, *236*
transverse cervical nerve, *34*
transverse costal facet, *267*
transverse costal process, *267*
transverse fascia, *288*
transverse foramen, *267*
transverse ligament, *216*
transverse plane, *5, 6, 6*
transverse process, 266, *266, 267*
transverse subtalar joint, *237*, 318
transverse tarsal joint, *233*, 234, *237*, 318
transversospinalis muscles, 282
transversus abdominis muscle, *82*, 275, 276, *284, 288*, 292, *292*
transversus thoracis muscle, 276, 284, *285*
trapezium bone, 125, *125*
trapezius muscle, *23, 24*, 59, 62, *63*, 64, *66, 66–67, 82, 83*, 108, *109*, 276, *277*
trapezoid bone, 125
trapezoid ligament, *58*
Trendelenburg gait, 200
triceps brachii muscle, *23, 82, 83*, 108, *108, 109*, 112, 116, *116*
    lateral head, *24, 109, 111, 116*
    long head, *24*, 81, *109, 111, 116*
    medial head, *111, 116*
triceps extension, 163, *163*
triceps surae muscle, 238
triquetrum bone, 125, *125*
trochanter, *10*
    greater, *2, 176*, 177
    lesser, *2, 176, 177, 177*
trochlea, *104*
trochlear notch, *104*
trochoginglymus joint, 217
trochoid joint, *14*, 106, 269
trochoidal joint, 13
true (vertebrosternal) ribs, 266, *268*
trunk and spinal column, 265–293
    exercises for, muscular analysis of, 297–310
    joints, 269
    movements, 272, *272–273*
    muscles, 273–276, *274–275*
    nerves, 276
    range-of-motion, 318
tubercle, *10*
    adductor, *176*
    Gerdy's, *176, 177*, 215, *216*, 217
    greater, *2*, 77, *77*
    lesser, *2*, 77, *77*
tuberosity, *10*
    calcaneal, *257*
    deltoid, 77, *77*
    gluteal, *177*

ischial, *2*, 176, *176, 177*
metatarsal, *258*
radial, *2*, 103, *104*
tibial, *2, 176*, 215, *216, 240*
ulnar, *104*

U

ulna, *2, 7*, 103, *104, 109*, 125, *126*, 135
ulnar artery, *131, 152*
ulnar collateral ligament, 105, *105*
ulnar deviation, *127*, 129, *129*, 130
ulnar flexion, 17, 130
ulnar nerve, *34, 109, 131*, 136, *136, 152*
ulnar tuberosity, *104*
umbilicus, *288*
unipennate muscles, 25, 26, *26*
upper extremity
    exercises, muscular analysis of, 157–171
    range-of-motion, 316–317
upward rotation, 17, 59, *60*, 61, *63*
upward tilt, 62

V

Valsalva maneuver, 160
vastus intermedius muscle, *23, 183*, 184, *184, 185*, 193, 217, 219, 220, *221*, 222, *222*, 224, *224*
vastus lateralis muscle, *23, 182, 183*, 184, *184, 185, 189*, 193, 217, 219, 220, *221*, 222, *222, 223, 223*, 239
vastus medialis muscle, *23, 182, 183*, 184, *184, 185*, 193, 217, 219, 220, *221*, 222, *222*, 225, *225*
vastus medialis obliquus muscle, 225
velocity, 51
ventral, 4
vertebrae, *7*, 265–266, *270*
    articular facets, *267, 269*
    cervical, *2*, 265, 266, *267*
    lumbar, *2, 34*, 265, *266, 267*
    thoracic, *2, 34*, 265, *266, 267, 268*
vertebral border, *2*
vertebral column, *2*
    bones, 265–266, *266, 267*
    muscles, 276, 282, *282, 283*
vertebral foramen, 266, *267*
vertebral (floating) ribs, 266, *268*
vertebrochondral (false) ribs, 266, *268*
vertebrosternal (true) ribs, 266, *268*
vertical axis, *5, 6, 6*
vertical jump, 222
volar, 4
voluntary movement, neural control of, 33–35

W

walking, phases of, 231, *232*
water, in bones, 9
weight-training exercises, 298–299
wheels, and axels, 50, *50*
wind-up phase. *See* preparatory phase
Wrisberg, ligament of, *216*
wrist, 124–153, *126*, 127
    bones, *125*, 125–126
    movements, 17, 129–130, *129–130*
    muscles, *131*, 131–135, *132–134*, 137–152, *153*
    nerves, 136, *136*
    range-of-motion, 127, *127*, 317

X

xiphoid process, *2*, 266, *268*

Y

Y ligament. *See* iliofemoral ligament
yellow marrow, 8

Z

zona orbicularis, *178*
zygomatic bone, *2*